Elbow Arthroscopy

In-Ho Jeon • Erica Kholinne
Jae-Man Kwak
Editors

Elbow Arthroscopy

Principles and Practical Techniques

Springer

Editors
In-Ho Jeon
Department of Orthopaedic Surgery
Asan Medical Center, University of
Ulsan College of Medicine
Seoul, Republic of Korea

Erica Kholinne
Faculty of Medicine
Universitas Trisakti
Jakarta, Indonesia

Jae-Man Kwak
Department of Orthopedic Surgery
Uijeongbu Eulji Medical Center, College
of Medicine, Eulji University
Uijeongbu, Republic of Korea

ISBN 978-981-95-3731-0 ISBN 978-981-95-3732-7 (eBook)
https://doi.org/10.1007/978-981-95-3732-7

This Springer imprint is published by the registered company Springer Nature Singapore Pte Ltd.
The registered company address is: 152 Beach Road, #21-01/04 Gateway East, Singapore 189721, Singapore

Contents

Part I

Introduction

History of Elbow Arthroscopy

1

In-Ho Jeon

1 Background

Elbow arthroscopy was long considered as a procedure of extreme risk due to the limited intra-articular space, complex anatomy, and proximity of major nerves. These challenges contributed to a significant delay in the widespread adoption of elbow arthroscopy, long after the routine implementation of knee and shoulder arthroscopy. Over time, however, the development of innovative techniques and the refinement of surgical instruments transformed elbow arthroscopy into a safe and essential operative modality. Its progression from a cautiously approached procedure to a standard component of orthopedic practice has been driven by a series of pivotal advancements.

2 Early Challenges

Although arthroscopy was first pioneered in the early twentieth century by Kenji Takagi and Eugen Bircher, their initial efforts were primarily directed toward the knee joint. The application of arthroscopy to the elbow was delayed for many years, largely due to a range of anatomical and technical challenges:

- *Limited intra-articular space:* The elbow's intra-articular volume is very small, severely limiting instrument maneuverability.
- *Complex anatomy:* Three articulations (humeroulnar, humeroradial, and proximal radioulnar) share one single capsule, complicating access.
- *Narrow safety margins:* Major nerves run close to the joint, leaving only tiny "safe" zones for portal placement.

These factors rendered even diagnostic elbow arthroscopy challenging until advancements in visualization and instrumentation significantly improved procedural feasibility.

3 Pioneering Era (1980s)

By the early 1980s, James R. Andrews, Bernard Morrey, and Shawn O'Driscoll, the pioneering surgeons, performed the first elbow arthroscopies using small scopes with primitive fiber-optic imaging and no fluid irrigation. Their early attempts were limited to simple diagnostic exams or loose body removal. Limited intra-articular space and rudimentary instrumentation frequently led to poor visualization and a high rate of complications; however, early pioneers successfully demonstrated the feasibility of the procedure and established the foundational safe portal techniques.

I.-H. Jeon (✉)
Department of Orthopedic Surgery, Asan Medical Center, University of Ulsan College of Medicine, Seoul, Republic of Korea

I.-H. Jeon et al. (eds.), *Elbow Arthroscopy*, https://doi.org/10.1007/978-981-95-3732-7_1

4 Technical Refinements (1990s)

During the 1990s, several advances greatly improved elbow arthroscopy:

- *Better tools:* Smaller angled scopes and miniaturized instruments (motorized shavers, RF probes) improved access and precision.
- *"Safe" portal mapping:* Surgeons like O'Driscoll defined safe portal sites (e.g., the posterolateral "soft spot") to avoid nerve injury.
- *Fluid irrigation:* Continuous pressurized fluid pumps kept the joint distended and clear, dramatically improving visibility.

These advancements have expanded the scope of conditions that can be effectively managed through arthroscopic techniques. By the late 1990s, surgeons could address common elbow problems such as *tennis elbow*, synovial plicae, and post-traumatic stiffness arthroscopically. Initial clinical studies by Morrey et al. indicated that these techniques were effective in reducing pain and enhancing range of motion, with a low incidence of complications.

5 Widespread Adoption (2000s)

By the early 2000s, elbow arthroscopy had achieved widespread clinical acceptance, supported by studies reporting excellent outcomes and relatively low complication rates, averaging approximately 5%. Outcomes of arthroscopic surgery is comparable to that of open surgery with quicker recovery. With the increased availability of specialized training and growing surgical experience, the indications for elbow arthroscopy expanded to include the release of post-traumatic contractures, excision of inflammatory synovitis, and removal of loose bodies in arthritic elbows. By 2010, these once-experimental procedures had become one of the routine procedures.

6 Modern Advances (2010s)

Over the past decade, elbow arthroscopy has been increasingly employed to address more complex pathologies, enabling surgeons to perform procedures arthroscopically that were previously deemed too challenging or high-risk, including:

- *Severe contractures:* Arthroscopic circumferential capsular release (pioneered by In-Ho Jeon) and excision of heterotopic bone to restore motion in stiff elbows.
- *Instability repairs:* Arthroscopic reconstruction of the lateral ulnar collateral ligament for posterolateral rotatory instability, aided by fluoroscopy.

The introduction of modern high-definition arthroscopes and advanced imaging modalities such as 3D CT and MRI has markedly improved visualization and intra-articular navigation, enabling surgeons to safely access and assess even the most constrained elbow joints with greater confidence.

7 Remaining Challenges and Lessons

Despite great advancement elbow arthroscopy remains as a challenging procedure:

- *Nerve injury risk:* Major nerves remain at risk of injury.
- *Steep learning curve:* Mastery demands in-depth anatomical knowledge and considerable practice.
- *Residual stiffness:* Scar tissue can still limit motion even after a successful release.

Comprehensive training and a thorough understanding of elbow anatomy remain essential to ensure procedural safety and optimal outcomes.

8 Conclusion

The evolution of elbow arthroscopy has shown innovative surgeons overcame anatomical barriers. What was once considered a high-risk and infrequently performed procedure has evolved into a refined, evidence-based surgical technique. Each milestone—from better tools and safer portals to expanded indications and improved outcomes—made the technique safer and more effective. Emerging technologies—including artificial intelligence, robotics, and biologic therapies—hold the potential to further advance elbow arthroscopy. Building upon prior innovations, these developments are expected to enhance surgical precision and enable more personalized treatment strategies.

Basic Anatomy of the Elbow

2

Jae-Man Kwak and Erica Kholinne

1 Introduction

Understanding the anatomy of the elbow is fundamental to ensuring safe and effective arthroscopic procedures [1]. The elbow joint, due to its compact structure and close proximity to critical neurovascular structures, presents unique challenges in arthroscopic surgery [2]. Successful elbow arthroscopy requires not only surgical expertise but also precise knowledge of the anatomical landmarks that guide portal placement. This chapter provides a comprehensive overview of the elbow's anatomy, highlighting the key osseous and soft tissue structures that are essential for accurate portal placement and minimizing potential complications during elbow arthroscopy [10].

2 General Elbow Anatomy

The elbow joint is a complex synovial hinge joint that connects the upper arm (humerus) to the forearm (radius and ulna). It consists of three distinct articulations: the humeroulnar joint (between the trochlea of the humerus and the trochlear notch of the ulna), the humeroradial joint (between the capitellum of the humerus and the radial head), and the proximal radioulnar joint (between the radial head and the radial notch of the ulna) (Fig. 2.1). These three components are enclosed within a single joint capsule, enabling both flexion-extension and pronation-supination movements.

Ligamentous structures are vital in maintaining elbow joint stability [3]. The medial (ulnar) collateral ligament complex and the lateral collateral ligament complex support the joint during dynamic motion. The annular ligament encircles the radial head, stabilizing it against the ulna and allowing smooth rotational movements. The primary stabilizer includes anterior band of the mcl, LCL complex, and ulnohumeral joint articulation [4–9]. Radiocapitellar articulation, common extensor, and flexor tendon group contribute the elbow stability as secondary stabilizer (Figs. 2.2, 2.3 and 2.4).

Musculature around the elbow includes the flexor-pronator mass arising from the medial epicondyle and the extensor-supinator mass from the lateral epicondyle. Key muscles influencing elbow movement include the biceps brachii (flexion and supination), triceps brachii (extension), brachialis (flexion), and the pronator teres and supinator (rotation).

Understanding the relationship between these anatomical structures and the overlying surface anatomy is essential for both diagnostic evalua-

J.-M. Kwak (✉)
Department of Orthopedic Surgery, Uijeongbu Eulji Medical Center, College of Medicine, Eulji University, Uijeongbu, Republic of Korea

E. Kholinne
Faculty of Medicine, Universitas Trisakti, Jakarta, Indonesia

I.-H. Jeon et al. (eds.), *Elbow Arthroscopy*, https://doi.org/10.1007/978-981-95-3732-7_2

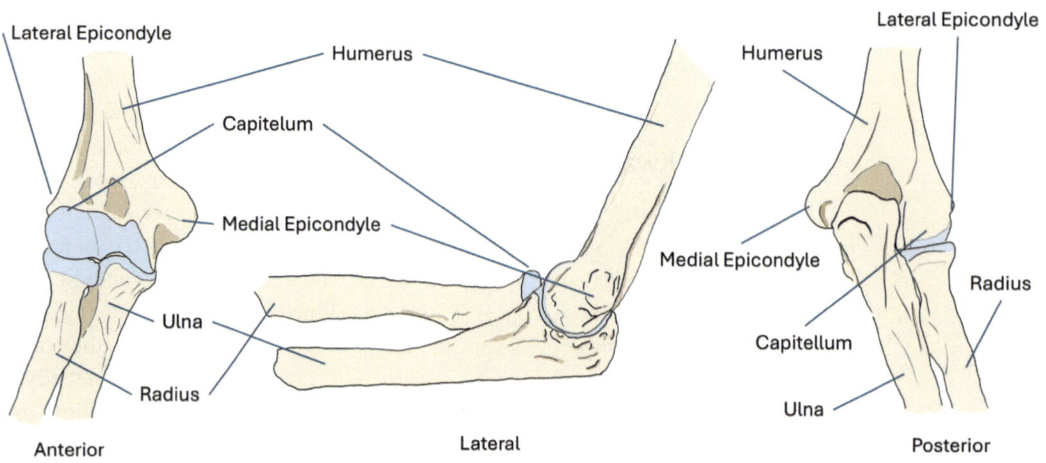

Fig. 2.1 Elbow joint articulation and bony landmark

Fig. 2.2 Elbow stabilizing structures

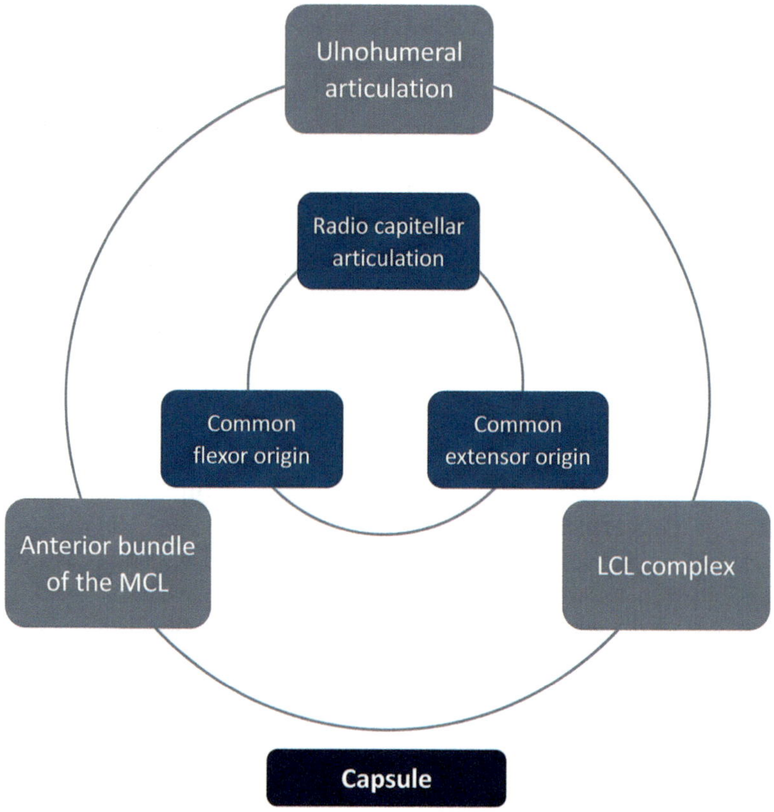

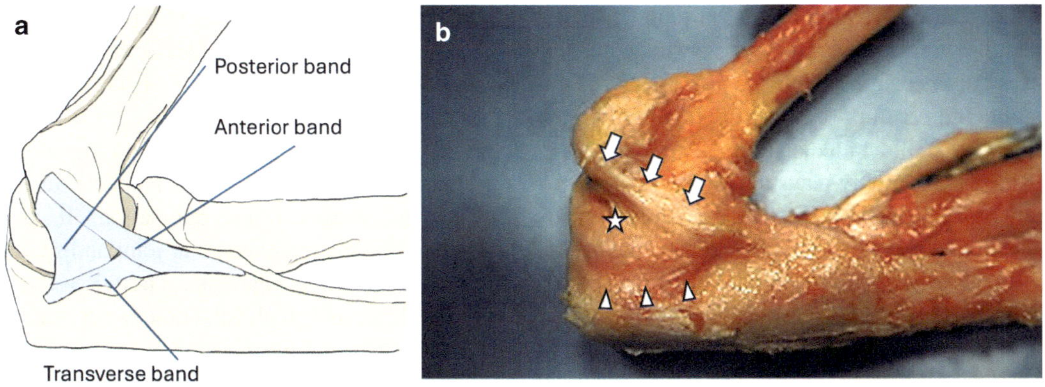

Fig. 2.3 MCL (medial collateral ligament): (**a**) Schematic image of medial collateral ligament of the elbow. (**b**) Cadaveric image. The arrow indicates the anterior band, the asterisk represents the posterior band, and the triangle denotes the transverse band

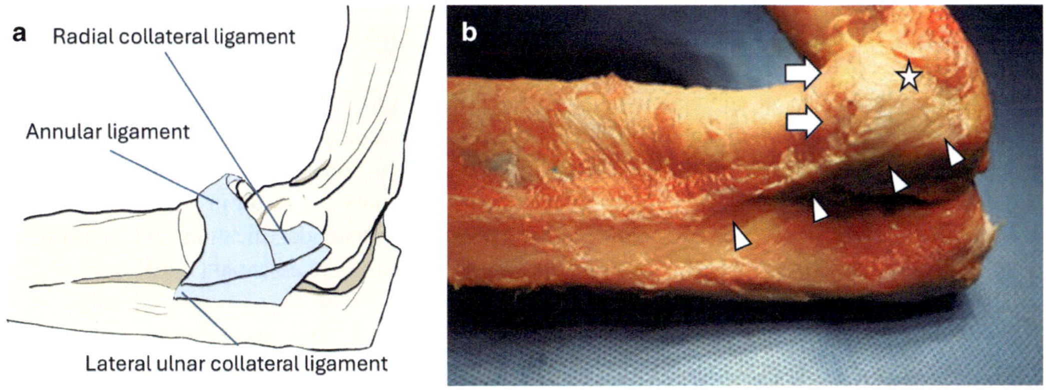

Fig. 2.4 LCL (lateral collateral ligament) complex. (**a**) Schematic image of lateral collateral ligament of the elbow. (**b**) Cadaveric image. The arrow indicates the annular ligament, the asterisk represents the radial collateral ligament, and the triangle denotes the lateral ulnar collateral ligament [6]

tion and surgical intervention, especially in arthroscopic procedures where precise portal placement is critical.

3 Anatomical Considerations for Elbow Arthroscopy

The elbow joint is a compact joint with close proximity of critical neurovascular structures. Unlike larger joints, the elbow has limited working space, making a detailed understanding of surface anatomy critical for procedural safety. A thorough palpation and marking of anatomical landmarks are mandatory before initiating arthroscopy.

A critical consideration in elbow arthroscopy is the close proximity of major neurovascular structures, including the ulnar nerve, radial nerve, median nerve, and brachial artery, which all course near the anterior, posterior, and lateral aspects of the joint. These structures are particularly vulnerable due to the limited soft tissue coverage and the narrow operative field, increasing the risk of iatrogenic injury if portals are improperly placed.

Additionally, the working space inside the elbow is limited, especially in the presence of joint contracture, synovitis, or intra-articular pathology such as loose bodies or osteophytes. This confined space demands precise instrumentation and careful triangulation, highlighting the importance of detailed anatomical knowledge.

Surface anatomy plays a pivotal role in ensuring procedural safety. A comprehensive understanding of bony landmarks such as the lateral epicondyle, medial epicondyle, olecranon, radial head, and ulnar border is essential. Palpation and marking of these anatomical landmarks prior to arthroscopic portal placement are not optional—it is a mandatory step that provides orientation and minimizes the risk of neurovascular compromise.

Moreover, elbow positioning during the procedure significantly affects the location of adjacent neurovascular structures. For example, flexion of the elbow moves the ulnar nerve posteriorly and away from the medial portal sites, while forearm pronation or supination can shift the radial nerve's position, influencing the safety zone for lateral portal placement.

4 Bony Landmarks

Palpable bony prominences serve as essential guides for portal placement. The following structures should be clearly identified and marked preoperatively:

- Lateral epicondyle: Located on the lateral aspect of the distal humerus, it serves as a key reference for lateral portal placement. It is particularly useful in identifying the anterolateral and posterolateral portals. The lateral epicondyle is easily palpable and acts as an anchor point for muscle attachments.
- Medial epicondyle: Situated on the medial aspect of the distal humerus, it is a critical landmark for avoiding injury to the ulnar nerve, which runs posterior to it. It is also used as a reference for locating the anteromedial portal.
- Olecranon: The prominent posterior projection of the proximal ulna, the olecranon serves as the central reference point for posterior portal placement. It also provides orientation during intra-articular navigation of the posterior compartment.
- Radial head: Located just distal to the lateral epicondyle, the radial head is palpable during forearm pronation and supination. It aids in locating the radiocapitellar joint and serves as a guide for the anterolateral portal.
- Capitellum and trochlea: Though not readily palpable externally, these humeral articular surfaces are important intra-articular landmarks that help orient the surgeon during diagnostic arthroscopy.

5 Soft Tissue Landmarks and Neurovascular Structures

In addition to bony landmarks, soft tissue structures, particularly neurovascular elements, must be carefully considered. Inadvertent injury to these structures can result in significant morbidity. Preoperative identification and marking of these structures are essential [1, 10].

- Ulnar nerve: This nerve courses posterior to the medial epicondyle within the cubital tunnel. It is highly vulnerable during medial portal placement. Palpation of the ulnar groove allows accurate localization and avoidance during surgery.
- Radial nerve and posterior interosseous nerve (PIN): The radial nerve divides into superficial and deep branches at the level of the radial head. The deep branch, or PIN, enters the supinator muscle and lies close to the anterolateral portal site. Great care must be taken when establishing lateral portals [11] (Table 2.1).
- Median nerve and brachial artery: These structures traverse the cubital fossa, medial to the biceps tendon. They are at risk during anteromedial portal placement. Identifying the biceps tendon helps avoid these vital structures (Figs. 2.5 and 2.6).

Table 2.1 Radial Nerve Anatomical Relationships

Structure	Relationship to radial nerve
Brachialis muscle	Medial to the nerve
Brachioradialis muscle	Lateral to the nerve
Anterior elbow capsule	Directly deep/anterior to the nerve, separated by fat
Radial head/neck	Medial-posterior to the nerve as it approaches supinator
Supinator muscle	PIN enters between its two heads at the radial neck

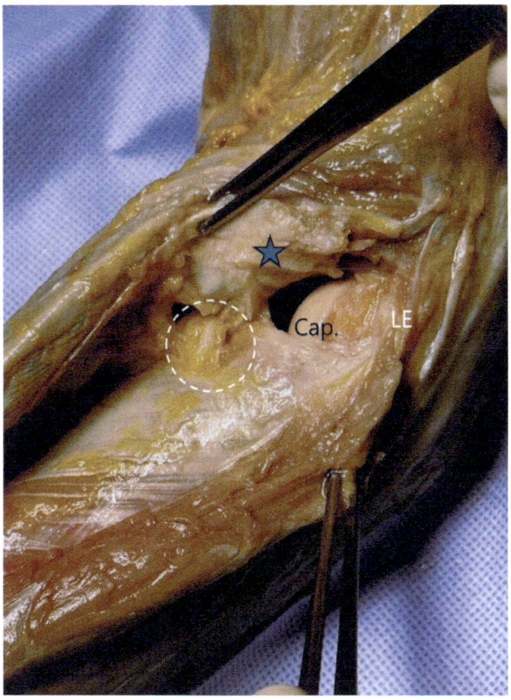

Fig. 2.5 Above the elbow, the radial nerve travels in the radial groove of the humerus, pierces the lateral intermuscular septum, and descends anterior to the lateral epicondyle. It then divides into a superficial sensory branch and a deep motor branch, the latter of which enters the supinator muscle by passing between its two heads. (White dotted line; radial nerve, blue star; ECRB with common extensor group; Cap.: capitellar lateral side; LE: lateral, epicondyle)

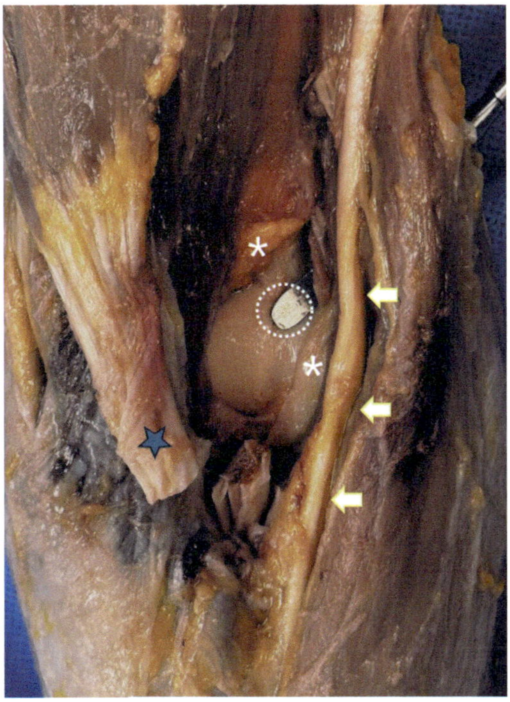

Fig. 2.6 After piercing the lateral intermuscular septum, the radial nerve runs between the brachialis medially and brachioradialis laterally. It lies just superficial to the anterior capsule of the elbow, close to the radial head, and divides into superficial and deep branches near the radial neck. The deep branch (PIN) then enters the supinator between its two heads. [Asterisk; capsule (cut), dotted line; proximal anterolateral portal, arrow; radial nerve, blue star; distal biceps tendon (cut)]

6 Conclusion

Mastery of the surface and internal anatomy of the elbow is indispensable for performing safe and effective arthroscopy. Precise preoperative identification and careful marking of bony and soft tissue landmarks enable the surgeon to navigate the joint with confidence. A structured and anatomical approach to portal placement not only prevents complications but also enhances surgical efficiency and outcomes. As techniques continue to evolve, a thorough understanding of elbow anatomy remains a cornerstone of successful arthroscopic intervention.

References

1. Hasan SS. Editorial Commentary: Avoiding Complications in Elbow Arthroscopy: Know the Indications, Learn the Anatomy, and Master a Safe Technique. Arthroscopy. 2023;39(11):2388–2391. https://doi.org/10.1016/j.arthro.2023.06.011. PMID: 37866876.
2. Martin S, Sanchez E. Anatomy and biomechanics of the elbow joint. Semin Musculoskelet Radiol. 2013;17(5):429–36. https://doi.org/10.1055/s-0033-1361587. Epub 2013 Dec 10. PMID: 24327407.
3. Safran MR, Baillargeon D. Soft-tissue stabilizers of the elbow. J Shoulder Elbow Surg. 2005;14(1 Suppl S):179S–185S. https://doi.org/10.1016/j.jse.2004.09.032. PMID: 15726079.
4. Regan WD, Korinek SL, Morrey BF, An KN. Biomechanical study of ligaments around the elbow joint. Clin Orthop Relat Res. 1991;(271):170–9. PMID: 1914292.
5. Alcid JG, Ahmad CS, Lee TQ. Elbow anatomy and structural biomechanics. Clin Sports Med. 2004;23(4):503–17, vii. https://doi.org/10.1016/j.csm.2004.06.008. PMID: 15474218.
6. Fuss FK. The ulnar collateral ligament of the human elbow joint. Anatomy, function and biomechanics. J Anat. 1991;175:203–12. PMID: 2050566; PMCID: PMC1224480.
7. Morrey BF, An KN. Functional anatomy of the ligaments of the elbow. Clin Orthop Relat Res. 1985;(201):84–90. PMID: 4064425.
8. Hannouche D, Bégué T. Functional anatomy of the lateral collateral ligament complex of the elbow. Surg Radiol Anat. 1999;21(3):187–91. https://doi.org/10.1007/BF01630899. PMID: 10431332.
9. Cohen MS, Hastings H 2nd. Rotatory instability of the elbow. The anatomy and role of the lateral stabilizers. J Bone Joint Surg Am. 1997;79(2):225–33. PMID: 9052544.
10. Camp CL, Degen RM, Sanchez-Sotelo J, Altchek DW, Dines JS. Basics of Elbow Arthroscopy Part I: Surface Anatomy, Portals, and Structures at Risk. Arthrosc Tech. 2016;5(6):e1339-e1343. doi: 10.1016/j.eats.2016.08.019. PMID: 28560134; PMCID: PMC5439187.
11. Chaware PN, Santoshi JA, Pakhare AP, Rathinam BA. Risk of nerve injury during arthroscopy portal placement in the elbow joint: A cadaveric study. Indian J Orthop. 2016;50(1):74–9. https://doi.org/10.4103/0019-5413.173510. PMID: 26952128; PMCID: PMC4759879.

Arthroscopic Setup and Equipment

3

Guido Fierro and Gabriela Gómez Romero

1 Preoperative Setup

The setup plays a critical role in overcoming the inherent challenges of the elbow's complex anatomy. After regional and/or general anesthesia is administered, the process starts with the application of a tourniquet, which can be either sterile or nonsterile, set to at least 100 mmHg above the patient's systolic blood pressure, with the authors recommending a target of 250 mmHg. Depending on how the patient is positioned, the forearm is wrapped with an elastic bandage from just below the elbow to the fingers to minimize swelling and fluid extravasation [1].

Before proceeding, all bony landmarks of the elbow are carefully palpated and marked on the skin, including the ulnar nerve, which is identified, marked, and assessed for stability. This is crucial, especially before making medial portal incisions, as the surgeon must determine whether the ulnar nerve is stable or subluxating [1]. To prevent pressure ulcers during surgery, essential supplies include padding materials such as foam or gel cushions to redistribute pressure, and positioning devices to reduce prolonged pressure on vulnerable areas. Protective dressings, like hydrocolloid or silicone-based materials, are also used to cushion bony prominences. Additionally, ensuring proper patient positioning during lengthy procedures is crucial for minimizing pressure ulcer risk. These supplies work together to protect the skin and underlying tissues from the sustained pressure that can lead to ulcer formation during surgery [2].

Once the tourniquet is inflated, joint distention is performed by insufflating the elbow with 15–30 mL of sterile saline through the lateral "soft spot," which is bordered by the radial head, lateral epicondyle, and olecranon tip. Sterile saline insufflation can be performed through the posterior portal, which is a straightforward, safe, and reliable location for this procedure. This distention increases the space within the joint, allowing for safer entry of arthroscopic instruments by moving neurovascular structures away from the joint. Care is taken to avoid overdistending the joint, as this could lead to capsular rupture, poor visualization, and fluid extravasation during the procedure [1, 3].

An elevated gravity bag is frequently adequate to achieve the required pressure for the surgical procedure, given that the pressure demand is reduced due to the use of a tourniquet. Two bags of Ringer's lactate or saline solution chosen by the surgeon are necessary to ensure continuous flow during the switch from one bag to the other during surgery

G. Fierro (✉)
Departamento de Ortopedia y Traumatología, Fundación Santa Fe de Bogotá, Hospital Serena del Mar, Universidad de los Andes, Bogotá, Colombia

Universidad de los Andes, Facultad de Medicina, Bogotá, Colombia

G. G. Romero
Departamento de Ortopedia y Traumatología, Fundación Santa Fe de Bogotá, Bogotá, Colombia

I.-H. Jeon et al. (eds.), *Elbow Arthroscopy*, https://doi.org/10.1007/978-981-95-3732-7_3

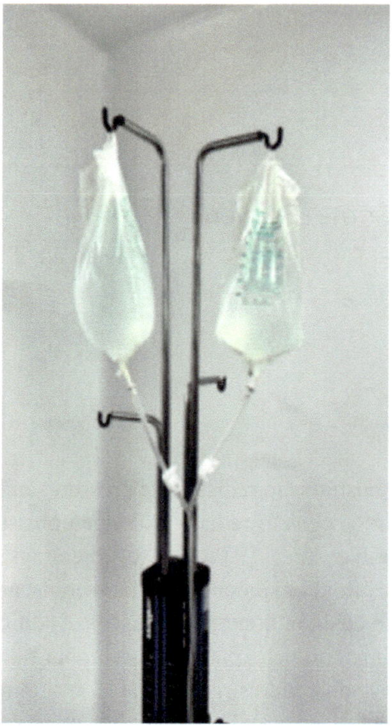

Fig. 3.1 Two elevated fluid bags

Table 3.1 List of setup requirements for arthroscopic elbow surgery

Set up requirement	Description
Tourniquet	The tourniquet should be applied at least 100 mmHg above the patient's systolic blood pressure, with the authors recommending a target of 250 mmHg, the forearm should be wrapped to minimize swelling, followed by joint distention with sterile saline to safely create space for arthroscopic instruments, ensuring neurovascular structures are protected
Marked bony landmarks	All bony landmarks of the elbow, including the ulnar nerve, are carefully palpated, marked, and assessed for stability to ensure safe medial portal incisions and prevent nerve injury
Skin protection	To prevent pressure ulcers during surgery, a combination of padding materials, protective dressings, and proper patient positioning is essential to protect vulnerable areas and prevent tissue damage from sustained pressure

(Fig. 3.1). This approach maintains an adequate operative field while minimizing complications associated with excessive or insufficient pressure. If an infusion pump is used, it is recommended to keep the pump pressure below 30 mmHg to avoid overdistension of the joint capsule and fluid extravasation into the soft tissues [1].

The extremity is sterilely prepared and draped, allowing for free manipulation during surgery. This meticulous setup ensures that the surgeon can safely navigate the elbow joint while minimizing the risk of neurovascular injury and optimizing surgical outcomes (Table 3.1).

2 Patient Positioning

For elbow arthroscopy, patients can be positioned in one of three ways: supine, prone, or lateral decubitus [4]. Each position offers advantages and disadvantages, depending on the surgical needs, anesthesia requirements and patient anatomy. In all cases, the capacity of free range of motion in flexion/extension and easy access to anterior and posterior compartment is mandatory.

Prone Position Described by Poehling in 1989, the prone position involves placing the patient on their chest with the nonoperative arm supported and the operative arm hanging freely (Fig. 3.2).

This position provides excellent access to the posterior compartment of the elbow without the need for traction, and allows for easy manipulation of the arm. A key advantage is that flexion of the elbow helps neurovascular structures shift anteriorly, reducing the risk of injury during portal creation. The surgeon should ensure there is space between the elbow and the operating table, allowing an easy manipulation of the arm. However, this position requires general anesthesia in the vast majority of the cases and poses challenges for airway access. Converting to an open procedure is also more difficult compared to the supine position, requiring additional support for the arm while the shoulder is rotated externally or internally to access the lateral or medial compartments [5].

Some devices have been described to enhance movement and improve radiological visualization when the patient is in this position. These tools are specifically designed to facilitate more precise adjustments and provide clearer imaging results, thereby contributing to more effective and accurate surgical outcomes. Some of these devices are readily available in operating rooms, while others can be fabricated using basic materials, such as PVC (polyvinyl chloride) pipes, as illustrated in Fig. 3.3. The use of these devices should be accompanied by protective gels to safeguard the skin and provide support for the arm over the PVC pipe [6].

Lateral Decubitus Position Introduced by O'Driscoll and Morrey in 1993, the lateral decubitus position involves turning the patient onto their side after anesthesia is administered. The operative arm is placed in 90° of flexion on a padded arm holder (Fig. 3.4.). This position offers the advantages of prone positioning while maintaining easier airway access. However, this position requires a padded arm holder and can complicate conversion to an open procedure compared to the supine position. Nevertheless,

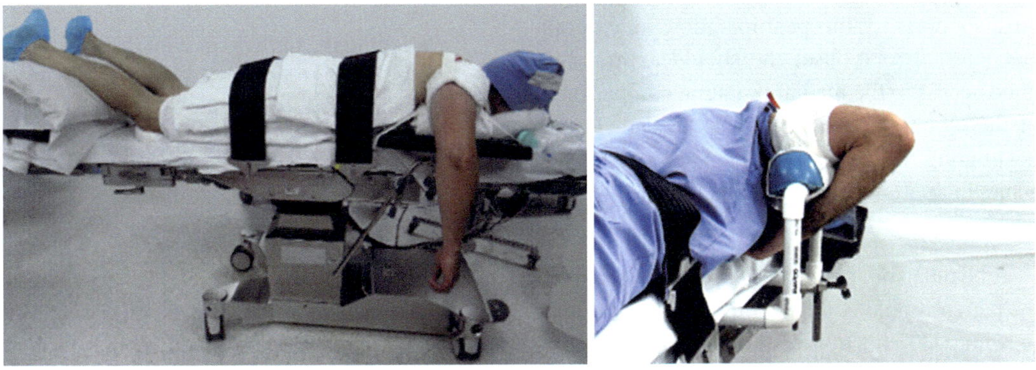

Fig. 3.2 Patient positioned in prone position

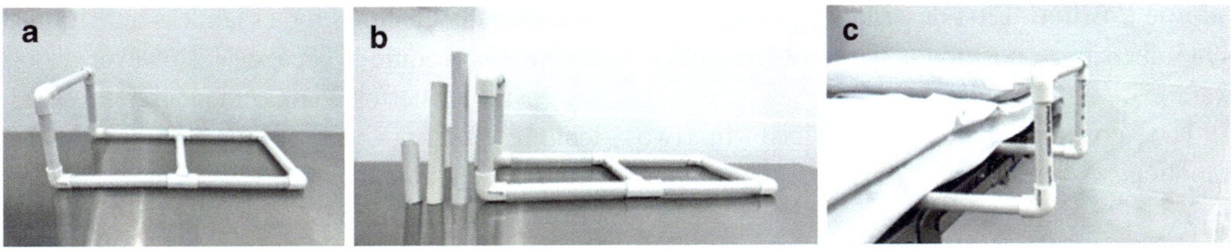

Fig. 3.3 (**a**) Elbow support device. (**b**) Support device with three vertical risers of different lengths. (**c**) Support device in place under the surgical table mattress

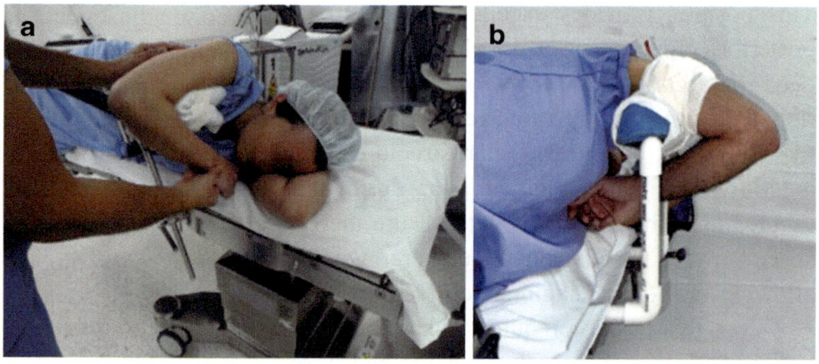

Fig. 3.4 (**a**) Patient positioned in lateral decubitus position with partial flexion range of motion. (**b**) Patient positioned in lateral decubitus position using the support device with full range of motion

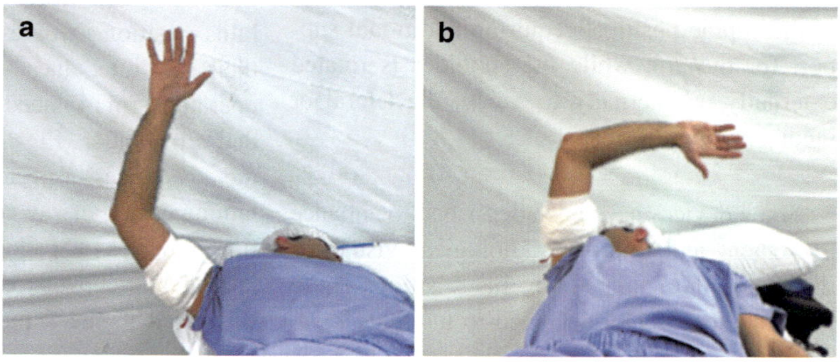

Fig. 3.5 (**a**) The patient is positioned supine with the elbow flexed to 70–90° and the shoulder abducted to 90° in the coronal plane. (**b**) The patient is positioned supine with the shoulder flexed to 90°

most supports for this position allow for external and internal rotation of the shoulder, providing good access to the medial or lateral compartment of the elbow if open surgery is needed. Proper positioning of the arm holder is crucial for achieving optimal elbow flexion [5, 7].

A beanbag or appropriate supports to maintain the patient stable in the lateral decubitus position or with a 20° tilt toward the surgeon is mandatory. The arm support must be sufficiently padded to prevent skin damage during surgery as previously established.

Supine Position First described by Andrews in 1985, the supine position is the most straightforward [5].

The position can be described in two variations:

1. *First variation:* The elbow is flexed to an angle between 70° and 90°, and the shoulder is abducted to 90° in the coronal plane, aligning the upper arm with the side of the body (Fig. 3.5a).
2. *Second variation:* The shoulder is flexed to 90°, bringing the arm forward in front of the body, while the elbow remains flexed at 90° (Fig. 3.5b).

When using the supine position, a mechanical arm holder or traction system is necessary. The arm holder should be positioned on the opposite side of the bed from the surgical site (e.g., the right side of the bed when operating on the left elbow).

This position is favored for its simplicity, clear anatomical orientation, and easy airway access. Additionally, it allows for a seamless transition to an open procedure if necessary. However, working in the posterior compartment is more challenging. The drawback of this position is that it brings the anterior neurovascular structures closer, theoretically increasing the risk of injury to them. Consequently, this position is less commonly used today than the other two and requires a more complex traction device [8] (Table 3.2).

Table 3.2 Advantages and disadvantages of each of the positions in which the patient may be positioned

Position	Advantages	Disadvantages
Prone	Provides excellent access to the posterior compartment of the elbow and reduces the risk of neurovascular injury by allowing the flexion of the elbow, which shifts neurovascular structures anteriorly. It enables free elbow movement across a wide range of flexion	Requires general anesthesia, complicates airway management, and makes it more challenging to convert to an open procedure if needed
Lateral decubitus	It provides superior airway access compared to the prone position, and the use of a padded bolster under the arm allows for unrestricted elbow flexion, which is crucial for optimal visualization and manipulation during surgery. The position also facilitates access to both the anterior and posterior compartments of the elbow, with the possibility of a slight 20° tilt toward the surgeon to prevent compression of the antecubital fossa. A traction device is not required	The airway may be less accessible compared to the supine position This position can complicate conversion to open surgery, especially on the medial side, and requires careful patient stabilization to ensure proper access and avoid impeding the surgical field Improper positioning can compromise access to the anterior elbow A beanbag or suitable supports are essential to keep the patient in the right position
Supine	Rapid positioning, favorable airway access for anesthetists, and simplified orientation for the surgeon It also facilitates easy conversion to an open procedure if necessary, particularly by dismantling the traction device and repositioning the limb. The use of a pneumatic or mechanical arm holder allows for effective stabilization and safe portal placement by shifting neurovascular structures anteriorly	A mechanical traction device is required Need for a dedicated assistant to stabilize the limb when not using an arm holder, and challenges in accessing the posterior compartment, which can make the procedure more complex The arm may feel unstable if not properly positioned and secured

3 Operating Room Setup

Patient should be positioned with the operative arm draped over a padded gutter. The anesthetic machine should be positioned near the patient's head, while the screen should be positioned directly in front of the surgeon's operating area. The surgeon should stand on the axillary side and the scrub team should be positioned right beside the surgeon (Fig. 3.6). This triangulation closely mirrors that used in shoulder arthroscopy, providing a familiar setup for the surgeon. The distance between the surgeon's direct view of the elbow and the screen should be minimized. Although a setup has been described where the screens are moved toward the patient's head, with the anesthetic machine also positioned at the head and the scrub team directly in front of the surgeon while the surgeon stands on the axillary side of the arm, the previously described setup is more advantageous as it allows for versatile approaches from the lateral, medial, and posterior sides of the elbow during arthroscopy, without the need for the surgeon to move within the surgical area [9].

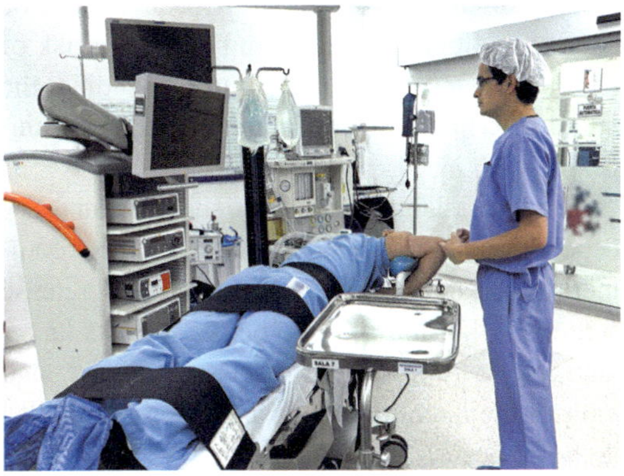

Fig. 3.6 Operating room setup, anesthetic machine positioned near the patient's head, screen positioned directly in front of the surgeon's operating area, scrub team positioned right beside the surgeon

4 Instrumentation

The arthroscopy tower should meet the minimum image quality standards commonly available in current systems. An image capture system is recommended to document the surgery for patient communication, as well as academic and legal purposes.

Elbow arthroscopy utilizes a standard 4.0-mm, 30° lens, which provides excellent visualization of the joint. In certain cases, such as in adolescent patients or when accessing smaller spaces like the lateral compartment, a smaller 2.7 mm arthroscope may be employed. The 70° lens is rarely used due to its limited availability in most hospitals, and its function can often be substituted with modifications to the technique using a 30° lens. However, the 70° lens has been described as enhancing visualization in certain areas or allowing the lateral portals to remain free as working portals while providing a lateral view from the posterior portal [5].

The use of smooth cannulas without side vents is crucial to prevent fluid extravasation into the soft tissues, which can lead to complications such as compartment syndrome. The most commonly used cannulas are short, with a diameter of no more than 6.5 mm. Soft or long cannulas are not utilized in elbow arthroscopy. Trocars should be conical and blunt-tipped to minimize the risk of neurovascular or articular injury, avoiding the initial insertion of sharp-pointed forceps for tunnel creation [3, 5].

The tip diameter of the shaver can vary depending on the procedure, with the most commonly used being 3.5 mm. In stiff elbow release surgery, a 4.0 mm tip may be used, as its larger diameter allows for faster tissue capture and reduces the likelihood of tissue becoming lodged in the device.

For effective procedure execution, a variety of handheld and motorized instruments are employed, including curettes, grasping forceps, basket, shaver, Jelco with suture, arthroscopic crochet, shavers, and burrs (Fig. 3.7). Careful control of fluid pressure, either by gravity or a mechanical pump, as discussed previously, is essential to maintain joint distention while

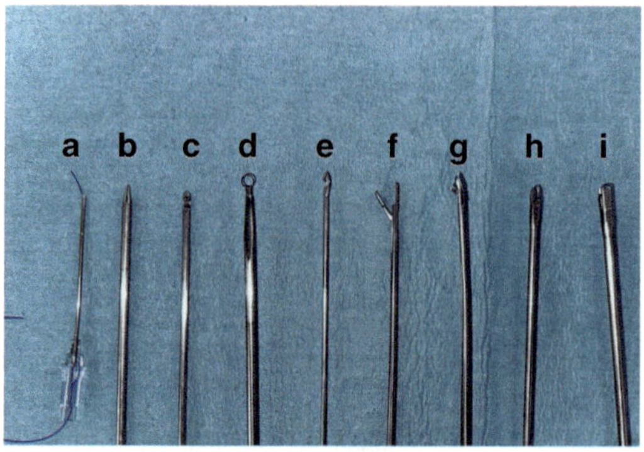

Fig. 3.7 Most frequently used instruments in elbow arthroscopy: A. Jelco No: 14 with and without prolene suture. B. Switching stick. C. Knot pusher. D. Arthroscopic curette. E. Crochet hook. F. Grasper. G. Biter or basket. H. Recovery grasper. I. Cutter

reducing the risk of fluid leakage into surrounding tissues. This approach ensures the integrity of the joint capsule during surgery, allowing for optimal visualization and maneuverability of instruments [1, 10].

As mentioned previously, before starting surgery, the joint must be insufflated with 15–30 mL of the surgical solution through the soft spot or posterior portal using a syringe with a Jelco to displace neurovascular structures from the surgical area. The use of shaver suction should be approached with caution. Options include using the shaver without suction to allow fluid to escape solely due to intra-articular pressure or connecting the suction at low power and applying it intermittently to avoid reducing the volume of intra-articular fluid [1, 3].

The instrument setup varies depending on the surgery being performed, with some instruments being basic and others specific to each procedure. The basic instruments include a switching stick, shaver, and a No. 14 Jelco for insufflating the solution before accessing the elbow.

For epicondylitis, an arthroscopic shaver and curette are used, which, due to the superficial nature of the tissue to be debrided, can often be a standard open surgery curette. If suture passage is required to close the debrided space of the extensor carpi radialis brevis (ECRB) or if the surgeon prefers to close the capsule after surgery, a Jelco with Prolene No. 01 and suture retrievers or a crochet hook are necessary [11].

For arthroscopic stiff elbow release surgery, it is often necessary to use retractors through accessory portals to separate the capsule and improve visualization. Basket forceps are used for the controlled cutting and removal of the joint capsule, while grasper forceps are employed for the removal of loose bodies. A 4.5 mm drill bit is required to create the pilot hole for the Outerbridge-Kashiwagi procedure, along with an arthroscopic burr for bone remodeling, the Outerbridge-Kashiwagi procedure, and the removal of osteophytes. Radiofrequency ablation is not commonly used and should be considered only according to the surgeon's preference [12].

If ulnar nerve exploration and repair are required before arthroscopic surgery, the instrument setup should include small basic retractors or drains to keep the ulnar nerve identified and protected during the arthroscopic procedure to avoid injury [13].

Lastly, for posterolateral elbow instability surgery, a No. 14 Jelco with a Prolene No. 01 suture is required for precise passage of the super-suture at the desired location. A crochet hook is used to retrieve the sutures beneath the skin, allowing them to be tied through the portal [14] (Table 3.3).

Ultimately, part of the success of arthroscopic elbow surgery is heavily dependent on meticulous preoperative setup, precise patient positioning, and the proper use of specialized instrumentation. Each step, from the application of the tourniquet to the careful management of fluid pressure, plays a critical role in optimizing surgical outcomes and minimizing complications. The detailed attention to the patient's anatomy and the specific challenges posed by elbow arthroscopy underscores the importance of using the correct equipment and positioning strategies. By adhering to these protocols, surgeons can achieve better visualization, reduce the risk of neurovascular injury, and enhance overall patient recovery.

Table 3.3 Arthroscopic elbow surgeries and the specific instruments required for each procedure

Surgery	Instruments
Epicondylitis surgery	Arthroscopic shaver, a curette (which can often be a standard open surgery curette), and, if suture passage is required, a Jelco with Prolene No. 01 along with suture retrievers or a crochet hook
Stiff elbow release surgery	Retractors for capsule separation, basket forceps for controlled cutting and removal of the joint capsule, grasper forceps for loose body removal, a 4.5 mm drill bit and arthroscopic burr for the Outerbridge-Kashiwagi procedure, with radiofrequency ablation being optional based on the surgeon's preference
Exploration and repair of the ulnar nerve	Small basic retractors or drains to keep the ulnar nerve identified and protected during the arthroscopic procedure
Posterolateral elbow instability surgery	No. 14 Jelco with a Prolene No. 01 suture for precise passage of the super-suture at the desired location and a crochet hook to retrieve the sutures beneath the skin

References

1. Abboud JA, Ricchetti ET, Tjoumakaris F, Ramsey ML. Elbow arthroscopy: basic setup and portal placement. J Am Acad Orthop Surg. 2006;14(5):312–8.
2. Speth J. Guidelines in practice: prevention of perioperative pressure injury. AORN J. 2023;118(1):37–44.
3. Bennett JM. Elbow arthroscopy: the basics. J Hand Surg Am. 2013;38(1):164–7.
4. Kholinne E, Jeon I h, Kwak JM. Basic to advanced elbow arthroscopy: the history, basic set up, and indications. Clin Shoulder Elbow. 2024;27(3):386–95.
5. Clark SM. Elbow arthroscopy: anatomy, setup, portals, and positioning. In: Wrist and elbow arthroscopy. New York, NY: Springer New York; 2015. p. 349–55.
6. Miller GK. An inexpensive support for prone or lateral decubitus elbow arthroscopy and open elbow surgery. Arthrosc Tech. 2017;6(4):e1411–4.
7. Camp CL, Degen RM, Dines JS, Altchek DW, Sanchez-Sotelo J. Basics of elbow arthroscopy part III: positioning and diagnostic arthroscopy in the lateral decubitus position. Arthrosc Tech. 2016;5(6):e1351–5.

8. Camp CL, Degen RM, Dines JS, Sanchez-Sotelo J, Altchek DW. Basics of elbow arthroscopy part II: positioning and diagnostic arthroscopy in the supine position. Arthrosc Tech. 2016;5(6):e1345–9.
9. Sinha A, Pydah SKV, Webb M. Elbow arthroscopy: a new setup to avoid visual paradox and improve triangulation. Arthrosc Tech. 2013;2(2):e65–7.
10. Dodson CC, Nho SJ, Williams RJ, Altchek DW. Elbow arthroscopy. J Am Acad Orthop Surg. 2008;16(10):574–85.
11. Terra BB, Rodrigues LM, Filho AN, de Almeida GDB, Cavatte JM, De Nadai A. Arthroscopic treatment for chronic lateral epicondylitis. Revista Brasileira de Ortopedia (English Edition). 2015;50(4):395–402.
12. Sanchez-Sotelo J. Arthroscopic management of elbow stiffness. J Exp Orthop. 2021;8(1):97.
13. Park SE, Bachman DR, O'Driscoll SW. The safety of using proximal anteromedial portals in elbow arthroscopy with prior ulnar nerve transposition. Arthroscopy. 2016;32(6):1003–9.
14. Anakwenze OA, Kancherla VK, Iyengar J, Ahmad CS, Levine WN. Posterolateral rotatory instability of the elbow. Am J Sports Med. 2014;42(2):485–91.

Surgical Anatomy and Portal Placement

4

Min Jong Park

1 Anatomy Surrounding the Elbow Joint

The elbow joint is formed by the distal articular surface of the humerus, the proximal ulna, and the radial head. Functionally, the elbow can be divided into three joints: the ulnohumeral joint, the radiocapitellar joint, and the proximal radioulnar joint. These three joints share a common synovial cavity, encapsulated within a single joint capsule. The anterior and posterior regions of the elbow are covered by a relatively simple joint capsule, while the medial and lateral sides are reinforced by the medial and lateral collateral ligaments. Surrounding the radial head is the annular ligament, which is part of the lateral collateral ligament complex.

The elbow joint is surrounded by several muscles, with important nerves and blood vessels situated closely, increasing the risk of neurovascular injury during arthroscopy compared to other joints [1, 2]. The primary consideration when developing arthroscopic portals is to find safe entry points that minimize the risk of damaging these neurovascular structures. Before discussing the arthroscopic portals, it is essential to review the anatomy surrounding the elbow (Fig. 4.1).

M. J. Park (✉)
Department of Orthopaedic Surgery, Samsung Medical Center, Sungkyunkwan University School of Medicine, Seoul, South Korea
e-mail: mjp3506@skku.edu

Anterior to the joint capsule, the brachialis muscle covers most of the capsule. Medially, the pronator teres, part of the common flexor muscles, is located, with the remaining flexor muscles positioned away from the capsule. Lateral to the brachialis are the brachioradialis, extensor carpi radialis longus (ECRL), and extensor carpi radialis brevis (ECRB). When the lateral capsule is removed during arthroscopy, the brachioradialis and ECRL, composed mainly of muscle fibers, are distinguishable from the ECRB, which originates from the lateral epicondyle and is closer to the capsule as a tendon structure. The extensor digitorum communis (EDC) lies posterior to the ECRB, with its origin merging with the ECRB into a conjoint tendon.

The brachial artery and median nerve are situated in front of the brachialis muscle. These important structures lie between the pronator teres and the tendon of the biceps brachii, with the brachial artery positioned medially to the median nerve. The radial nerve, located between the brachialis and brachioradialis, divides into the deep radial nerve (or posterior interosseous nerve) and the superficial radial nerve. The superficial radial nerve, a sensory nerve, is positioned anteriorly and farther from the joint, while the deep radial nerve, responsible for wrist and finger extension, runs just above the brachialis muscle, making it susceptible to injury during arthroscopy due to its proximity and limited mobility. It is crucial to avoid passing instruments anterior to

I.-H. Jeon et al. (eds.), *Elbow Arthroscopy*, https://doi.org/10.1007/978-981-95-3732-7_4

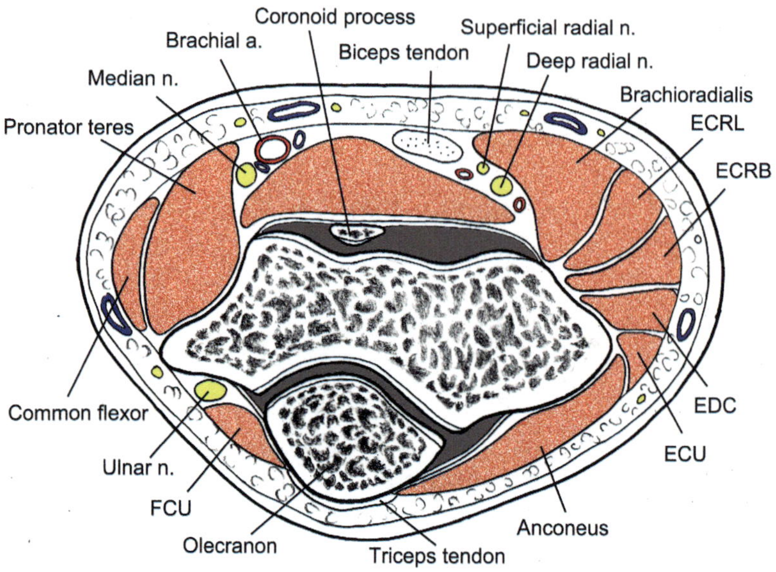

Fig. 4.1 For safe elbow arthroscopy, it is essential to know the anatomy surrounding the elbow

the brachialis muscle, as this poses a significant risk to the neurovascular structures.

Posteriorly, the elbow joint is safer for arthroscopic entry on the lateral side, as no major neurovascular structures pass through this region. However, on the medial side, the ulnar nerve runs close to the joint capsule, making this area particularly vulnerable. The triceps muscle is located above the olecranon, and the anconeus muscle covers the lateral joint capsule, allowing relatively safe access to the joint from any point. There is no completely safe method to enter the joint medially because the ulnar nerve is closely positioned on the medial side within the cubital tunnel. Therefore, it is advised not to attempt portal entry on the medial side of the olecranon and to avoid approaching the medial capsule during arthroscopy. If instruments must be used in this area, it is essential to remember that the ulnar nerve lies just beyond the capsule.

2 Indications and Relative Contraindications for Arthroscopic Elbow Surgery [3, 4] (Table 4.1)

Table 4.1 Indications and contraindications of elbow arthroscopy [5]

Indication	Contraindication
1. Loose body removal 2. Synovectomy 3. Septic arthritis lavage and debridement 4. Contracture release 5. Lateral epicondylitis release 6. Osteoarthritis—Excision of the osteophyte 7. Osteochondritis dissecans of the capitellum 8. Radial head excision 9. Assisted reduction and fixation of fractures 10. Posterior elbow impingement 11. Posterolateral synovial plica syndrome 12. Olecranon bursitis 13. Elbow instability (LUCL repair, rare)	*Relative* 1. Prior elbow surgery 2. Previous elbow trauma 3. Previous subcutaneous transposition of the ulnar nerve 4. Severe posttraumatic/degenerative arthritis 5. Ulnar nerve entrapment distal to elbow joint *Absolute* 1. Previous submuscular/intramuscular transposition of the ulnar nerve

3 Portals for Elbow Arthroscopy

3.1 Anterior Portals for Elbow Arthroscopy

Anteromedial Portal This portal is established 1.0–1.5 cm distal and 1.0–1.5 cm anterior to the easily palpable medial epicondyle, entering parallel to the joint line (Fig. 4.2). It was used as the standard medial portal when elbow arthroscopy was first introduced. Although this portal is advantageous for those unfamiliar with arthroscopy due to its straightforward direction, it requires penetrating the common flexor muscles and places the median nerve and brachial artery at significant risk. The portal should be made directly through the joint capsule, and extreme caution is necessary to avoid passing over the brachialis muscle, which could result in damage to the median nerve.

Proximal Anteromedial Portal This portal is created 1.5–2.0 cm proximal and 1.0–1.5 cm anterior to the medial epicondyle [6]. A cord-like medial intermuscular septum can be palpated proximal to the medial epicondyle. The insertion point is selected just anterior to this septum. After penetrating the skin, the portal is directed obliquely distally and laterally along

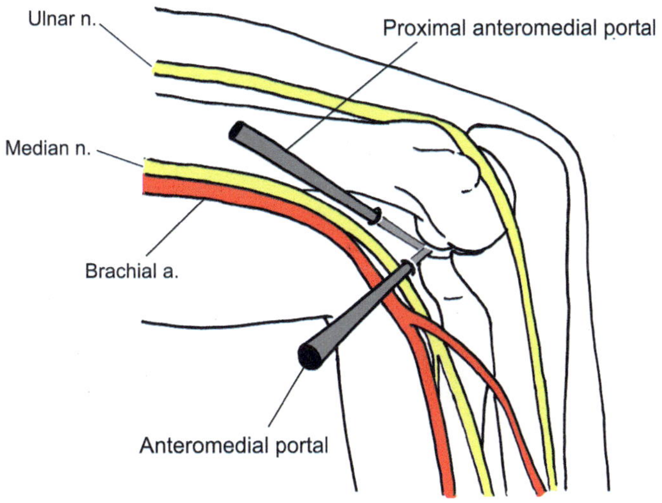

Fig. 4.2 Anteromedial portal and proximal anteromedial portal. The proximal anteromedial portal is more commonly used

the anterior surface of the humerus until it enters the joint capsule (Fig. 4.2). This portal, which follows the anterior humeral surface just above the origin of the common flexor muscles, is easier to insert than the anteromedial portal which requires penetration of the flexor muscles. Moreover, this approach is farther from the median nerve and brachial artery, reducing the risk of injury compared to the anteromedial portal. Nevertheless, it's important to maintain close contact with the anterior humeral surface to penetrate the joint capsule directly, avoiding the risk of advancing too far anteriorly and causing nerve injury. Additionally, care must be taken to avoid the ulnar nerve, which lies just behind the medial intermuscular septum. As the ulnar nerve can sublux anteriorly when the elbow is flexed, it is essential to palpate and verify its location before proceeding. The proximal anteromedial portal is now more commonly used as the standard portal.

Anterolateral Portal When approaching the anterior joint space from the lateral side, the primary concern is avoiding injury to the radial nerve, especially the deep radial nerve or posterior interosseous nerve. This nerve is thin, has limited mobility, and is susceptible to injury from direct trauma or traction, which can lead to significant functional impairment.

This portal is aligned with the radiocapitellar joint line, entering the anterior space 1.0–1.5 cm distal and 1.0 cm anterior to the lateral epicondyle. The portal passes through the extensor muscles directly into the joint space (Fig. 4.3) [7]. Although this portal is advantageous due to its straightforward entry parallel to the joint line, it is essential to remember that the deep radial nerve is in close proximity during insertion. If the joint capsule is not penetrated directly after passing through the extensor muscles, there is a high risk of damaging the deep radial nerve. A safer and easier alternative is to first create a medial portal and then use a Wessinger rod (switching stick) to create the lateral portal using the inside-out technique.

Proximal Anterolateral Portal This portal is created by making a skin incision 1.5–2 cm proximal and 1–1.5 cm anterior to the lateral epicondyle. The portal is directed slightly downward, following the anterior surface of the humerus to penetrate the joint capsule (Fig. 4.3). Initially, the anterolateral portal was the standard; however, the risk associated with its proximity to the deep radial nerve necessitated the development of a

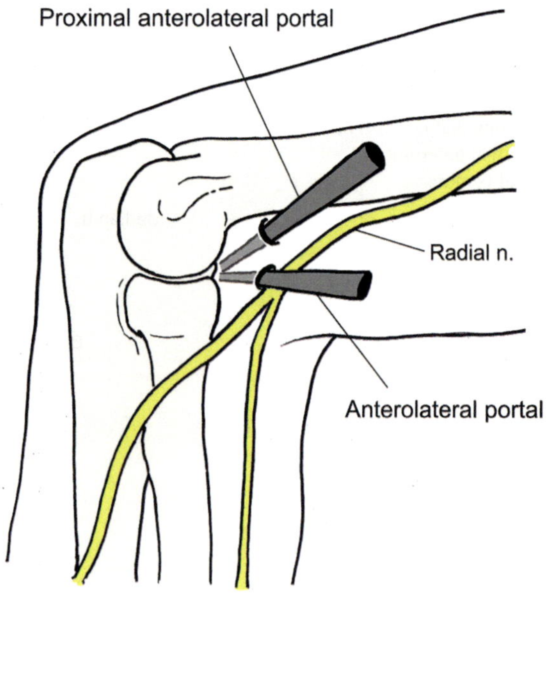

Fig. 4.3 Anterolateral portal and proximal anterolateral portal. The proximal anterolateral portal is more commonly used

safer alternative. Cadaveric studies have shown that the closer the portal is to the distal end, the closer it gets to the radial nerve [8, 9]. Conversely, the more proximal the approach, the farther it is from the nerve. Consequently, the proximal anterolateral portal is now more commonly used as the standard lateral portal. Despite being relatively safer, this portal still carries the risk of nerve injury, so careful attention must be paid to avoid proceeding outside the joint capsule during insertion. After penetrating the skin, the humeral bone should be palpated immediately, and the joint capsule should be punctured immediately after following the anterior surface of the bone to ensure the brachialis muscle provides a protective buffer for the radial nerve.

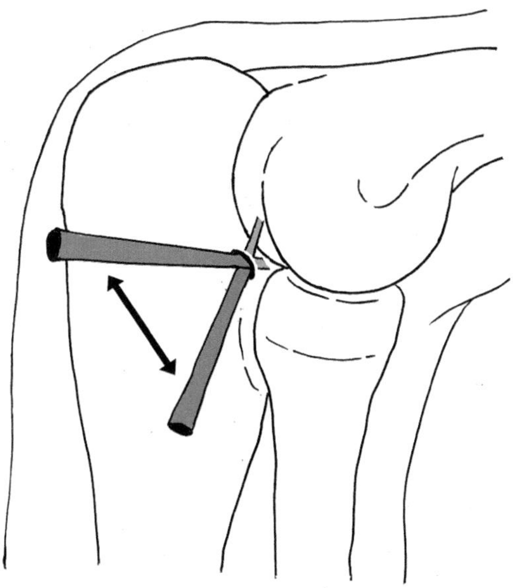

Fig. 4.4 Soft spot portal (straight lateral portal or midlateral portal)

3.2 Posterior Portals for Elbow Arthroscopy

Soft Spot Portal The soft spot portal is the most straightforward and safest entry point into the elbow joint. It is located at the center of the triangle formed by the lateral epicondyle, olecranon, and radial head, commonly referred to as the "soft spot" (Fig. 4.4). This portal is also known as the straight lateral portal or midlateral portal. It serves as the initial point for saline infusion at the start of arthroscopy. Upon penetrating the skin, the instrument directly enters the joint space. When saline is injected without resistance and flows easily anteriorly, it confirms accurate placement. Upon penetrating the joint capsule, the instrument is positioned just above the radial head, allowing visualization of the capitellum and proximal radioulnar joint. From this point, it is possible to advance anteriorly into the anterior joint space or ascend along the lateral gutter, adjacent to the lateral border of the olecranon, to reach the olecranon fossa. However, the lateral gutter has a narrow space, making passage of the arthroscope difficult. Forcing instruments through this space should be avoided, which can damage the articular cartilage.

Posterolateral Portal The posterolateral portal is the most commonly used entry point for accessing the posterior joint space (Fig. 4.5). The insertion point is approximately 4–5 cm proximal to the most prominent part of the olecranon, corresponding to the lateral border of the triceps muscle. To accurately determine this point, palpate the proximal boundary of the olecranon to locate the olecranon fossa, then select a site slightly proximal and just lateral to the lateral border of the triceps. From this location, the instrument is directed obliquely downward beneath the triceps into the joint space. A significant advantage of this portal is the absence of major neurovascular structures lateral to the triceps, allowing for safe portal creation.

Posterior Central Portal Also known as the transtriceps portal or straight posterior portal, the posterior central portal involves direct entry into the olecranon fossa through the central portion of the triceps muscle. Similar to the posterolateral portal, the insertion point is slightly proximal to the olecranon fossa at the posterior midline. The instru-

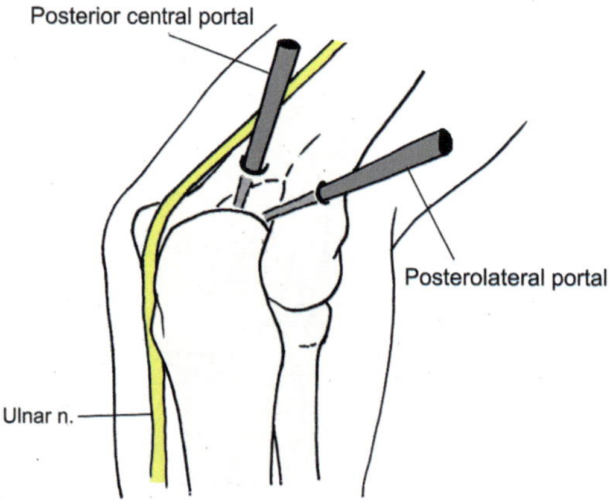

Fig. 4.5 Posterolateral portal and posterior central portal

ment is advanced distally towards the olecranon fossa (Fig. 4.5). When inserting an arthroscope or instruments through this portal towards the medial side of the olecranon tip, it is crucial to remember that the ulnar nerve lies just outside the joint capsule in the medial gutter. Advancing instruments distally through this area poses a risk of ulnar nerve injury and should be approached with caution.

Accessory Lateral Portal Along the lateral border of the triceps muscle, extending distally past the lateral border of the olecranon to the soft spot, additional accessory portals can be established as needed without concern for neurovascular injury. Since instruments can easily enter the joint space by penetrating the capsule at any point along this path, various accessory portals can be created. However, the lateral gutter corresponding to this area is extremely narrow, necessitating meticulous instrument handling to avoid damaging the articular cartilage. To access the posterior aspect of the radial head, an accessory portal is typically created 1–1.5 cm proximal to the soft spot. Combined with the soft spot portal, arthroscope and instruments can be alternately inserted through these portals to perform necessary procedures (Fig. 4.6).

While the posteromedial portal has also been described in literature, its use is rare due to the immediate proximity of the ulnar nerve, posing a significant risk. If the posteromedial portal must be employed, the safest approach involves making a small skin incision, carefully dissecting the soft tissue to partially expose the ulnar nerve, and inserting instruments under direct visualization of the nerve.

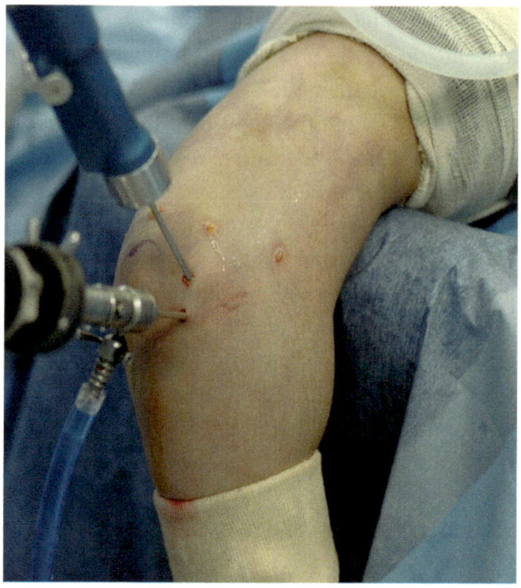

Fig. 4.6 Posterior radiocapitellar space can be accessed by using accessory lateral portal and soft spot portal

4 Author's Basic Techniques

The 30° arthroscope is predominantly used, while the 70° scope can be used in selected cases. A 2.9 mm arthroscope is usually used for both anterior and posterior spaces. In some patients, a smaller (2.4–2.7 mm) arthroscope is selectively needed in the lateral gutter and the posterior radiocapitellar joint, where the space is extremely narrow.

4.1 Preparation for Arthroscopy

Anesthesia General anesthesia or brachial plexus block can be used. However, arm blocks, including brachial plexus blocks, have the drawback of prolonged anesthesia, which prevents immediate postoperative nerve function checks.

During regional block anesthesia, the patient is usually awake, which can be uncomfortable, especially if the surgery requires the patient to lie on their side or stomach for about an hour. Intravenous sedation is often used to enhance comfort during the procedure. If the patient struggles with the position or experiences pressure pain, converting to general anesthesia is challenging. Therefore, general anesthesia is generally preferable and safer for elbow arthroscopy.

Patient Positioning The patient's position for elbow arthroscopy varies according to the surgeon's preference. The three possible positions are the supine (lying on the back), lateral decubitus (lying on the side), and prone (lying on the stomach). The supine position, though it requires securing the arm, offers easy joint adjustment and familiar joint orientation for the surgeon, making it suitable for beginners. In contrast, the lateral decubitus and prone positions provide better stability and access to the posterior joint space, but require careful positioning to avoid pressure-related complications. In the prone position, the chest should be cushioned with pads to avoid compression, and care must be taken to prevent pressure on the anterior superior iliac spine (ASIS) and the anterior knee skin. The lateral decubitus position, easier for maintaining the airway, requires precautions to protect the non-operative arm and the skin between the knees and ankles. Using a bean bag is ideal for maintaining stable positioning (Fig. 4.7a). Experienced surgeons may prefer the lateral decubitus or prone positions for their ease of access and comfortable positioning. A significant drawback is the difficulty in converting to open surgery, if necessary, such as in transposing the ulnar nerve or dealing with fractures. Therefore, careful consideration is required when choosing the position, especially if an open surgical approach may be needed.

Tourniquet and Other Preparations The tourniquet should be applied as proximally as possible on the upper arm to avoid interfering with the surgery. A sterile tourniquet is recommended to ensure sufficient surgical area while draping. The tourniquet pressure should be maintained at 200–250 mmHg after squeezing the upper limb. Keeping the compression bandage in place from just below the surgical site to the fingertips during the procedure followed by release of the bandage can help reduce postoperative swelling and soft tissue pressure caused by extravasation of irrigation saline during the procedure (Fig. 4.7b).

4.2 Step-by-Step Procedures

The following description assumes the lateral decubitus or prone position, with the surgical arm draped over a support attached to the side of the operating table.

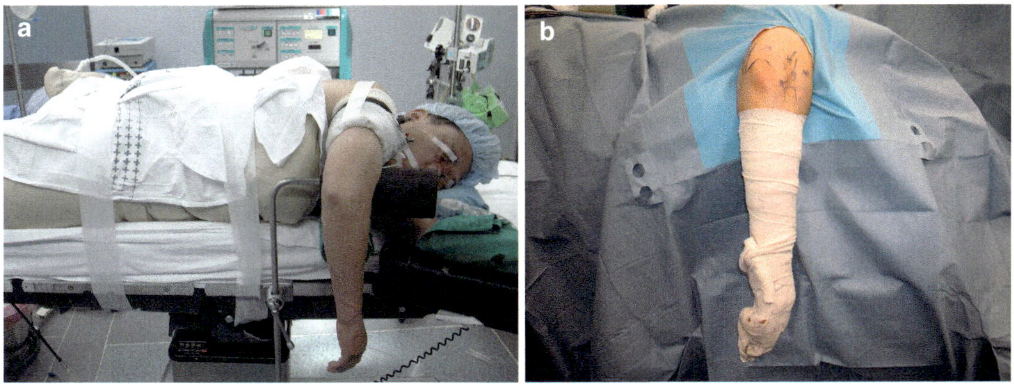

Fig. 4.7 Lateral decubitus position for elbow arthroscopy

Marking Anatomical Landmarks Before inserting the arthroscope, it is crucial to mark the anatomical landmarks to avoid difficulties in accessing the joint and to reduce the risk of nerve injury. Typically, the medial and lateral epicondyles, the olecranon tip, and the radial head (palpated while rotating the forearm) are marked (Fig. 4.8).

Accessing the Anterior Joint Space of Ulnohumeral Joint Arthroscopy typically begins with the anterior joint space. Approaching from the side at an angle is required to avoid critical nerves and blood vessels, making the creation of the anterior portal more challenging than the posterior. To facilitate portal creation, the joint capsule should be distended by injecting saline through the soft spot, usually 20–25 cc, using a 30 cc syringe. Care must be taken not to overinflate the joint capsule, which could cause it to rupture. Injecting saline into the joint space can expand the joint cavity, making the joint capsule taut. This not only facilitates the creation of an entry point but also moves the nerves and blood vessels located anterior to the joint capsule further away, providing a safer environment for the procedure (Fig. 4.9).

The choice of the initial entry point for arthroscopy through the anterior portal varies among surgeons and may also differ depending

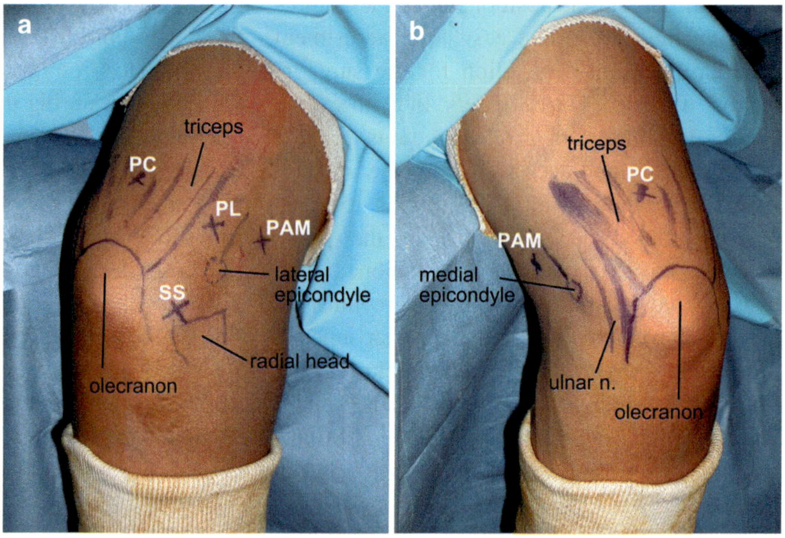

Fig. 4.8 Marking of anatomical landmarks and portals used for arthroscopy

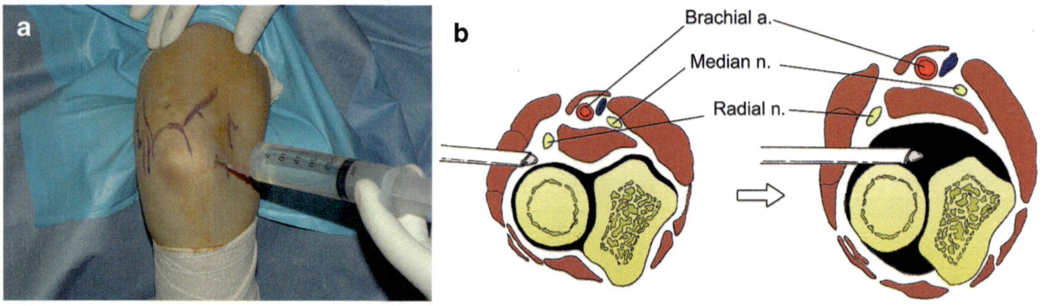

Fig. 4.9 Before establishing the portals, joint capsule is distended by injecting saline through the soft spot (**a**). Injection of saline can expand the joint cavity, making the joint capsule taut and moving the neurovascular structures further away from the joint (**b**)

on the surgical procedure. The most common choice is the proximal anteromedial portal. This portal is generally preferred because it offers a safer approach compared to the lateral side, where the deep radial nerve is in close proximity. If the surgeon chooses to create the proximal anteromedial portal first, a small skin incision of about 5 mm is made at the marked point using a No. 11 or 15 blade. A straight mosquito is then inserted, ensuring that the tip of the mosquito contacts the humerus, passing anterior to the medial intermuscular septum. It is crucial to avoid the ulnar nerve, which passes posterior to the medial intermuscular septum. The medial intermuscular septum is typically thick and taut, like a tendon, and can be easily palpated or felt with the tip of the mosquito. Once the tip of the straight mosquito is placed against the humerus, it should be advanced toward the joint at an angle of approximately 45° downward along the anterior surface of the humerus. The surgeon will clearly feel the mosquito penetrate the taut joint capsule. This moment is critical in creating the portal, as failure to accurately enter the joint space can lead to ongoing difficulties when inserting instruments during the surgery.

One common reason for the mosquito slipping anterior to the joint capsule is the concern about injuring the median nerve or brachial artery located anteriorly. This concern may lead to starting the insertion too close to the medial intermuscular septum, thus not achieving the minimal angle necessary to enter the joint space. Therefore, the anterior portal should be initiated 1.0–1.5 cm anterior to the medial intermuscular septum. Another important tip is that the mosquito's tip should contact the surface of the humerus immediately after passing the anterior aspect of the medial intermuscular septum (Fig. 4.10). Considering that the portal should pass through the most medial point of the anterior joint capsule, if the mosquito contacts the humeral surface after passing the medial border, it may have already missed the intended penetration point of the joint capsule. This mistake often occurs when the skin incision is made too far anteriorly. If there is no distinct feeling of piercing the joint capsule after contacting the bone surface and slightly advancing with the mosquito, it is likely that the mosquito has passed anterior to the joint capsule. In such cases, the surgeon should avoid forcing the mosquito forward or repeatedly attempting in the same direction, as this increases the risk of nerve or vascular injury.

Once the mosquito has penetrated the joint capsule and entered the joint space, the surgeon should slightly open the mosquito's handles to widen the capsule's opening. If saline begins to leak out, this indicates successful entry into the joint space. The mosquito is then removed, and the arthroscopic sheath (cannula) with an obturator (blunt trocar) is inserted along the same path. If the obturator tip contacts the hard surface of the bone, this confirms correct entry into the joint space; otherwise, it may have exited the joint, requiring reassessment. The obturator is

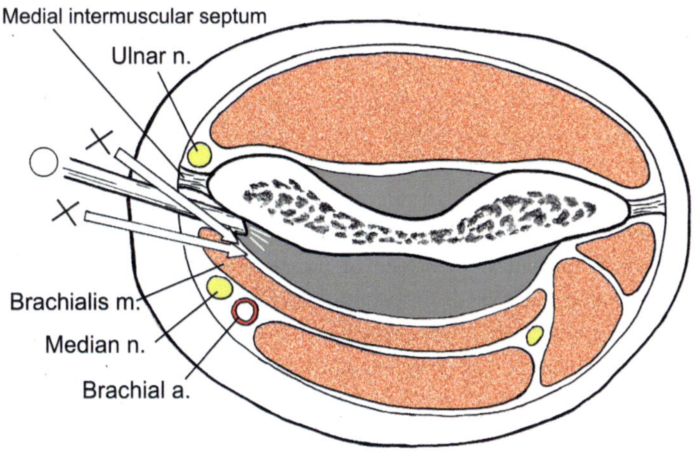

Fig. 4.10 Developing the successful anterior portals requires the mosquito's tip contacting the surface of the humerus immediately after passing the anterior aspect of the medial intermuscular septum. It should pass through the most medial point of the anterior joint capsule

then removed, and irrigation saline is introduced through the sheath before inserting the arthroscope. Opening the saline flow before inserting the arthroscope helps preventing air from entering the joint. Once the arthroscope is inserted through the medial portal, the radial head on the lateral side is usually the first visible structure, providing a reference for orienting the procedure. The radial head can be easily identified by rotating the forearm.

There are two primary methods for creating the lateral portal. The first involves creating the lateral portal in the same sequence as the medial portal, while observing through the arthroscope inserted via the medial portal. The second method uses an inside-out technique with a switching stick, known as the Weissinger rod. Initially, the inside-out technique was widely used to avoid deep radial nerve injury, but with the increasing use of the proximal anterolateral portal, this technique has been less commonly used. When using a switching stick, the lateral portal is created in a straight line from the medial portal, resulting in a more traditional anterolateral portal or a slightly more distal portal than the proximal anterolateral portal.

The proximal anterolateral portal enters the joint space above the radial head, and this area should be visualized through the arthroscope inserted via the medial portal. By pressing the marked skin insertion point with a finger, the surgeon can approximate where the lateral portal will enter the joint space. Although using a needle to confirm the exact location is an option, it is not recommended to prevent potential injury to the nearby radial or subcutaneous nerves. If the insertion point seems appropriate, a small skin incision is made, and a straight mosquito is inserted, similar to the medial portal. The mosquito should immediately contact the humerus surface after passing through the skin, and advancing obliquely downward at approximately 45° along the anterior surface of the bone, the surgeon can observe the mosquito pushing the lateral superior part of the joint capsule. Just as with the medial portal, it is crucial that the mosquito follows the most lateral edge of the humerus down the anterior surface to ensure it penetrates the joint capsule properly. Failing to do so risks the mosquito passing anterior to the joint capsule, which increases the likelihood of injuring the deep radial nerve and makes it difficult to enter the joint space. As with all arthroscopic surgeries, establishing an accurate portal path at the start is crucial for successful operation. Once the mosquito has successfully penetrated the joint capsule, the handles are widened to enlarge the capsule's opening. The main procedure usually starts with a shaver removing the synovium obstructing the view.

Accessing the Posterior Joint Space The posterior aspect of the elbow joint is approached through the space between the tip of the olecranon and the olecranon fossa with the elbow flexed at 90°. Among the standard portals, it is generally advisable to create the posterolateral portal first. The posterolateral portal is created by entering towards the olecranon fossa from the lateral edge of the triceps muscle. This approach is relatively straightforward and safe, as there are no significant structures at risk in this area. The skin incision should be made 2–3 cm proximal to the proximal border of the olecranon, angled slightly downward toward the olecranon fossa. While the use of a needle is generally discouraged when creating anterior portals due to the risk of nerve injury, it can be helpful for determining the optimal location when creating posterior portals. After making the skin incision, a mosquito is inserted underneath the triceps muscle and advanced into the olecranon fossa. The posterior joint capsule is thinner and looser than the anterior capsule, which may cause the mosquito to push the capsule instead of piercing it. Therefore, the mosquito should be advanced firmly until it contacts the bony surface of the olecranon fossa, and then the mosquito's handles should be opened widely to create a sufficiently large opening in the capsule. If the capsule is not adequately penetrated, the arthroscope or instruments may catch on the capsule, making it difficult and frustrating to insert them into the joint space. After inserting the arthroscope, the first step is to identify the olecranon tip to establish a sense of location and orientation.

The posterior central portal is created at the same level as the posterolateral portal, at the midpoint of the triceps muscle. To confirm the exact location, a needle can be inserted into the joint while viewing through the posterolateral arthroscope. After making a skin incision, a mosquito is used to penetrate the triceps muscle and the joint capsule, advancing into the joint space. Once it is confirmed that the tip of the mosquito has entered the joint, the mosquito's handles should be opened to widen the portal. Given the orientation of the muscle fibers in the triceps, it may be most effective to open the handles vertically. Once the portal is established, the first step is usually insertion of a shaver to clear the view.

Accessing the Posterior Joint Space of the Radiocapitellar Joint The posterior joint space between the radial head and the capitellum is connected anteriorly to the anterior space and extends superiorly along the lateral border of the olecranon to the posterior space. However, it is technically very difficult to observe the posterior aspect of the radiocapitellar joint using arthroscope inserted through the standard anterior and posterior portals. Therefore, creating a direct portal to access this area is the most feasible approach. The safest and easiest point of entry into the posterior space of the radiocapitellar joint is the "soft spot," which can be easily palpated with the elbow flexed at 90°. This spot is located between the radial head, capitellum, and the lateral border of the olecranon. Inserting the arthroscope through this soft spot allows direct access to the posterior space of the radiocapitellar joint. The process of creating a portal at the soft spot is similar to that of other portals. First, a needle is inserted to confirm that the entry path is clear of bony obstacles and that it is directed correctly. Once the optimal site is identified, a small incision is made, and a mosquito is inserted to establish the portal. If an additional portal is required for surgical manipulation, instruments can be inserted through either the posterior central portal or the posterolateral portal to access the joint via the lateral gutter. However, except in cases where the synovial membrane is lax, such as in patients with rheumatoid arthritis, the narrow space of the lateral gutter makes it difficult to pass through. Forcing instruments through this space can cause damage to the articular cartilage. Therefore, it is preferable to create an accessory lateral portal along the lateral border of the olecranon. When determining the location of the accessory portal, it is important to avoid placing it too close to the existing portals, as this can make instrument handling difficult and increase the risk of damaging the arthroscope. Ideally, the accessory portal should be placed at least 1.5 cm away from the main portal (Fig. 4.6). The easiest method is to insert a needle while visualizing with the arthroscope in soft spot, directing the needle downward to find the optimal site for incision, then inserting a mosquito to establish the portal.

Other Basic Techniques When using irrigation fluid, it is preferable to control the pressure by adjusting the height of the saline bag rather than using a mechanical pump. Excessive pressure can lead to extravasation of fluid outside the joint capsule, increasing tissue pressure and potentially causing complications. Conversely, insufficient pressure may fail to distend the joint capsule adequately, making manipulation more difficult. The use of an outflow portal may be necessary to maintain a clear field of vision, but it should be regulated appropriately. Keeping the outflow open can prevent sufficient distension of the capsule, making surgical procedures more challenging. In a practical sense, the outflow and mechanical pump are rarely used in most procedures.

One of the most challenging aspects of elbow arthroscopy is maintaining adequate space within the joint, as the joint capsule is relatively lax compared to other joints, making it difficult to keep the capsule distended. This is particularly important in areas where important nerves are located close to the capsule, as sufficient space is critical to avoid nerve injury. The introduction of intra-articular retractors has been highlighted as a useful method to assist in these situations. A retractor can be inserted through an extra portal to provide traction of the capsule, or it can be inserted alongside the arthroscope or instruments through a standard portal.

If significant bleeding is expected after synovectomy or osteophyte removal, it is advisable to insert a Hemovac drain. Under arthroscopic visualization through the anterior portal, the outflow sheath can be advanced anteriorly through the soft spot portal, and the trocar can be removed to insert the Hemovac tube (Fig. 4.10). It is crucial to use a Hemovac tube that is sturdy and resistant to breakage. If the tube becomes caught within the joint, elastic one can be stretched and cut inside the joint. Finally, the portal incisions are sutured, and the elastic bandage wrapped around the forearm during surgery is released to allow extravasated saline to spread, reducing postoperative swelling. The procedure is completed with a compression dressing, removal of the tourniquet, and application of a splint if necessary (Fig. 4.11).

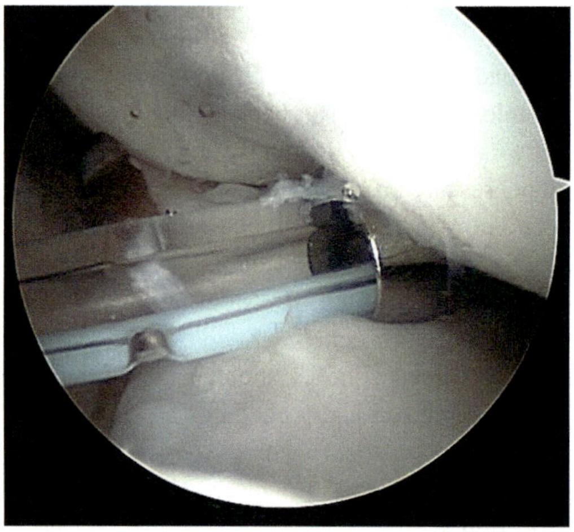

Fig. 4.11 The suction drain is inserted from the soft spot portal and advanced anteriorly through the space between the radial head, capitellum, and coronoid

References

1. Kelly EW, Morrey BF, O'Driscoll SW. Complications of elbow arthroscopy. J Bone Joint Surg Am. 2001;83(1):25–34. https://doi.org/10.2106/00004623-200101000-00004.
2. Lynch GJ, Meyers JF, Whipple TL, Caspari RB. Neurovascular anatomy and elbow arthroscopy: inherent risks. Arthroscopy. 1986;2(3):190–7. https://doi.org/10.1016/s0749-8063(86)80067-6.
3. O'Driscoll SW, Morrey BF. Arthroscopy of the elbow. Diagnostic and therapeutic benefits and hazards. J Bone Joint Surg Am. 1992;74(1):84–94.
4. Steinmann SP. Elbow arthroscopy: where are we now? Arthroscopy. 2007;23(11):1231–6. https://doi.org/10.1016/j.arthro.2007.08.008.
5. Kholinne E, Jeon IH, Kwak JM. Basic to advanced elbow arthroscopy: the history, basic set up, and indications. Clin Shoulder Elb. 2024;27(3):386–95. https://doi.org/10.5397/cise.2023.01032.
6. Poehling GG, Whipple TL, Sisco L, Goldman B. Elbow arthroscopy: a new technique. Arthroscopy. 1989;5(3):222–4. https://doi.org/10.1016/0749-8063(89)90176-x.
7. Andrews JR, Carson WG. Arthroscopy of the elbow. Arthroscopy. 1985;1(2):97–107. https://doi.org/10.1016/s0749-8063(85)80038-4.
8. Field LD, Altchek DW, Warren RF, O'Brien SJ, Skyhar MJ, Wickiewicz TL. Arthroscopic anatomy of the lateral elbow: a comparison of three portals. Arthroscopy. 1994;10(6):602–7. https://doi.org/10.1016/s0749-8063(05)80055-6.
9. Stothers K, Day B, Regan WR. Arthroscopy of the elbow: anatomy, portal sites, and a description of the proximal lateral portal. Arthroscopy. 1995;11(4):449–57. https://doi.org/10.1016/0749-8063(95)90200-7.

Part II

Tendinopathy

5 Arthroscopic Release of the Extensor Carpi Radialis Brevis

Erica Kholinne and Jae-Man Kwak

1 Background

The initial management of tennis elbow is nonsurgical. The condition usually resolves on its own, with 70–80% of patients experiencing relief within 1 year [1]. Treatment options may include modifying activities, doing stretching exercises, using forearm counterforce bracing, receiving steroid injections, and doing low-resistance muscle conditioning. While these measures can improve pain and grip strength, there is limited scientific evidence on their long-term effects on tennis elbow.

Various surgical procedures have been used to treat lateral epicondylitis, such as epicondylectomy, debridement of degenerative ECRB and EDC tendon tissue, denervation of the lateral epicondyle, removal of intraarticular capsular folds, and division of the annular ligament. Studies have supported the effectiveness of open debridement of degenerative ECRB and EDC tendon tissue alone or combined with partial epicondylectomy [2]. Recently, a less invasive arthroscopic approach to tendon debridement has become well known due to improved understanding of elbow anatomy and advances in arthroscopic techniques.

Baker et al. later reported successful outcomes with arthroscopic debridement in 40 patients (42 elbows) with recalcitrant lateral epicondylitis [3]. Using a standard medial portal for viewing and a superior lateral portal for debridement, they often used a burr to decorticate the lateral epicondyle. Subsequent reports and long-term follow-ups consistently show favorable results with this arthroscopic approach [4].

2 Anatomical Consideration

The extensor carpi radialis longus (ECRL) and extensor carpi radialis brevis (ECRB) have a distinct anatomical relationship at the elbow. The ECRL lies over the proximal part of the ECRB, requiring anterior elevation of the ECRL to view the superficial surface of the ECRB. These two structures are separated by a thin layer of areolar connective tissue. The origin of the ECRL is entirely muscular, located along the lateral supracondylar ridge of the humerus, forming a triangular shape with the apex pointing proximally. In contrast, the ECRB has a purely tendinous origin. Although it blends with the extensor digitorum communis (EDC), it can be separated

Supplementary Information The online version contains supplementary material available at https://doi.org/10.1007/978-981-95-3732-7_5.

E. Kholinne (✉)
Faculty of Medicine, Universitas Trisakti, Jakarta, Indonesia
e-mail: erica@trisakti.ac.id

J.-M. Kwak
Department of Orthopedic Surgery, Uijeongbu Eulji Medical Center, College of Medicine, Eulji University, Uijeongbu, Republic of Korea

I.-H. Jeon et al. (eds.), *Elbow Arthroscopy*, https://doi.org/10.1007/978-981-95-3732-7_5

from the EDC back to the humerus through dissection from distal to proximal along the tendon's undersurface. The ECRB originates beneath the most distal point of the lateral supracondylar ridge, with a diamond-shaped footprint measuring about 13 by 7 mm [5]. At the radiocapitellar joint level, the ECRB is closely positioned to the underlying anterior capsule of the elbow joint but can be easily separated at this point. Based on this anatomical information, an arthroscopic technique for lateral epicondylitis has been developed.

3 Indications and Relative Contraindications for Arthroscopic Elbow Surgery

The generally accepted indications for arthroscopic ECRB release surgery are as follows:

Indications	Contraindications
3.1 Patient underwent nonoperative measures that included rest, activity modification, counterforce bracing, nonsteroidal anti-inflammatory medication, and steroid injections 3.2 Patient was without improvement after nonoperative treatment for at least 6 months 3.3 *Atypical lateral epicondylitis:* Patients whose pain is located in the posterior recess or under the radial head, or those who experience clicking on pronation and supination of the elbow. This condition may involve snapping elbow or plica syndrome, making arthroscopic evaluation essential for diagnosing and treating intraarticular problems [6] 3.4 *Patients with inadequate outcomes from open procedures:* Individuals who have undergone a previous open resection of the extensor carpi radialis brevis (ECRB) and remain symptomatic may have underlying intraarticular pathology that needs to be addressed arthroscopically [7]	The generally accepted relative contraindications for arthroscopic elbow surgery are as follows [8]: Prior elbow surgery Previous elbow trauma Previous transposition of the ulnar nerve The operating surgeon should be mindful that any variation from normal anatomy can affect safe portal placement. For patients with ulnar nerve subluxation, a preoperative elbow ultrasound can be useful to determine the nerve's path. The procedure can still be performed, provided that the ulnar nerve remains within the ulnar groove throughout the procedure

4 Surgical Technique

Ideal positioning for elbow arthroscopy should allow 360° access to the elbow and free elbow flexion during surgery. There are three standard positions for elbow arthroscopy settings: supine, prone, and lateral decubitus [8]. The technique with the patient in the supine, prone, and lateral decubitus is essentially the same. The arthroscopic procedure can be performed under regional block or general anesthesia. The elbow joint is examined under anesthesia for instability because it is not uncommon for a lateral epicondylitis patient to present with concomitant instability. Repeated steroid injection to the lateral side with excessive lateral loading from daily activity may propagate this [9]. The hand and forearm should be wrapped with an elastic bandage to limit fluid extravasation. Additionally, a sterile pneumatic tourniquet should be placed proximally around the arm. It is advisable to make preoperative anatomical markings, such as identifying bony landmarks (lateral and medial epicondyles, radial head, and olecranon tip), as well as marking the course of the ulnar nerve before starting the surgery. An 18-gauge needle is inserted into the lateral soft spot, and the elbow joint is insufflated with 10–20 mL of sterile saline (Fig. 5.1).

The proximal anteromedial portal is created through a stab incision 2 cm proximal to the medial epicondyle, just anterior to the medial intermuscular septum (Fig. 5.2). Subcutaneous tissue is spread with a hemostat clamp, and the anterior joint compartment is penetrated with a blunt obturator or a switching stick (Fig. 5.3).

Blunt trocar is preferable to avoid cartilage injury during insertion aiming at the radial head. The obturator is exchanged for a standard 4.0 mm 30° offset arthroscope, and gravity inflow of sterile saline is established. If a mechanical pump is used, fluid pressure may be kept by gravity inflow or at <40 mmHg.

The proximal anterolateral portal is created using an outside-in technique (Fig. 5.4). The skin is punctured with an 18 gauge needle 1–2 cm proximal to the lateral epicondyle. Once the correct angle and position are confirmed arthroscopically, the viewing portal is created and the

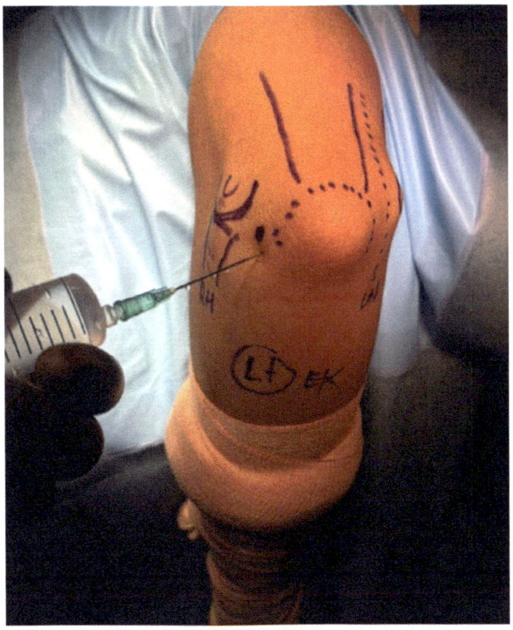

Fig. 5.1 Injection of 10–20 mL of saline through the soft spot located by palpation using the following bony landmarks: radial head, lateral epicondyle, and tip of the olecranon

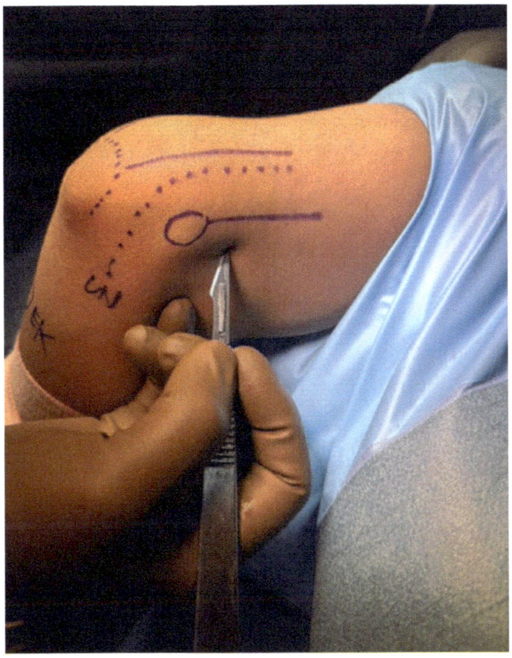

Fig. 5.2 The viewing portal was made using a blade

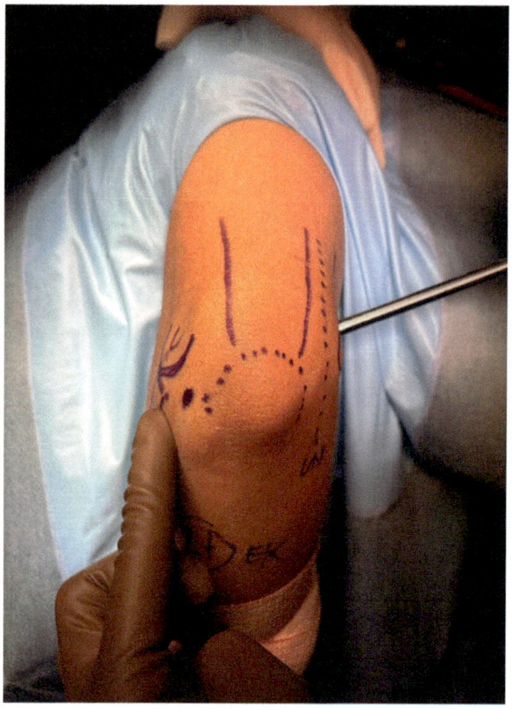

Fig. 5.3 A blunt trocar was used to penetrate the joint, which was aimed at the radial head

radiocapitellar joint is visualized. The hallmark pathology of lateral epicondylitis was systematically described using the classification by Baker et al. which are type I lesion (intact capsule), type II lesion (linear capsular tear) (Fig. 5.5), or a type III lesion (complete capsular tear) [3].

A motorized shaver is inserted into the lateral working portal, and a partial lateral capsulectomy is performed to visualize the underlying extensor muscles (Fig. 5.6) fully. The ECRB was resected to the point of its origin—the humeral lateral epicondyle. The resection is carried out proximally toward the supracondylar humeral ridge and distally from the top of the capitellum to the middle point of the radiocapitellar joint. The process should be completed when tendon fiber from the extensor carpi radialis longus is visible. An arthroscopic electrocautery device may be used concurrently with a motorized shaver to perform the debridement. During the procedure, care must be taken to avoid injury of the lateral collateral ligament by staying anteriorly to the equator of the radial head.

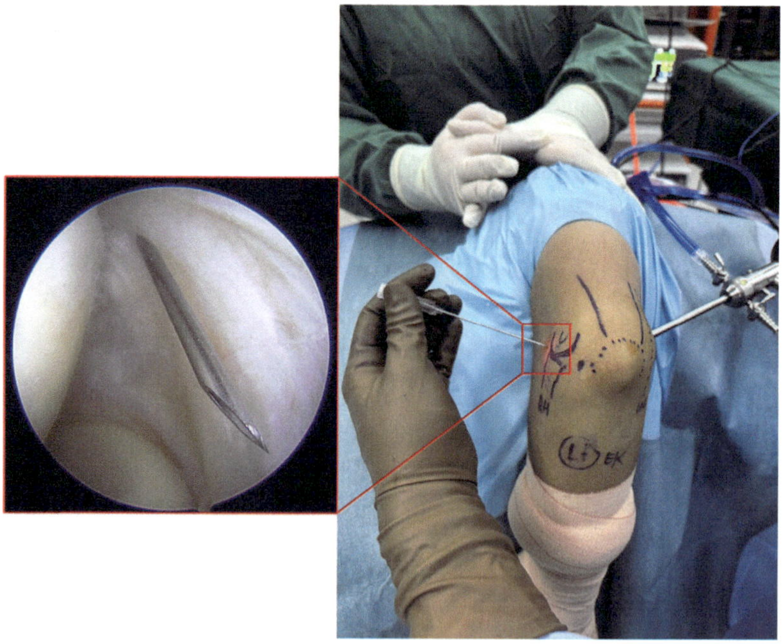

Fig. 5.4 The outside-in technique was used to create the working portal with an 18 G needle to confirm the trajectory

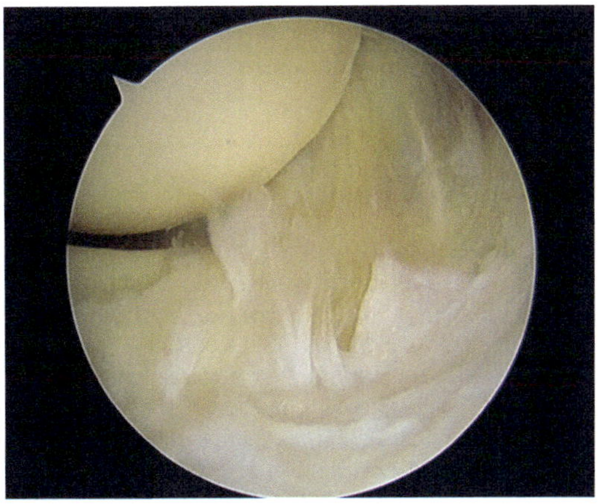

Fig. 5.5 Type II lesion with partial tear of the capsule viewed from proximal anteromedial portal

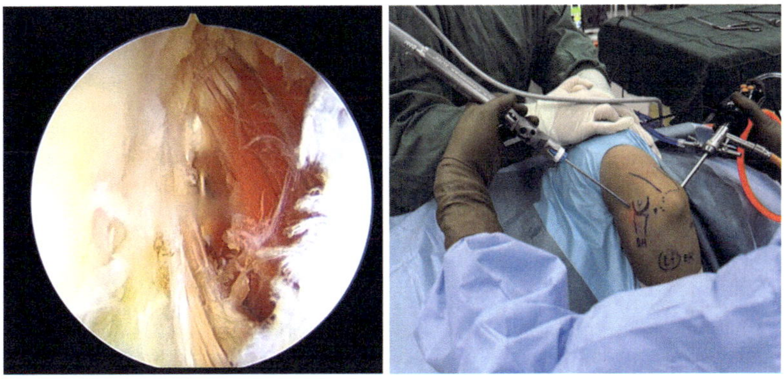

Fig. 5.6 A motorized shaver was used to debride the capsule and ECRB to the origin until the ECRL muscle fiber is visualized

5 Pearls and Pitfalls

1. Anatomic studies have demonstrated that a complete resection of the ECRB origin is safe if the dissection does not extend posterior to a line bisecting the radial head. In this way, the lateral ligamentous structures are protected without resulting in iatrogenic posterolateral rotatory instability.
2. Decortication of the bone may result in postoperative bony tenderness.
3. Third, a posterolateral compartment should be inspected for posterolateral synovitis or a thickened plica, which can be a pain generator. A preoperative evaluation usually shows posterolateral pain at the terminal elbow extension.

6 Complications of Arthroscopic Tennis Elbow Surgery [10]

While no specific reports detail complications for arthroscopic tennis elbow release surgery, a comprehensive meta-analysis of 95 studies, including 14,289 elbow arthroscopic procedures, identified an overall complication rate of 11.0%. The most frequent complications were elbow stiffness (4.5%), attributed to variations in follow-up duration, definitions, and patient characteristics; nerve injuries (3.4%), notably ulnar nerve injuries (2.6%) and lateral antebrachial cutaneous nerve (LABCN) injuries (1.0%), linked to prior trauma, previous surgeries, rheumatoid arthritis, and contracture; and infections (1.55%), which, although relatively low, were influenced by factors like advanced age, high BMI, smoking, diabetes, and the use of intra-articular corticosteroids.

References

1. Kalainov DM, Makowiec RL, Cohen MS. Arthroscopic tennis elbow release. Tech Hand Up Extrem Surg. 2007;11(1):2–7. https://doi.org/10.1097/01.bth.0000248358.06825.98.
2. Boyer MI, Hastings H 2nd. Lateral tennis elbow: is there any science out there? J Shoulder Elb Surg. 1999;8(5):481–91. https://doi.org/10.1016/s1058-2746(99)90081-2.
3. Baker CL Jr, Murphy KP, Gottlob CA, Curd DT. Arthroscopic classification and treatment of lateral epicondylitis: two-year clinical results. J Shoulder Elb Surg. 2000;9(6):475–82. https://doi.org/10.1067/mse.2000.108533.
4. Kholinne E, Singjie LC, Anastasia M, Liu F, Anestessia IJ, Kwak JM, et al. Comparison of clinical outcomes after different surgical approaches for lateral epicondylitis: a systematic review and meta-analysis. Orthop J Sports Med. 2024;12(5):23259671241230291. https://doi.org/10.1177/23259671241230291.
5. Cohen MS, Romeo AA. Open and arthroscopic management of lateral epicondylitis in the athlete. Hand Clin. 2009;25(3):331–8. https://doi.org/10.1016/j.hcl.2009.05.003.
6. Jeon IH, Kwak JM, Zhu B, Sun Y, Kim H, Koh KH, et al. Arthroscopic modified Bosworth procedure for refractory lateral elbow pain with Radiocapitellar joint snapping. Orthop J Sports Med. 2020;8(6):2325967120929929. https://doi.org/10.1177/2325967120929929.
7. Kholinne E, Jeon IH, Kwak JM. Basic to advanced elbow arthroscopy: the history, basic set up, and indications. Clin Shoulder Elb. 2024;27(3):386–95. https://doi.org/10.5397/cise.2023.01032.
8. Kholinne E, Kim M-S, Jeon I-H, Mah ET. Anatomy and portals in elbow arthroscopy. In: Doral MN, Karlsson J, editors. Sports injuries. Berlin, Heidelberg: Springer Berlin Heidelberg; 2024. p. 1–9.
9. Kholinne E, Liu H, Kim H, Kwak JM, Koh KH, Jeon IH. Systematic review of elbow instability in association with refractory lateral epicondylitis: myth or fact? Am J Sports Med. 2021;49(9):2542–50. https://doi.org/10.1177/0363546520980133.
10. Ahmed AF, Alzobi OZ, Hantouly AT, Toubasi A, Farsakoury R, Alkhelaifi K, et al. Complications of elbow arthroscopic surgery: a systematic review and meta-analysis. Orthop J Sports Med. 2022;10(11):23259671221137863. https://doi.org/10.1177/23259671221137863.

Arthroscopic Release of Pathologic Plica

6

Yi Lu

1 Background

Synovial plica is a prominent synovial fold attached to the capsule, present in 86–100% of individuals [1]. It most commonly extends into the posterior and posterolateral aspects of the radiocapitellar joint, covering approximately 18% of the radial head [2–4] (Fig. 6.1).

From a histological point of view, synovial plica is generally described as a structure mainly made up of fibroadipose tissue with moderate vascularization and plenty of nerve endings in its periphery (Fig. 6.2).

However, it can become symptomatic in 7.2–8.7% of elbow arthroscopies with a thickened synovial plica in the radiocapitellar joint covering more than 30% of the radial head [1]. Symptomatic plica occurs when chronic inflammation, secondary to trauma or overuse, leads to fibrosis, resulting in a thickened or hardened tissue fold that becomes compressed between the radial and humeral heads during joint movement (Fig. 6.3).

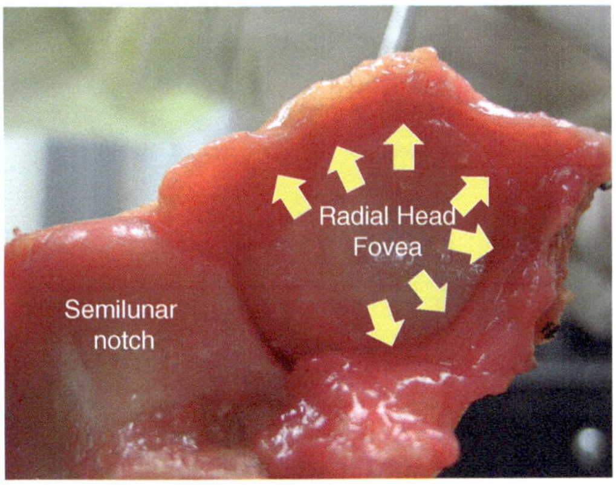

Fig. 6.1 Anatomy of Plica

Supplementary Information The online version contains supplementary material available at https://doi.org/10.1007/978-981-95-3732-7_6.

Y. Lu (✉)
Department of Sports Medicine, Beijing Ji Shui Tan Hospital, Capital Medical University, Beijing, China

I.-H. Jeon et al. (eds.), *Elbow Arthroscopy*, https://doi.org/10.1007/978-981-95-3732-7_6

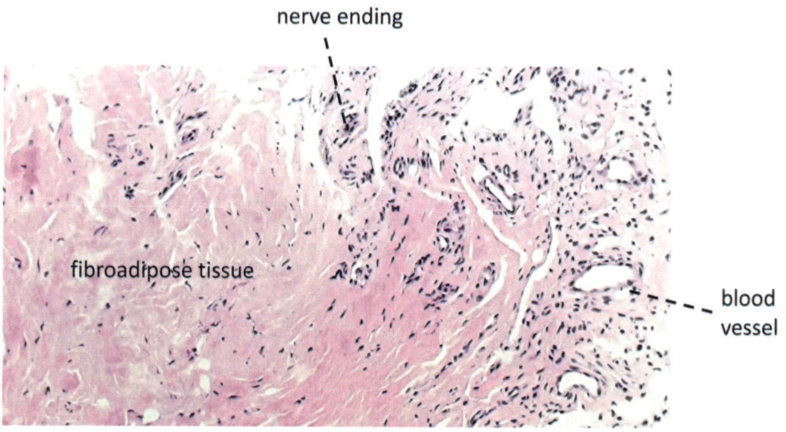

Fig. 6.2 Histological view of synovial plica, a structure mainly made up of fibroadipose tissue with moderate vascularization and plenty of nerve endings in their periphery

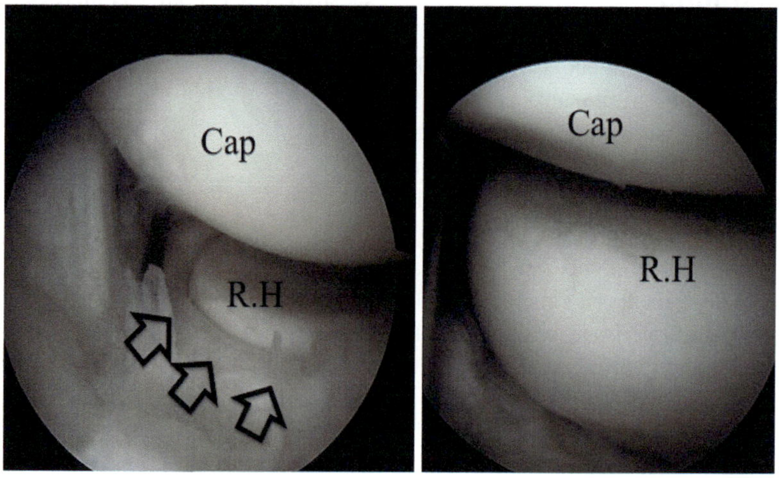

Fig. 6.3 Thickened synovial plica impinging in the radiocapitellar joint at extension (right) and flexion (left), in other words, snapping meniscocapsular complex

2 Clinical Manifestations

Symptomatic synovial plica (SSP) can occur at any age. There are no significant differences between men and women. The patient typically presents with chronic, repetitive injury or a single traumatic episode [1].

The most common and obvious presentation is pain, snapping and catching of the elbow. However, the symptoms of a symptomatic synovial plica in the radiocapitellar joint are often nonspecific and can mimic other conditions, such as tennis elbow, loose bodies, early degenerative changes, osteochondritis dissecans, or posterolateral rotatory instability [5].

Thus, certain characteristics may aid in its differential diagnosis [6]. Patients commonly report lateral elbow pain, which is typically aggravated at the extremes of motion or terminal extension [7]. During physical examination, tenderness may be present around the radiocapitellar joint (RCJ), lateral epicondyle, or the soft spot. Additionally, a painful snapping sensation during passive or active movement occurs in approximately 45% of cases. This snapping typically occurs when the elbow is flexed about 90° to 100° in pronation (Video 6.1) [8]. Some individuals may also experience joint locking with mild motion limitation.

3 Imaging

The most commonly used diagnostic imaging tool is MRI, in which synovial plica appears as a band of low signal intensity within the high-signal joint fluid. A synovial fold thickness greater than 3 mm was considered a pathologic plica (Fig. 6.4) [9–11].

In ultrasonography, the morphology of the SSP appears as a triangular structure with hypoechoic borders between the capitellum and the radial head, exhibiting an isoechoic consistency similar to muscles and distinct from other periarticular structures (Fig. 6.5). Pathological fold usually shows larger fibrotic change and impinges on the limits of motion, with evident impingement on dynamic testing (Video 6.1). Ultrasonography is commonly used to diagnose synovial plica and differentiate it from other pathologies, such as tendinopathy, loose bodies, impinging osteophytes, and snapping triceps.

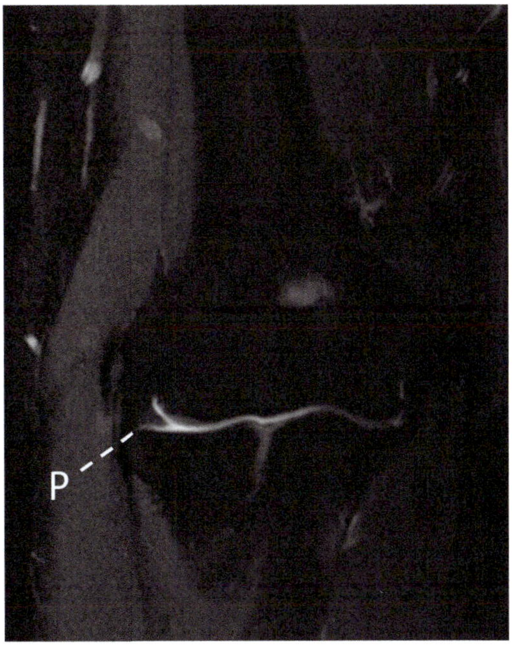

Fig. 6.4 Synovial plica from MRI/T2 showed a band of low signal intensity within the high signal intensity of joint fluid. *P* plica

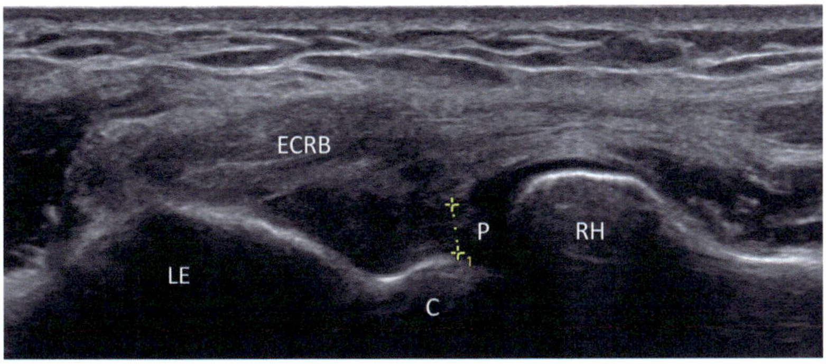

Fig. 6.5 Synovial plica from ultrasound showed a triangular structure surrounded by hypoechoic borders between the capitellum and the radial head and isoechoic with muscle. *C* capitellum, *ECRB* extensor carpi radialis brevis, *LE* lateral epicondyle, *RH* radial head, *P* plica

4 Indications and Contraindications for Arthroscopic Plica Releasing (Table 6.1)

Table 6.1 Indications and contraindications

Indications	Contraindications
1. Patients with persistent pain and mechanical symptoms, such as repeated snapping or locking on the lateral/posterior/posterolateral side of the elbow, which are unresponsive to nonoperative treatments 2. Combined with other problems such as recalcitrant lateral epicondylitis	1. Never receive nonoperative treatments before 2. An incidental finding on MRI without any symptoms or discomfort 3. Untreated or uncontrolled arthritis (RA, OA, etc.) 4. Unknown synovitis or infection

5 Step-by-Step Procedure

5.1 Preparation

The patient is placed in the lateral decubitus position under general anesthesia, according to the surgeon's preference. A tourniquet is applied, and a standard 4.0–mm, 30° arthroscope is used. The use of a pump is not routinely recommended. Although some surgeons suggest inflating the joint with saline using a syringe and needle through the soft spot to facilitate joint penetration, this technique has not been routinely adopted in plica release procedures.

5.2 Portal Setup

Four portals are routinely used. Diagnostic arthroscopy is performed through the soft spot portal as a standard viewing portal. An accessory posterolateral portal is established as the working portal. These two portals can be alternated to release most part of the plica on the posterior and posterolateral aspects of the joint.

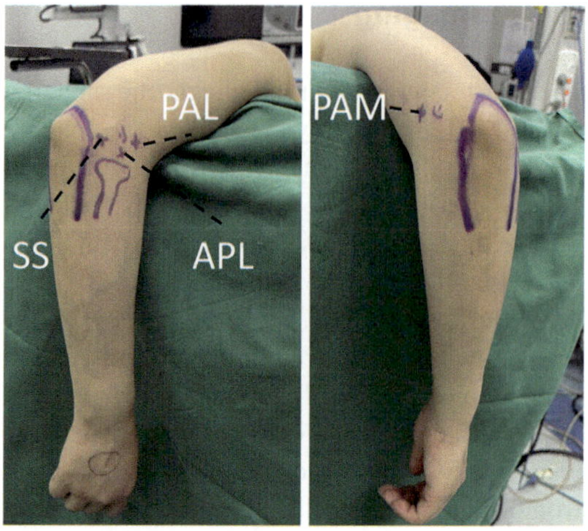

Fig. 6.6 Routinely portals set up for synovial plica releasing. *APL* accessory posterolateral portal, *PAM* proximal anteromedial portal, *PAL* proximal anterolateral portal, *SS* soft spot portal

To release the plica on the anterior aspect of the joint, the proximal anteromedial and proximal anterolateral portals are commonly used, although some surgeons prefer using the anteromedial or anterolateral portals (Fig. 6.6).

5.3 Plica Releasing

The camera is introduced through soft spot portal. A variable amount of soft tissue is usually in the way precluding proper visualization. This tissue, which forms part of the plica, can be safely debrided using a shaver (Fig. 6.7).

The plica is usually well visualized when elbow flexion exceeds 90° to 100°. A capsule rent on the lateral capsule near the radiocapitellar joint may be observed as part of the pathological changes. Observing the altered position of the plica with flexion and extension provides absolute confirmation of the diagnosis. The relationship of the plica to the radial head and radiocapitellar joint is carefully evaluated for any impingement or interference during elbow motion and forearm rotation (Fig. 6.8).

The synovial plica around the lateral aspect of the joint is debrided with a 4.5 mm motorized

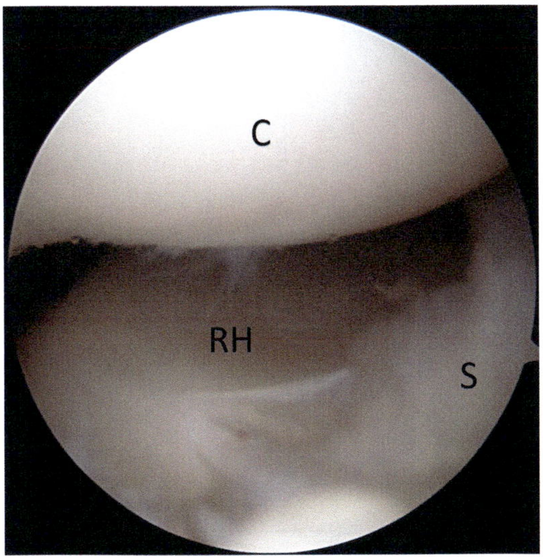

Fig. 6.7 When the camera introduced through soft spot portal, a variable amount of soft tissue is usually in the way precluding proper visualization. *C* capitellum, *RH* radial head, *S* synovium

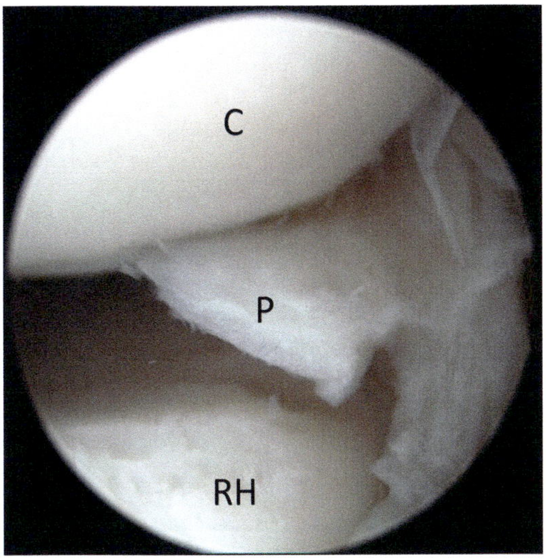

Fig. 6.8 The plica in lateral aspect of the joint looks like capsular rent as part of the pathologic changes. (Viewed from the soft spot portal. *C* capitellum, *RH* radial head, *P* plica)

shaver through accessory posterolateral portal. All plica tissue in this area should be thoroughly removed. Plica release is continued until no soft tissue remains interposed between the radial head and the humeral capitellum throughout the full range of pronation-supination and flexion-extension (Fig. 6.9).

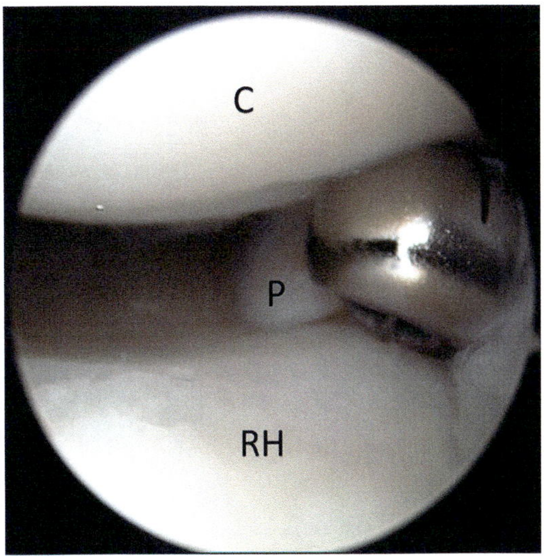

Fig. 6.9 The synovial plica was removed with a 4.5 mm motorized shaver. (Viewed from the soft spot portal. *C* capitellum, *RH* radial head, *P* plica)

Radiofrequency devices, such as ArthroCare, may be used for capsular shrinkage to potentially prevent plica recurrence, though this technique is based on personal experience and lacks evidence-based validation (Fig. 6.10).

Special attention is required when debriding the capsule, especially lateral to the radial head, to avoid damaging the lateral collateral ligament or annular ligament (Fig. 6.11).

To achieve complete plica release, the viewing and working portals can be exchanged, with the camera in the accessory posterolateral portal and the shaver introduced through the soft spot portal. The articular surfaces of the lateral olecranon, lesser sigmoid notch and proximal radioulnar joint are visualized and evaluated. The posterior joint is then cleared of synovitis or any residual plica using a shaver (Fig. 6.12).

Attention is then turned to the anterior compartment of the joint. The proximal anterolateral and proximal anteromedial portals are established separately as the viewing and working portals, which may be alternated as needed. The anterior plica is identified as a fibrous band covering a variable portion of the anterior radial head, extending from the lateral capsule to the anterior capsule medial to the radial head.

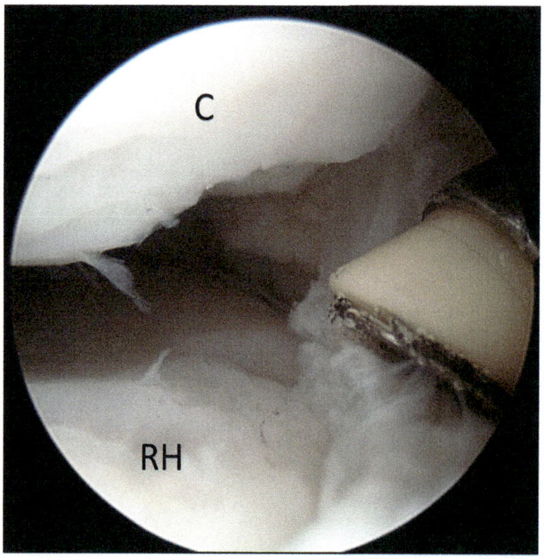

Fig. 6.10 Radiofrequency device can be used to perform capsule shrinkage. Viewed from the soft spot portal. *C* capitellum, *RH* radial head

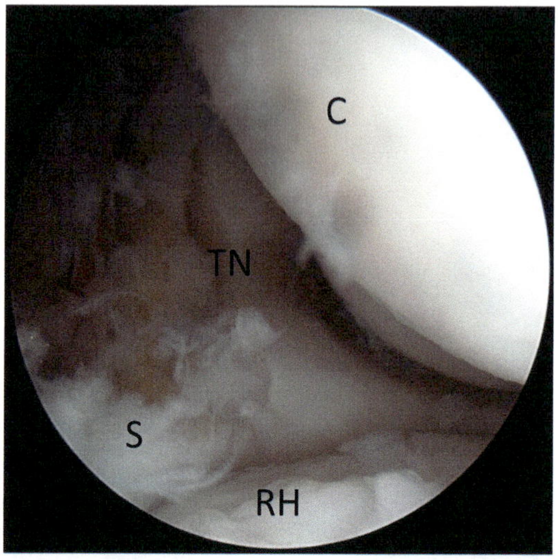

Fig. 6.12 With portal exchanging, most of plica can be removed on the posterior compartment of the joint. (Viewed from the accessary posterolateral portal. *C* capitellum, *RH* radial head, *S* synovium, *T* trochlear notch)

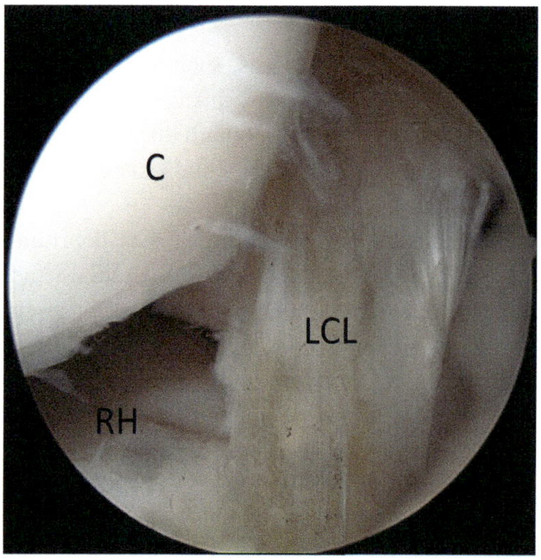

Fig. 6.11 According to anatomical closure, avoiding releasing too much to damage lateral collateral ligament. (Viewed from the soft spot portal. *C* capitellum, *LCL* lateral collateral ligament, *RH* radial head)

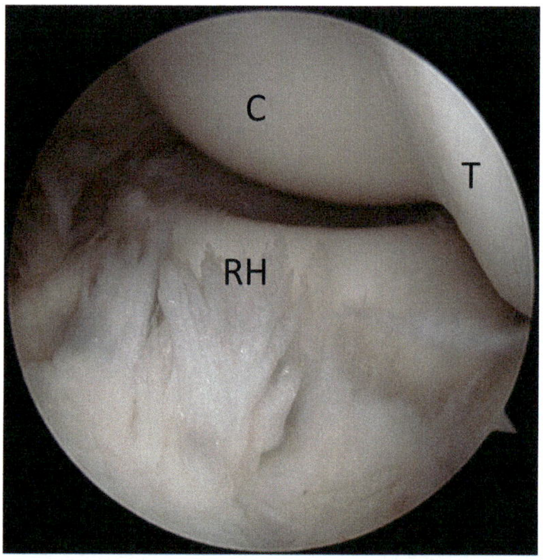

Fig. 6.13 The plica in the anterior compartment of the joint. (Viewed from the proximal anteromedial portal. *C* capitellum, *RH* radial head, *T* trochlea)

Resection of the plica in the anterior compartment is performed using a shaver and/or a radiofrequency device under direct visualization, with the goal of exposing at least two-thirds of the anterior articular surface of the radial head (Figs. 6.13 and 6.14).

Careful debridement should be performed with the jaws of the shaver oriented toward the humerus and never directed anteriorly, to avoid perforation of the anterior capsule. The posterior interosseous nerve lies just behind the capsule, anterior to the radial head and neck.

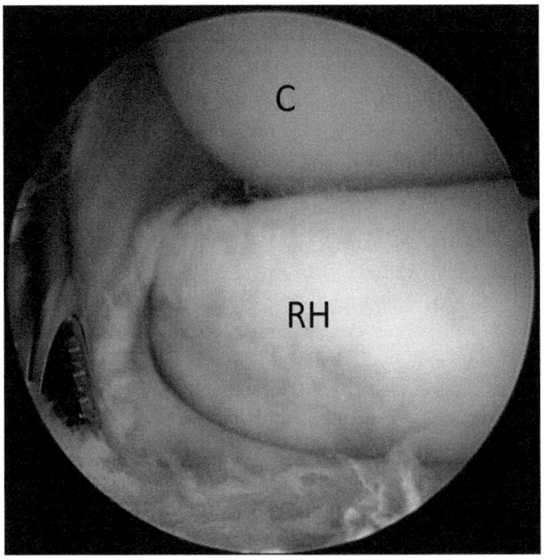

Fig. 6.14 The plica in anterior compartment of the joint is removed with shaver through proximal anterolateral portal under direct visualization with camera in proximal anteromedial portal. *C* capitellum, *RH* radial head

5.4 Combined Lesions

The combined lesions, such as chondromalacia, osteochondral lesions on the radial head, cartilage erosion of the capitellar or trochlea, ECRB degeneration may be encountered in patients with synovial plica. It is important not to overlook a thorough examination of the entire joint. Additional debridement or other necessary procedures should be performed as indicated. Any associated intra-articular pathology can be addressed during the same surgical session.

6 Pitfalls of the Procedure

1. Inaccurate portal placement may result in a lack of appreciation of the extent of the pathology.
2. Excessive releasing of plica (particularly when the shaver passes posterior to the meridian of the radial head) might damage the lateral ulnar collateral ligament, potentially resulting in posterolateral rotatory instability of the elbow.
3. Excessive release of the plica can damage the annular ligament and lead to proximal radio-ulnar joint (PRUJ) instability.
4. Take care to protect neural structures during anterior plica release. Injury to the posterior interosseous nerve (PIN), which lies anterior to the radial head, must be avoided.
5. Do not neglect the combined injury or disease, such as lateral epicondylitis and chondromalacia of the radial head and capitellum.

Do not overlook associated injuries or conditions, such as lateral epicondylitis, chondromalacia of the radial head, or capitellar chondromalacia.

7 Key Points

1. MRI can identify a synovial fold in most patients. However, a thorough examination and clinical correlation are required. If these factors are overlooked, diagnosing SSP prior to surgery may be challenging.
2. Complete plica release may not be possible from a single portal. Be prepared to employ several portals to adequately visualize and release the plica when necessary.
3. The soft spot portal may be the most effective for diagnosing and visualizing the releasing procedure. However, evaluating the whole procedure through different portal is mandatory.
4. Release the plica as much as we can, but keep important structures, such as articular ligament, lateral collateral ligament, and PIN intact.

Video 6.2 (Surgical procedure, by Prof. Lu Yi)

References

1. Lubiatowski P, Wałecka J, Dzianach M, Stefaniak J, Romanowski L. Synovial plica of the elbow and its clinical relevance. EFORT Open Rev. 2020;5(9):549–557. Published 2020 Sep 30.
2. Koh S, Morris RP, Andersen CL, Jones EA, Viegas SF. Ultrasonographic examination of the synovial

fold of the radiohumeral joint. J Shoulder Elb Surg. 2007;16(5):609–15.
3. Awaya H, Schweitzer ME, Feng SA, et al. Elbow synovial fold syndrome: MR imaging findings. AJR Am J Roentgenol. 2001;177(6):1377–81.
4. Steinert AF, Goebel S, Rucker A, Barthel T. Snapping elbow caused by hypertrophic synovial plica in the radiohumeral joint: a report of three cases and review of literature. Arch Orthop Trauma Surg. 2010;130(3):347–51.
5. Bjerre JJ, Johannsen FE, Rathcke M, Krogsgaard MR. Snapping elbow—a guide to diagnosis and treatment. World J Orthop. 2018;9(4):65–71.
6. Park KB, Kim SJ, Chun YM, Yoon TH, Choi YS, Jung M. Clinical and diagnostic outcomes in arthroscopic treatment for posterolateral plicae impingement within the radiocapitellar joint. Medicine (Baltimore). 2019;98(18):e15497.
7. Clarke RP. Symptomatic, lateral synovial fringe (plica) of the elbow joint. Arthroscopy. 1988;4(2):112–6.
8. Antuna SA, O'Driscoll SW. Snapping plicae associated with radiocapitellar chondromalacia. Arthroscopy. 2001;17(5):491–5.
9. Bonczar M, Ostrowski P, Bednarz W, Wojciechowski W, Walocha J, Koziej M. Synovial plica of the elbow—detailed measurements and how to implicate its relevance in clinical practice. Int Orthop. 2023;47(4):1031–9.
10. Ruiz de Luzuriaga BC, Helms CA, Kosinski AS, Vinson EN. Elbow MR imaging findings in patients with synovial fringe syndrome. Skeletal Radiol. 2013;42:675–80.
11. Kholinne E, Nanda A, Liu H, Kwak JM, Kim H, Koh K-H, Jeon IH. The elbow plica: a systematic review of terminology and characteristics. J Shoulder Elb Surg. 2021;30(5):185–98.

7 Arthroscopic and Minimally Invasive Management of Medial Epicondylitis

Takashi Oda

1 Anatomy of the Medial Elbow [Background]

The intramuscular septa between the pronator teres (PT), flexor carpi radialis (FCR), palmaris longus (PL), and flexor digitorum superficialis (FDS) collectively form the anterior common tendon [1]. This anterior common tendon attaches to the medial epicondyle and the anterior joint capsule of the elbow, encompassing the attachment of the anterior oblique ligament. The intramuscular septum between the FDS and flexor carpi ulnaris (FCU) constitutes the posterior common tendon that attaches to the inferior surface of the medial epicondyle and the medial joint capsule. Approximately 50–75% of the proximal segment of the anterior oblique ligament comprises an intermixture of common tendons and fibers [2].

Supplementary Information The online version contains supplementary material available at https://doi.org/10.1007/978-981-95-3732-7_7.

T. Oda (✉)
Department of Orthopedic Surgery, Hokkaido Saiseiaki Otaru Hospital, Otaru, Japan

2 Indications of Arthroscopic Surgery for Medial Epicondylitis (Table 7.1)

Table 7.1 Indications for arthroscopic release of the flexor-pronator origin in the treatment of medial epicondylitis [3–5]

Indication	Contraindication
1. Patients whose symptoms persist despite 6 months or more of conservative therapy 2. Patients experiencing severe exertional pain, spontaneous pain, or nocturnal pain 3. Patients with concurrent progressive ulnar neuropathy	Absolute 1. Patients who have undergone anterior transposition of the ulnar nerve Relative 2. Patients with anterior subluxation of the ulnar nerve during elbow flexion

3 Step-by-Step Procedure

3.1 Portals

The proximal medial portal serves as the primary working portal, while the anterolateral portal is utilized as a viewing portal. The proximal medial adjacent portal, which is established 1 cm proximal to the proximal medial portal by the outside-in technique, is used as a secondary working portal (Fig. 7.1a) [3, 6].

I.-H. Jeon et al. (eds.), *Elbow Arthroscopy*, https://doi.org/10.1007/978-981-95-3732-7_7

3.2 Intra-Articular Treatment

Using the anterolateral portal as the arthroscopic entry point, insert a 4-mm 30° oblique scope to observe the medial aspect of the anterior joint space. The visual field is secured by inserting a switching rod or probe via a proximal medial portal and retracting the anterior joint capsule anteriorly (Fig. 7.1a). Insert a shaver (3.5 mm full-radius cutter) or radiofrequency device through the proximal medial adjacent portal to initiate resection of the medial joint capsule, expanding the resection area distally while using the proximal edge of the coronoid fossa as a reference (Fig. 7.1b).

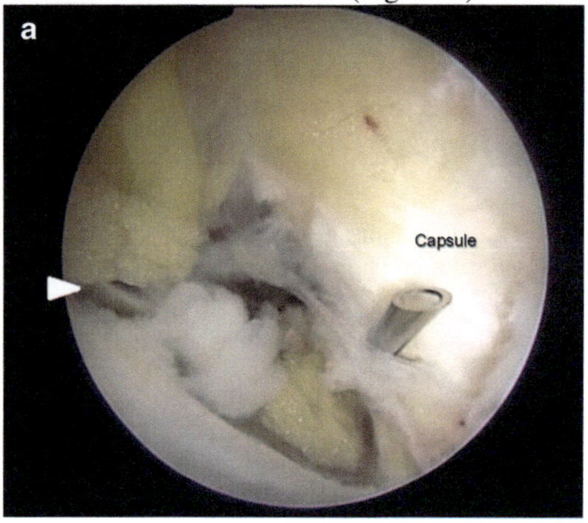

Fig. 7.1a The joint capsule is retracted anteriorly with a switching rod (indicated by the arrowhead) introduced through the proximal medial portal, while an epidural needle is inserted percutaneously 1 cm proximal to the proximal medial portal

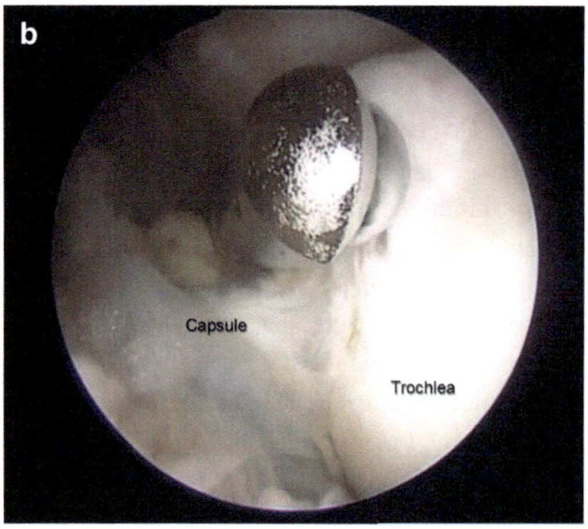

Fig. 7.1b The medial joint capsule is excised using a shaver

3.3 Release of Tendon Origin

Replace the arthroscope with a 70° oblique scope and identify the lateral margin of the origin of the flexor-pronator group, which attaches to the anterolateral surface of the medial epicondyle. Using a shaver or radiofrequency device, release the origin of the flexor-pronator muscle group subperiosteally from the anterior surface of the medial epicondyle (Fig. 7.1c).

Advance the incision at the tendon origin toward the medial side (Fig. 7.1d). The superior proximal edge of the articular cartilage of the

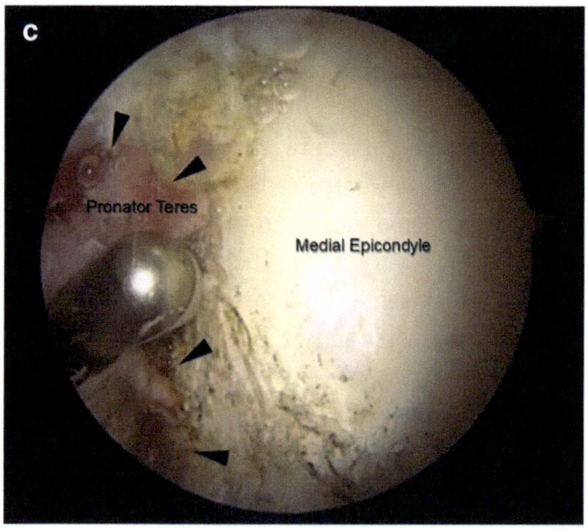

Fig. 7.1c The origin of the pronator teres muscle is released using a radiofrequency device

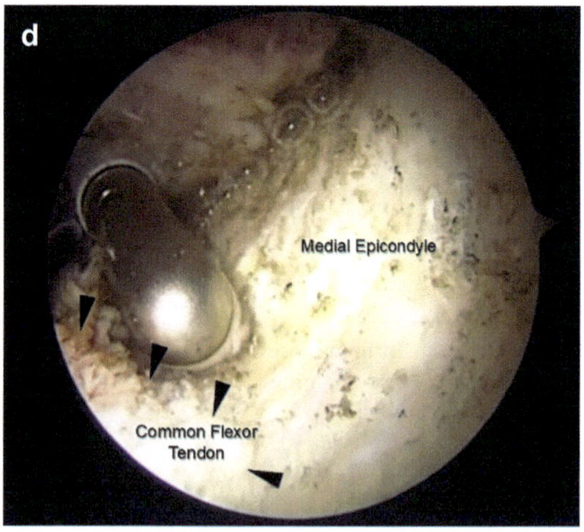

Fig. 7.1d The common tendon of the pronator-flexor group is detached from the anterior aspect of the medial epicondyle

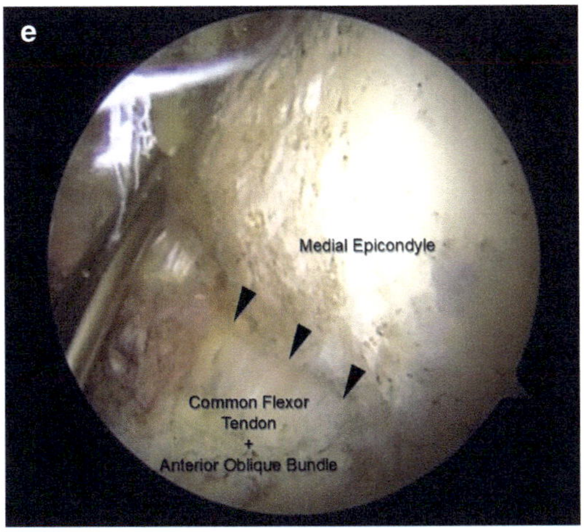

Fig. 7.1e Anterior surface of the medial epicondyle following the release of the common tendon origin of the pronator-flexor muscle

humeral trochlea serves as a rough guide to the distal end of the tendon origin at the medial epicondyle.

When the medial origin of the tendon is fully dissected, a "cliff view" [6] is observed, where the flat anterior surface of the medial epicondyle appears to descend precipitously at the medial edge, resembling a cliff (Fig. 7.1e).

4 Pitfalls of the Procedure

1. Take care to avoid cutting at the tip of the medial epicondyle, where the anterior oblique fibers of the ulnar collateral ligament are anchored. The mean distance between the resection site of the tendon attachment and the origin of the anterior oblique ligament was 8.3 mm [6]. Since it is difficult to clearly separate the common tendon and the anterior oblique ligament, care should be taken not to cut the tendon to the lower end of the medial epicondyle to which the ligament attaches.
2. The most critical complication in arthroscopic surgery for medial epicondylitis is intraoperative ulnar nerve injury. The average distance between the tendon attachment resection site and the ulnar nerve is 20.8 mm [6], indicating a low risk of ulnar nerve damage during arthroscopic procedures. However, the ulnar nerve may shift anteriorly and come into contact with the medial epicondyle when the elbow joint is flexed, necessitating careful assessment of this position prior to surgery.

5 Key Procedure

Supplementary Video. Arthroscopic release of the pronator-flexor origin from the medial epicondyle (left elbow)

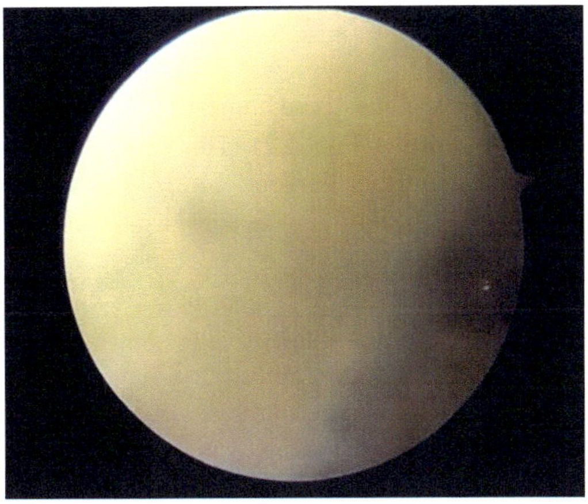

References

1. Otoshi K, Kikuchi S, Shishido H, Konno S. The proximal origins of the flexor-pronator muscles and their role in the dynamic stabilization of the elbow joint: an anatomical study. Surg Radiol Anat. 2014;36(3):289–94. https://doi.org/10.1007/s00276-013-1168-3.
2. Gabel GM, Morrey BF. Medial epicondylitis. In: Morrey BF, editor. The elbow and its disorders. Philadelphia, PA: Saunders Elsevier; 2009. p. 506–14.
3. Oda T, Wada T, Yamamoto O, Saito A, Kondo M. Arthroscopic release of the pronator-flexor origin for medial epicondylitis. Tech Should Elbow Surg. 2018;19(2):75–9. https://doi.org/10.1097/bte.0000000000000135.
4. do Nascimento AT, Claudio GK. Arthroscopic surgical treatment of medial epicondylitis. J Shoulder Elbow Surg. 2017;26(12):2232–5. https://doi.org/10.1016/j.jse.2017.08.019.
5. Kim BS, Jung KJ, Lee C. Open procedure vs. arthroscopic debridement for chronic medial epicondylitis. J Shoulder Elb Surg. 2023;32(2):340–7. https://doi.org/10.1016/j.jse.2022.09.018.
6. Zonno A, Manuel J, Merrell G, Ramos P, Akelman E, DaSilva MF. Arthroscopic technique for medial epicondylitis: technique and safety analysis. Arthroscopy. 2010;26(5):610–6. https://doi.org/10.1016/j.arthro.2009.09.017.

Part III

Trauma and Instability

8 Arthroscopic-Assisted Fracture Fixation of Radial Head Fracture

Panai Laohaprasitiporn and Gregory Bain

1 Introduction

1.1 Overview of Radial Head Fracture Treatment

Radial head fractures are common elbow injuries, frequently occurring due to falls onto an outstretched hand. The approach to managing these fractures depends on a variety of factors, including patient-specific considerations such as age, comorbidities, physical activity level, occupation, and hand dominance. Additionally, fracture characteristics—such as the number of fragments, the extent of displacement, and the timing of treatment post-injury—along with the presence of any associated injuries or instabilities, play a crucial role in determining the appropriate management of radial head fractures.

A widely utilized classification system for radial head fractures is the Hotchkiss modification of the Mason classification [1, 2]:

Type I: Non-displaced or minimally displaced fractures.

Type II: Displaced fractures more than 2 mm, motion may be mechanically blocked.

Type III: Comminuted fractures involving multiple fragments.

Type IV: Radial head fracture associated with elbow dislocation [3].

Nonoperative treatment is generally indicated for Mason type I radial head fractures. This approach involves initial immobilization using a sling or posterior splint, followed by early mobilization.

Operative management is recommended for fractures that are displaced and impede motion (Mason type II), comminuted fractures (Mason type III), as well as cases involving associated ligamentous injury or elbow dislocation. Surgical interventions may include open reduction and internal fixation to restore joint congruity and achieve stable fixation, allowing for early mobilization. In instances where the fracture is irreparable and comminuted, radial head excision and replacement may be necessary [4]. Additionally, arthroscopic-assisted reduction and fixation offer a minimally invasive option for selected cases, offering enhanced visualization that improves precision during fracture reduction. This technique also results in reduced soft tissue swelling and morbidity, thereby accelerating the recovery process.

P. Laohaprasitiporn
Department of Orthopaedic Surgery, Flinders University and Flinders Medical Centre, Adelaide, Australia

Department of Orthopaedic Surgery, Faculty of Medicine Siriraj Hospital, Mahidol University, Bangkok, Thailand

G. Bain (✉)
Department of Orthopaedic Surgery, Flinders University and Flinders Medical Centre, Adelaide, Australia
e-mail: greg@gregbain.com.au

I.-H. Jeon et al. (eds.), *Elbow Arthroscopy*, https://doi.org/10.1007/978-981-95-3732-7_8

2 Indications and Contraindications for Arthroscopic Management

2.1 Indications

- Mason type II fractures are well-suited for arthroscopic-assisted reduction and internal fixation (ARIF).
- In cases of an angulated pediatric radial neck fracture with incomplete ossification of the radial head, elbow arthroscopy can assist with fracture visualization and reduction [5].

2.2 Relative Contraindications

- Severe soft tissue swelling or impending compartment syndrome.
- Severely displaced or comminuted intra-articular fractures.
- Previous elbow injury, surgery or arthritis, producing deformity, contracture, or ulnar nerve entrapment.
- Neurovascular compromise requiring urgent exploration.

3 Preoperative Planning

3.1 Specific Patient Evaluation

In the acute setting, evaluating elbow motion and stability can be facilitated by aspirating hemarthrosis and injecting intra-articular lidocaine. This approach provides analgesia, allowing for a more accurate assessment, especially to identify if stiffness is due to pain or locked displaced fragments.

3.2 Imaging

- Anteroposterior, lateral, and Greenspan views of the elbow X-ray.
- A computed tomography (CT) scan with three-dimensional reconstructions is very useful for preoperative planning. It allows for a detailed assessment of intra-articular fracture morphology and assists in determining the optimal reduction techniques. Additionally, it can be used preoperatively to determine the trajectory and length of the screws. The CT scan is useful in identifying associated injuries, particularly coronoid process fractures and medial joint space widening, which may indicate medial collateral ligament injury.

3.3 Equipment

- A 4.0 mm, 30° arthroscope.
- A 4.0 mm, 70° arthroscope can be utilized for visualizing the capitellum and radial head from a posterior portal, especially when instrumentation is needed from the soft spot portal.
- A 2.7 mm, 30° arthroscope is an alternative for visualizing the posterior compartment.
- A 3.5 mm, full-radius shaver is employed for the removal of hematoma and debris.
- Retractors including switching sticks, interchangeable cannulas, and blunt freer-type dissectors can be used to protect neurovascular structures during instrument insertion and can assist in fracture reduction.
- Arthroscopic instruments including probe, grasper, and basket forceps. Sometimes, we may use a pituitary rongeur or small Hoke osteotome.
- K-wires may be used to assist with reduction and facilitate the placement of cannulated screws.
- Cannulated screws for internal fixation.
- Intraoperative imaging intensifier.

3.4 Applied Anatomy

The radial nerve perforates the lateral intermuscular septum 10 cm proximal to the lateral epicondyle and then enters the anterior compartment, lying between the brachialis and brachioradialis muscles. It passes through the radial tunnel, which extends 5 cm from the radiocapitellar joint to the proximal supinator muscle (Fig. 8.1). The tunnel's lateral wall is formed by the brachioradialis and extensor muscles, with the roof formed by the spiraling brachioradialis and the floor by the joint capsule and deep supinator (Fig. 8.2). The posterior interosseous nerve (PIN) lies near the radial head, crossing the radial neck at approximately 16.9 mm from the radial head surface in supination and 33.4 mm in pronation, when viewed from the anterior aspect. From the lateral view, it crosses at about 41.1 mm in supination and 61.8 mm in pronation [6] (Fig. 8.3).

The joint capsule at the lateral aspect of the elbow thickens to form the lateral collateral ligament complex, which consists of four distinct bundles: the lateral ulnar collateral ligament (LUCL), radial collateral ligament (RCL), annular ligament, and accessory lateral ulnar ligament. The lateral collateral ligament firmly attaches to the lateral epicondyle, which is the center of rotation, and can be viewed arthroscopically from the posterolateral portal through the lateral gutter of the elbow (Fig. 8.4).

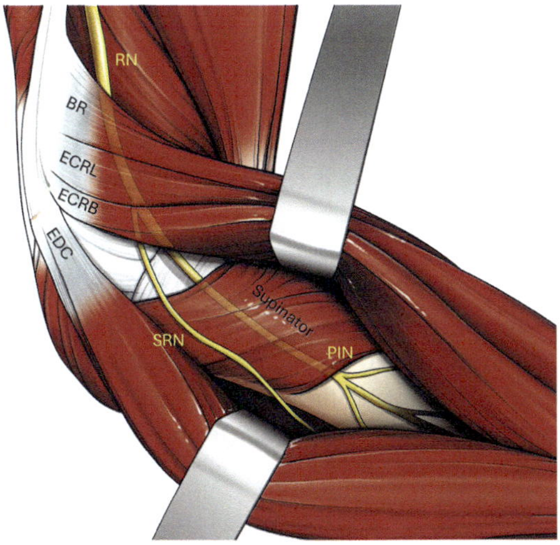

Fig. 8.1 The radial tunnel extends from the radiocapitellar joint to the proximal portion of the supinator muscle. This anatomical region encompasses the path of the radial nerve as it passes beneath the supinator muscle, particularly the Arcade of Frohse, a common site for compression. (*RN* Radial nerve, *PIN* Posterior interosseous nerve, *SRN* Superficial radial nerve, *BR* Brachioradialis, *ECRL* Extensor carpi radialis longus, *ECRB* Extensor carpi radialis brevis, *EDC* Extensor digitorum communis) (Copyright Dr. Gregory I. Bain and Max Crespi)

3.5 Patient Positioning and Anesthesia

3.5.1 Anesthesia

Elbow arthroscopy can be performed under either general or regional anesthesia. The use of regional anesthesia, while effective, may complicate postoperative neurological assessment.

3.5.2 Fluoroscopic Examination

Conducting a fluoroscopic examination after anesthesia is crucial to confirm the stability of the medial and lateral collateral ligaments, and to ensure that it is not compromised.

3.5.3 Lateral Decubitus Position

We typically use lateral decubitus position, as it provides optimal access to the elbow joint while minimizing the airway difficulties encountered with the prone position. Additionally, this position facilitates an easy conversion to an open procedure if necessary (Fig. 8.5).

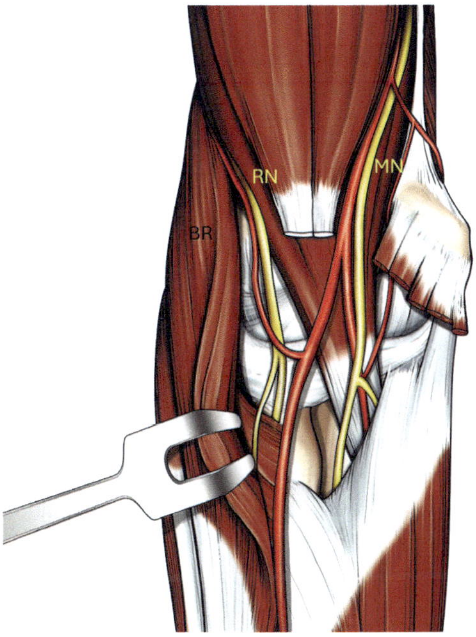

Fig. 8.2 The lateral wall of the radial tunnel is formed by the brachioradialis and extensor muscles, while the roof is created by the spiralling of the brachioradialis muscle. The floor of the tunnel consists of the joint capsule and the deep portion of the supinator muscle. (*RN* Radial nerve, *MN* Median nerve, *BR* Brachioradialis) (Copyright Dr. Gregory I. Bain and Max Crespi)

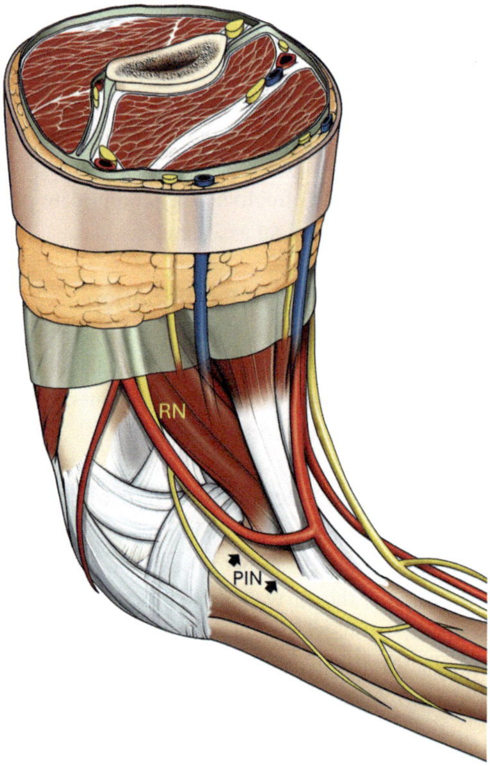

Fig. 8.3 The posterior interosseous nerve lies in close proximity to the radial head, where it crosses over the radial neck. (*RN* Radial nerve, *PIN* Posterior interosseous nerve) (Copyright Dr. Gregory I. Bain and Max Crespi)

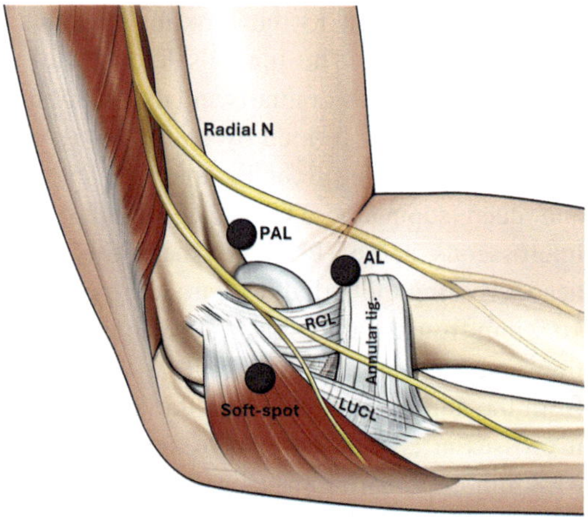

Fig. 8.4 From anterior compartment portals, the lateral collateral ligament is positioned posterior to the mid-portions of the capitellum and radial head. Its location relative to these structures is important to consider during arthroscopic procedures to avoid damaging the lateral collateral ligaments while gaining access to the radial head and capitellum for reduction and fixation of fractures. Caution is required when using the anterolateral portal, as the radial nerve lies in very close proximity to this portal. (*PAL* Proximal anterolateral portal, *AL* Anterolateral portal, *RCL* Radial collateral ligament, *LUCL* Lateral ulnar collateral ligament) (Copyright Dr. Gregory I. Bain and Max Crespi)

3.5.4 Supine Position

The supine position offers several advantages in surgical procedures. It features a straightforward setup and provides easy access to the airway for anesthesia. The anatomical structures are well-defined and easily oriented in this familiar anatomical alignment. Additionally, the supine position facilitates a seamless transition to an open procedure if necessary. However, the use of this position may necessitate the implementation of a hand and wrist holder that attaches to the operating table to stabilize the arm during the procedure. The posterior portals can be created by positioning the arm across the patient's body, thereby facilitating access to the posterior aspect of the elbow.

3.5.5 Prone Position

We avoid using the prone position for general anesthesia due to the challenge of limited airway access for the anesthesia team. We consider this position is reserved exclusively for bilateral elbow arthroscopy.

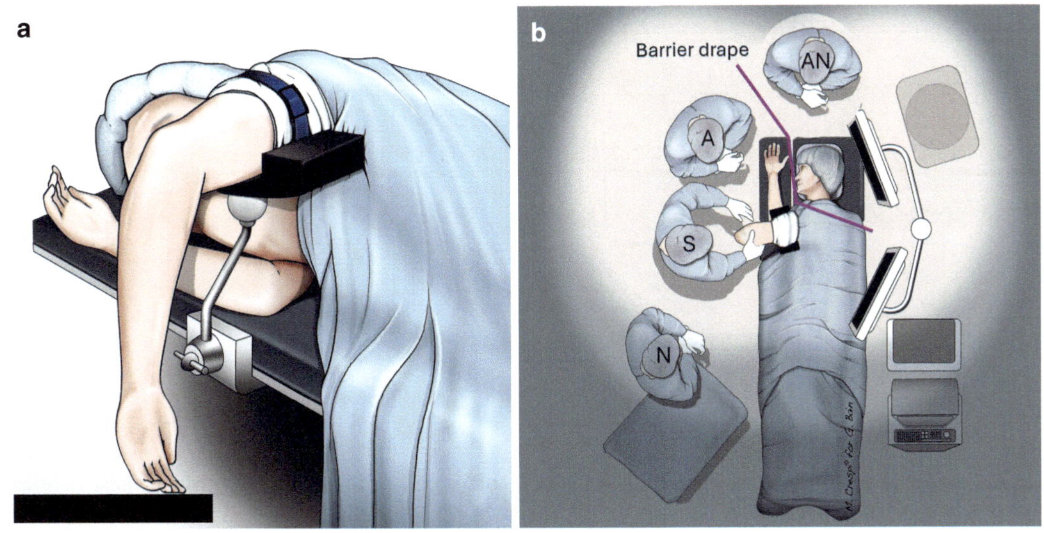

Fig. 8.5 Lateral decubitus position for elbow arthroscopy. (**a**) Arm holder and tourniquet are positioned as proximally as possible to provide full circumferential access to the elbow. (**b**) Room set up: The surgeon, assistant and nurse are positioned on the same side of the operative field. Alternatively, having the nurse on the opposite side of the table can help optimize space and improve workflow during the procedure. (*AN* Anaesthetist, *A* Assistant, *S* Surgeon, *N* Nurse) (Copyright Dr. Gregory I. Bain and Max Crespi)

4 Surgical Technique

4.1 Assessment of Ulnar Nerve Stability

Assessment of ulnar nerve subluxation can be performed by flexing and extending the elbow joint while palpating the ulnar nerve to identify if there is anterior subluxation of the ulnar nerve from its groove. Performing this maneuver is crucial to confirm the stability of the ulnar nerve, especially before placement of medial portals for elbow arthroscopy. If ulnar nerve subluxation is detected, ulnar nerve exploration can be performed prior to the placement of the medial portal to ensure the nerve's safety during the procedure.

4.2 Commonly Used Elbow Arthroscopy Portals for Radial Head Fracture Reduction and Fixation

The elbow joint can be conceptualized as a box, allowing for the insertion of the scope and working instruments from multiple angles, which facilitates comprehensive visualization and precise instrumentation (Fig. 8.6). The optimal position allows the scope to provide a panoramic view, while the working portal permits unhindered instrument management [7].

- The proximal anteromedial portal is commonly utilized as a viewing portal, as it provides optimal visualization of the anterior aspect of the radial head (Fig. 8.7).
- The proximal anterolateral portal can also be used as a viewing portal to visualize coronoid process and medial capsule; however, it is most frequently employed for instrumentation during radial head reduction and fixation (Fig. 8.4).
- The direct anterolateral portal is primarily used for instrumentation targeting the radial head (Fig. 8.8).
- The posterolateral portal and lateral gutter portals can be used for visualization of the posterior aspect of the radial head (Fig. 8.9).
- The soft-spot portal is versatile, serving both as a visualization portal and for instrumentation of the posterior aspect of the radial head.

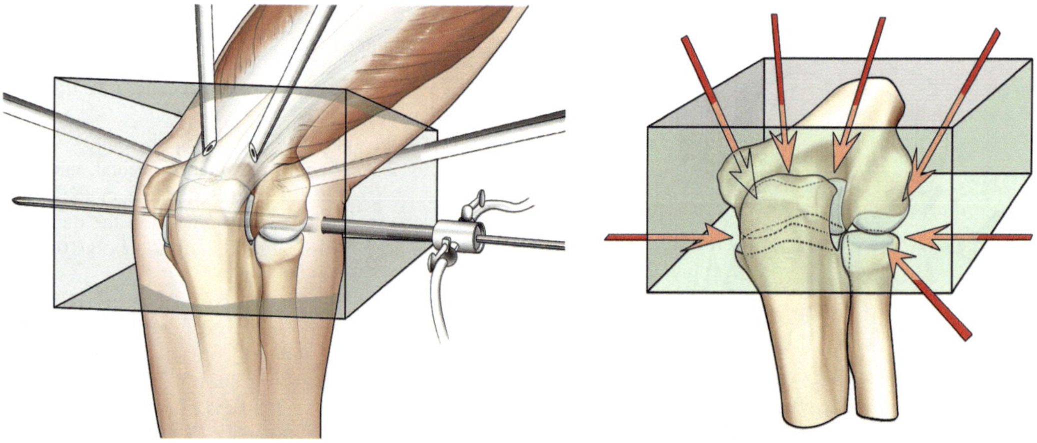

Fig. 8.6 The elbow joint can be conceptualized as a box-like structure, providing multiple points of entry for the insertion of the arthroscope and working instruments from various angles. This "box" concept is especially useful in arthroscopic-assisted surgeries, where optimal visualization and instrument control are crucial for successful outcomes. (Copyright Dr. Gregory I. Bain and Max Crespi)

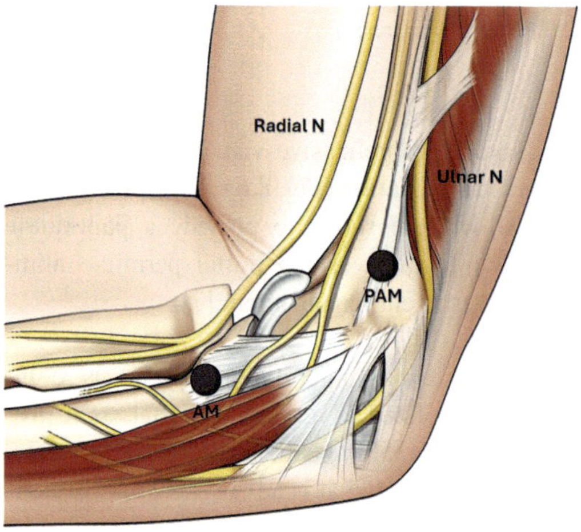

Fig. 8.7 Proximal anteromedial (PAM) and anteromedial (AM) portals. (Copyright Dr. Gregory I. Bain and Max Crespi)

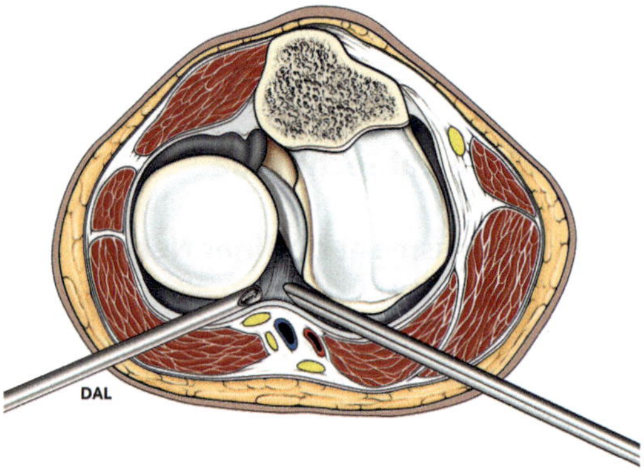

Fig. 8.8 The direct anterolateral (DAL) portal is primarily utilized for instrumentation targeting the radial head. (Copyright Dr. Gregory I. Bain and Max Crespi)

4.3 Dry Arthroscopy

In practice, a combination of dry and wet arthroscopy is often most effective. To minimize bleeding, we administer 1% lignocaine with adrenaline to the joint before introducing the scope and shaver. After debridement of the joint, the fluid is aspirated, allowing the procedure to continue under dry arthroscopy as much as possible. Dry arthroscopy offers several advantages [8]:

- *Enhanced tissue definition*: Dry arthroscopy provides better visualization of tissues, such as subtle synovitis, chondral damage, and partial ligament tears. This is due to the air-fluid interface reflecting light, enhancing detail, unlike wet arthroscopy, where fluid can obscure finer details.
- *Reduced intra-articular pressure*: Unlike wet arthroscopy, which distends tissues and compresses capillaries, dry arthroscopy preserves vessel visibility and allows better appreciation of synovitis.
- *Less swelling*: Dry arthroscopy causes less swelling compared to wet arthroscopy, which

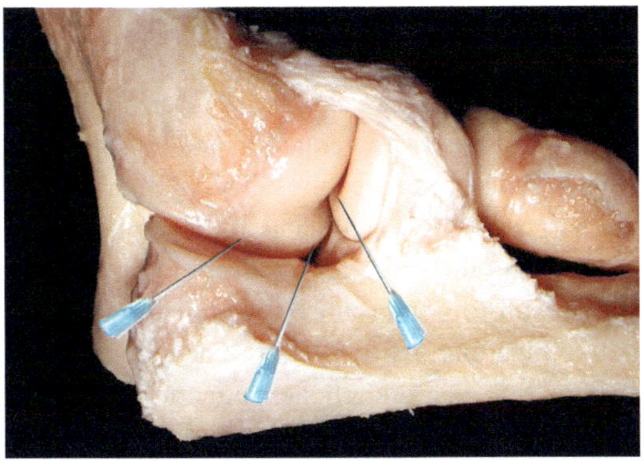

Fig. 8.9 Lateral gutter portals. This dissection of the lateral elbow shows how the outside-in techniques can be used to place portals anywhere along the lateral gutter. This is important to ensure the lateral working portals are precisely placed, in position and direction, to reduce and stabilise the radial head fracture. (Anatomical photograph courtesy of Dr. Amit Gupta)

leads to progressive swelling that limits safe working time and can compromise visualization.
- *Easier conversion to open surgery*: Dry arthroscopy avoids the fluid extravasation of wet procedures, making it easier to dissect and identify anatomic planes if conversion to open surgery is required.
- *Faster rehabilitation*: With less postoperative swelling in dry arthroscopy, patients experience less pain and faster mobilization, leading to quicker rehabilitation.

4.4 Fracture Reduction and Fixation

Step 1 Dry Arthroscopy For fractures, we routinely perform dry elbow arthroscopy for the initial arthroscopic examination, as it offers superior tissue definition. Additionally, dry arthroscopy extends the surgical working time by minimizing swelling and leads to reduced postoperative discomfort for the patient. The procedure typically begins with air insufflation using a 20 ml syringe through the olecranon fossa of the elbow. In the fracture case, we infiltrate 1% lignocaine with adrenaline to reduce any bleeding. The fluid displaces the capsule and surrounding neurovascular structures from the articular surface, making it easier to get in while reducing the risk of neurovascular injury [8].

Step 2 Diagnostic Arthroscope A viewing portal is established through either the proximal anteromedial or posterolateral portal. A standard diagnostic arthroscopy is then conducted to evaluate the coronoid process and the capsuloligamentous structures. The fracture is assessed for articular incongruity, fragment mobility, and any impingement that may restrict forearm rotation. The humeral origin of the lateral collateral ligament is also inspected and evaluated for any abnormalities.

Step 3 Working Portals Create working portals, optimally established through the middle anterolateral and soft-spot portals.

Step 4 Fracture Preparation and Reduction Remove hematoma and debris from fracture site using an arthroscopic shaver and grasper. Subsequently, the fracture fragments are reduced with the aid of a probe, grasper, or curved freer elevator to carefully manipulate the displaced fragments into alignment with the contour of the capitellum and the lesser sigmoid notch as a template for anatomical restoration. Additionally, a K-wire can be used as a joystick to assist in the fracture reduction. If the fracture is impacted or has undergone partial healing, the fragments may require disengagement using the freer elevator or a small osteotome for proper repositioning. Fluoroscopy is used to confirm the adequacy of the reduction.

Step 5 Fracture Fixation Position a spinal needle over the reduced radial head to identify the optimal position for internal fixation. A K-wire can be placed across the fracture site from either the anterolateral or soft-spot portal (Fig. 8.10). A percutaneous K-wire positioned parallel to the radiocapitellar joint as a reference may enhance the precision of placement of both the K-wire and the drill for subsequent insertion of cannulated screws [9]. To prevent rotation of the fragment, at least two K-wires should be placed prior to the

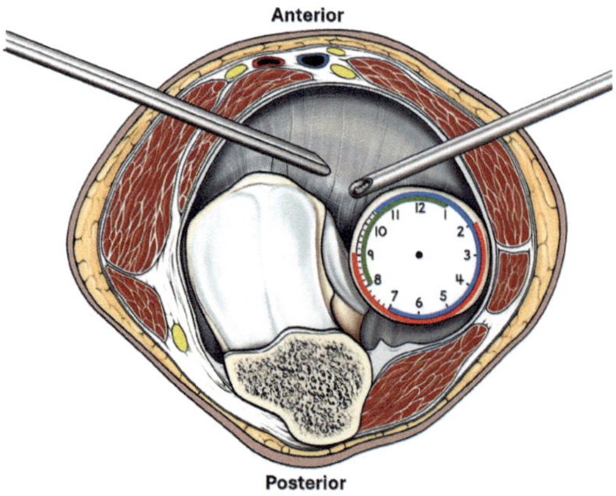

Fig. 8.10 Various working positions for arthroscopic fixation of radial head fractures are illustrated using a clock reference superimposed over the radial head, conventionally depicted in neutral forearm rotation. Based on the location of the radial fracture, three distinct arthroscopic working configurations can be selected: (1) Fractures involving the anteromedial portion of the radial head (green arc on the clock; 8 to 1 o' clock) can be addressed through an anteromedial working portal. (2) Fractures affecting the anterior and lateral portions of the radial head (blue arc; 10 to 7 o' clock) can be fixed using an accessory anterolateral working portal. (3) Fractures involving the posterior portion of the radial head (red arc; 2 to 9 o' clock) can be repaired through an accessory posterolateral working portal while viewing through the midlateral or posterolateral portal. (Copyright Dr. Gregory I. Bain and Max Crespi)

insertion of cannulated screws. Verify the fracture reduction and the trajectory of the fixation using an intraoperative fluoroscopy. Once confirmed, proceed with definitive fixation using absorbable pins or headless cannulated compression screws.

Step 6 Bone Grafting If Required If bone grafting is planned, an intra-articular fluid should be removed out before the graft is inserted.

Step 7 Final Assessment of Motion and Fluoroscopic Evaluation Assess the forearm rotation and elbow flexion under arthroscopy and fluoroscopy to ensure full motion of the elbow without any impingement.

4.5 Challenges

Several challenges can arise during elbow arthroscopic-assisted reduction and internal fixation of radial head fractures. The optimal timing for surgery is between 3 and 10 days postinjury. Performing the procedure within the first 3 days may result in compromised visualization due to active bleeding. After 10 days, partial healing of the fracture can complicate reduction and fixation. In most cases of acute radial head trauma, hemarthrosis can significantly hinder the surgeon's ability to visualize the fracture site. Keeping the inflow open allows the shaver to function effectively to irrigate the joint. Consequently, the elbow joint must be thoroughly irrigated with fluid, and the hematoma should be removed using an arthroscopic shaver. Clear visualization of the elbow joint is crucial before performing fracture reduction and fixation. While cautery can be used in a dry arthroscopy, it generates smoke, which can obscure the lens. Therefore, we prefer to use fluid when applying cautery.

The fluid helps distend the joint capsule, improving visualization. In dry arthroscopy, retractors are essential for maintaining joint space.

It is also critical to ensure precise trajectory of percutaneous K-wires and screws. Inaccurate placement may cause interference from extra-articular soft tissue, bend the K-wires, and ultimately make the procedure more challenging. This complication can be mitigated by using a spinal needle to mark the entry point and guide the direction prior to the insertion of K-wires and screws.

Preoperative confirmation of the ideal fluoroscopy placement in the operating room is crucial to avoid interference with arthroscopic equipment. Fluoroscopy can be positioned at the patient's head, with the C-arm angled 40°–60° above the patient to optimize screen visualization. The denser X-ray beam detector is placed near the patient's head. This setup enables simultaneous reduction and fixation while acquiring imaging in real time. The surgical field is then prepared using standard sterile technique, including draping over both the patient and the fluoroscopy equipment. This careful planning helps maintain optimal workflow during surgery [10].

Arthroscopic-assisted reduction and internal fixation is a time-sensitive procedure due to the potential for soft tissue swelling caused by fluid extravasation. It is essential for the surgeon to establish a time allocation for each step of the procedure to ensure efficiency. If the reduction is unsatisfactory and excessive time is being spent on the arthroscopic portion, conversion to an open procedure should be considered to achieve the primary goal—anatomical reduction of the intra-articular fracture and stable fixation.

5 Outcomes and Complications

5.1 Clinical Outcomes

Mid- to long-term results of an arthroscopic technique for the reduction and percutaneous fixation of Mason type 2 radial head fractures demonstrated good to excellent results in terms of pain relief, range of motion, and radiological assessments [11, 12]. Arthroscopic-assisted reduction and internal fixation (ARIF) of radial head fractures demonstrates superior patient functional outcomes compared to open reduction and internal fixation (ORIF) techniques. ARIF is associated with reduced elbow stiffness and fewer complications than ORIF [13]. The common complications of ORIF are persistent pain of elbow, crepitation during motion and limitation of forearm rotation. Notably, there was no significant difference in operative time between the two methods.

5.2 Possible Complications

5.2.1 Neurologic Injury

Potential complications specific to arthroscopic techniques include nerve injury, which can range from neuropraxia to neurotmesis. The nerves at risk include the ulnar nerve, particularly from anteromedial portal placement, and the radial nerve, which may be injured during instrumentation at the anterolateral portal.

Open identification of the ulnar nerve prior to the creation of an anteromedial portal significantly reduces the risk of ulnar nerve injury, particularly when the portal is placed more distally than usual. Another technique to prevent ulnar nerve injury during portal placement involves using the surgeon's thumb to stabilize the ulnar nerve, preventing subluxation and keeping it out of the pathway of the instruments being introduced into the proximal anteromedial portal (Fig. 8.11).

The radial nerve is situated in close proximity to the anterior capsule and the anterolateral portal, with the risk of injury increasing when the portal is positioned more distally. The classical anterolateral portal, located 3 cm distal and 1 cm anterior to the lateral epicondyle, should be avoided due to the high risk of radial nerve injury. Instead, the proximal anterolateral and accessory proximal anterolateral portals are considered safer alternatives.

5.2.2 Fluid Extravasation

Swelling is a significant risk factor, particularly when wet arthroscopy exceeds 60 min. Swelling can impair visualization by collapsing the surrounding soft tissues. Converting to open surgery after significant soft tissue swelling may result in more challenging dissection, altered anatomy, and potential wound healing complications. We recommend using dry arthroscopy as much as possible. However, if wet arthroscopy is necessary, fluid extravasation can be minimized by employing several strategies: using a fluid pump

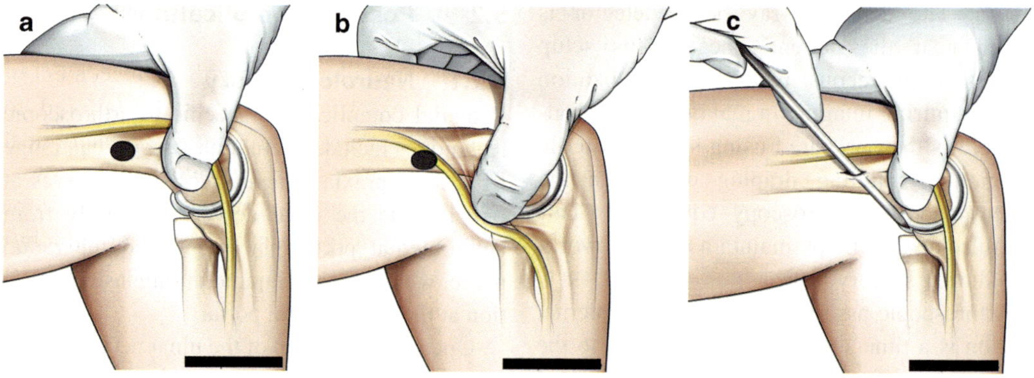

Fig. 8.11 Ulnar nerve stability. (**a**) in the normal situation the nerve is stable, behind the medial epicondyle. (**b**) If the nerve is unstable, this needs to be identified. (**c**) To prevent ulnar nerve injury during portal placement, the surgeon can use their thumb to stabilize the ulnar nerve, preventing subluxation and ensuring it remains out of the instrument pathway when accessing the proximal anteromedial portal. This technique helps to protect the ulnar nerve from inadvertent damage, which is particularly important due to its proximity to this portal. (Copyright Dr. Gregory I. Bain and Max Crespi)

set to a maximum pressure of 30 mmHg, using a gravity system or a modified pulsatile system, creating large arthroscopic portals to enhance fluid outflow from the joint, and utilizing non-fenestrated arthroscopic cannulae to prevent fluid leakage into the soft tissue.

6 Conclusion

Arthroscopic-assisted reduction and internal fixation (ARIF) of radial head fractures, particularly Mason type II fractures, has emerged as a highly effective minimally invasive treatment modality, offering several advantages over traditional open reduction and internal fixation (ORIF). The ARIF technique provides superior patient outcomes, with significant improvements in pain relief, range of motion, and overall functional recovery, while also reducing the risk of elbow stiffness and complications commonly associated with ORIF.

Despite these advantages, ARIF is not without its challenges. A thorough understanding of elbow joint anatomy, including the surrounding soft tissues, a detailed appreciation of the fracture pattern, and being advanced on the learning curve are essential for success in these procedures. The potential for nerve injury, particularly to the ulnar and radial nerves, underscores the importance of meticulous surgical planning and technique, including open ulnar nerve identification and careful portal placement. Additionally, the risk of fluid extravasation and subsequent swelling necessitates stringent fluid management protocols to maintain visualization and prevent complications that could complicate conversion to open surgery if required.

References

1. Hotchkiss RN. Displaced fractures of the radial head: internal fixation or excision? J Am Acad Orthop Surg. 1997;5(1):1–10.
2. Mason ML. Some observations on fractures of the head of the radius with a review of one hundred cases. Br J Surg. 1954;42(172):123–32.
3. Johnston GW. A follow-up of one hundred cases of fracture of the head of the radius with a review of the literature. Ulster Med J. 1962;31(1):51–6.
4. Ashwood N, Bain GI, Unni R. Management of Mason type-III radial head fractures with a titanium prosthesis, ligament repair, and early mobilization. J Bone Joint Surg Am. 2004;86(2):274–80.
5. Dawson FA, Inostroza F. Arthroscopic reduction and percutaneous fixation of a radial neck fracture in a child. Arthroscopy. 2004;20(Suppl 2):90–3.
6. Hackl M, Wegmann K, Lappen S, Helf C, Burkhart KJ, Müller LP. The course of the posterior interosseous nerve in relation to the proximal radius: is there a reliable landmark? Injury. 2015;46(4):687–92.

7. McGuire D, Bain G. Elbow arthroscopy—anatomy and portals. In: Pederzini L, Bain G, Safran M, editors. Elbow arthroscopy. ISAKOS: Springer; 2013.
8. Phadnis J, Bain G. Dry arthroscopy of the elbow. Arthrosc Tech. 2015;4(4):e335–9.
9. Camenzind RS, Cucchi D, Leschinger T, Hackl M, Müller LP, Wegmann K. Screw placement in arthroscopically assisted osteosynthesis of radial head fractures using a reference k-wire in the radiocapitellar joint: a cadaveric study. Arch Orthop Trauma Surg. 2023;143(7):4111–6.
10. Valencia M, Foruria AM. The role of arthroscopy in the management of adult elbow trauma. J Exp Orthop. 2023;10(1):144.
11. Michels F, Pouliart N, Handelberg F. Arthroscopic management of Mason type 2 radial head fractures. Knee Surg Sports Traumatol Arthrosc. 2007;15(10):1244–50.
12. Wang J, Qi W, Shen X, Tao S, Liu Y. Results of arthroscopic fixation of Mason type II radial head fractures using Kirschner wires. Medicine (Baltimore). 2018;97(12):e0201.
13. Guerra E, Marinelli A, Tortorella F, Flöter MDS, Ritali A, Sessa A, et al. Elbow arthroscopy for the treatment of radial head fractures: surgical technique and 10 years of follow up results compared to open surgery. J Clin Med. 2023;12(4)

Arthroscopic-Assisted Fixation of Capitellar Fracture

9

Erica Kholinne and Jae-Man Kwak

1 Background

Distal humeral fractures, including coronal shear fractures of the capitellum and trochlea, are uncommon injuries with various management options. These range from closed reduction and immobilization to open reduction with internal fixation (ORIF) and elbow arthroplasty for irreparable fractures [1–5]. Arthroscopic reduction and percutaneous screw fixation have emerged as effective options for simple fractures, offering advantages such as minimal soft tissue trauma and superior visualization [6–8]. Dubberley et al. classified capitellum and trochlea fractures into three main types: type 1 involves the capitellum with or without the lateral trochlear ridge, type 2 features a single fragment comprising the capitellum and trochlea, and type 3 involves separate fragments of the capitellum and trochlea. These types are further categorized based on the presence (subtype B) or absence (subtype A) of posterior condylar comminution, with subtype B posing limitations to arthroscopic fixation [2]. Dubberley et al. and Ring stress the importance of the integrity of the posterior condyle of the distal humerus when considering arthroscopic fixation [2, 4].

Specifically, patients may benefit from surgical intervention to achieve anatomic reduction and prevent complications such as joint stiffness, instability, and post-traumatic osteoarthritis. While open reduction offers precise fragment reduction, it carries risks such as fragment devascularization and periarticular soft tissue injury. Conversely, conservative treatments may result in displaced fragments, articular incongruity, and secondary instability. Arthroscopic techniques provide a minimally invasive alternative, combining the benefits of precise reduction with reduced risks of soft tissue damage and contracture. This chapter describes the arthroscopic management of coronal shear fractures, demonstrating its feasibility and effectiveness in treating a capitellum fracture with fragment fixation under arthroscopic control.

2 Indications for Arthroscopic Capitellum Fixation Surgery

The generally accepted indications for arthroscopic capitellum fracture fixation are as follows:

E. Kholinne (✉)
Faculty of Medicine, Universitas Trisakti, Jakarta, Indonesia
e-mail: erica@trisakti.ac.id

J.-M. Kwak
Department of Orthopedic Surgery, Uijeongbu Eulji Medical Center, College of Medicine, Eulji University, Uijeongbu, Republic of Korea

I.-H. Jeon et al. (eds.), *Elbow Arthroscopy*, https://doi.org/10.1007/978-981-95-3732-7_9

- Patient with displaced capitellum fracture type 1-A Dubberley classification.
- Patient with intact lateral collateral ligament complex.

The relative contraindications for arthroscopic elbow surgery include prior elbow surgery, previous elbow trauma, and a history of ulnar nerve transposition.

3 Surgical Technique

3.1 Preoperative Imaging

All patients underwent preoperative CT of the elbow, which is essential to define the fracture morphology and identify medial fracture lines directed towards the trochlea or impacted fractures with deformed osteochondral fragments, which can complicate reduction. The CT almost always reveals medial fracture lines (toward the trochlea) or impact lesions with osteochondral fragment deformity that make reduction challenging.

3.2 Patient Setup and Preparation

The patient is positioned on the operating table in a lateral decubitus position under general anesthesia. The arm is fastened to a padded bolster, with the shoulder raised to 90° and the elbow bent at 90°, allowing the hand to hang freely. Once the skin is prepared and draped, a sterile tourniquet is applied and inflated to 250 mm Hg after the limb has been exsanguinated. The water pump is adjusted to 30 mm Hg.

3.3 Portal Establishment and Assessment

Inject a 20 mL normal saline solution into the elbow joint through an 18-gauge needle at the "soft spot" (mid-lateral portal) to expand the joint. Establish the proximal anteromedial portal 2 cm above the medial epicondyle and 1–2 cm anterior to the medial intermuscular septum using a blunt trocar and a Wissinger rod. Perform diagnostic arthroscopy of the elbow with a 4.5 mm, 30° arthroscope starting with an assessment of the anterior portion of the joint and followed by establishing proximal anterolateral portal using the inside-out technique. Use an arthroscopic shaver to remove the hematoma, which enhances visualization of the fracture fragment (Fig. 9.1). The surgeon performs arthroscopic reduction by applying a distraction varus force and gradually extending the elbow. The surgeon repositions the fragment using a periosteal elevator while maintaining the elbow at a 90° flexion (Fig. 9.2).

Because visualization from the proximal anteromedial portal is often inadequate, the posterolateral portal is established to access the posterior compartment. This portal provides improved visualization, enabling precise observation of the fracture line with the elbow in 90° flexion (Fig. 9.3). In arthroscopic surgery, the anterior compartment and the posterolateral gutter must be thoroughly visualized. Relying solely on anterior or posterolateral portals is insufficient; instead, the arthroscope must be repositioned multiple times to achieve proper visualization and accurate fixation, making this procedure highly complex. The posterolateral gutter is debrided with a shaver to facilitate "transjoint visualization."

Afterward, the arthroscope is moved to the mid-lateral portal, providing a detailed view of the radiocapitellar joint, including the fracture line. A probe is inserted into the posterior elbow joint through the posterolateral portal to maintain the reduction (Fig. 9.4), alongside a periosteal elevator from the anterolateral portal.

While compressing the fragment with the periosteal elevator, the fragment is temporarily fixed with two 1.2 mm retrograde Kirschner wires. An image intensifier confirms anatomic reduction (Fig. 9.5).

Two percutaneous guide pins for 2.4 mm headless compression screws (DePuy Synthes) are inserted retrogradely under the direct control of both the image intensifier and the arthroscopic view (Fig. 9.6).

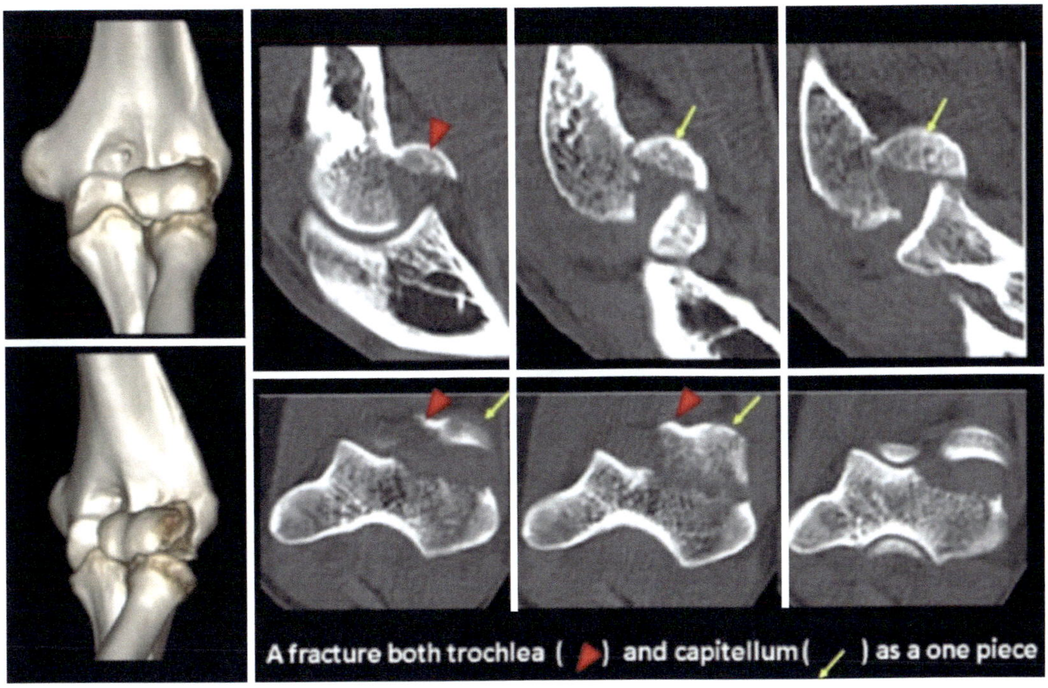

Fig. 9.1 CT scan illustrating a fracture line at the capitellum (yellow arrow) extending to the trochlea (red head arrow)

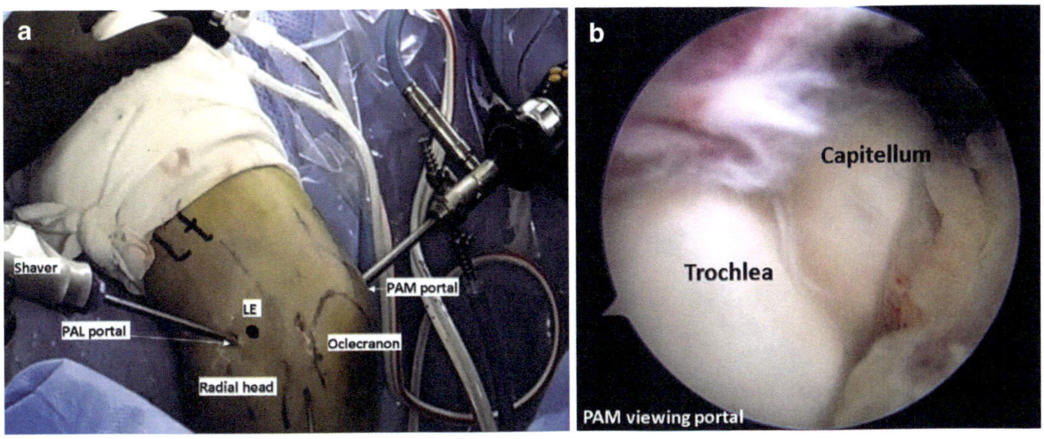

Fig. 9.2 The patient is positioned in the lateral decubitus position with the left elbow, and the proximal anteromedial portal is used for viewing. (**a**) The arthroscopic shaver is inserted through the working portal (proximal anterolateral portal). (**b**) The arthroscopic view reveals the fragment involving both the capitellum and trochlea (*LE* lateral epicondyle, *PAL* proximal anterolateral, *PAM* proximal anteromedial)

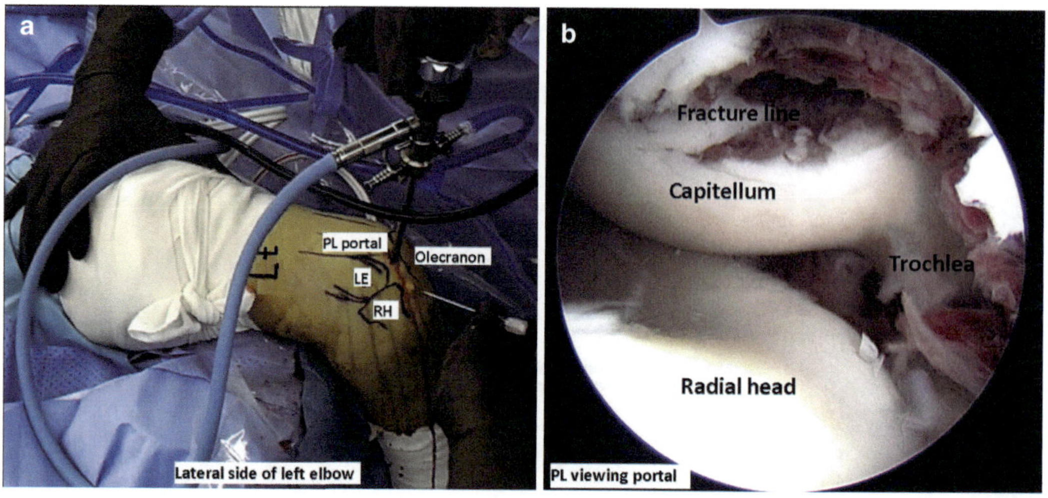

Fig. 9.3 The posterolateral portal is used to facilitate viewing of the posterolateral gutter. (**a**) An arthroscopic view of the posterior elbow chamber reveals the fragment involving the capitellum and trochlea, as seen from the posterolateral viewing portal after manipulative reduction (**b**) (*LE* lateral epicondyle, *PL* posterolateral, *RH* radial head)

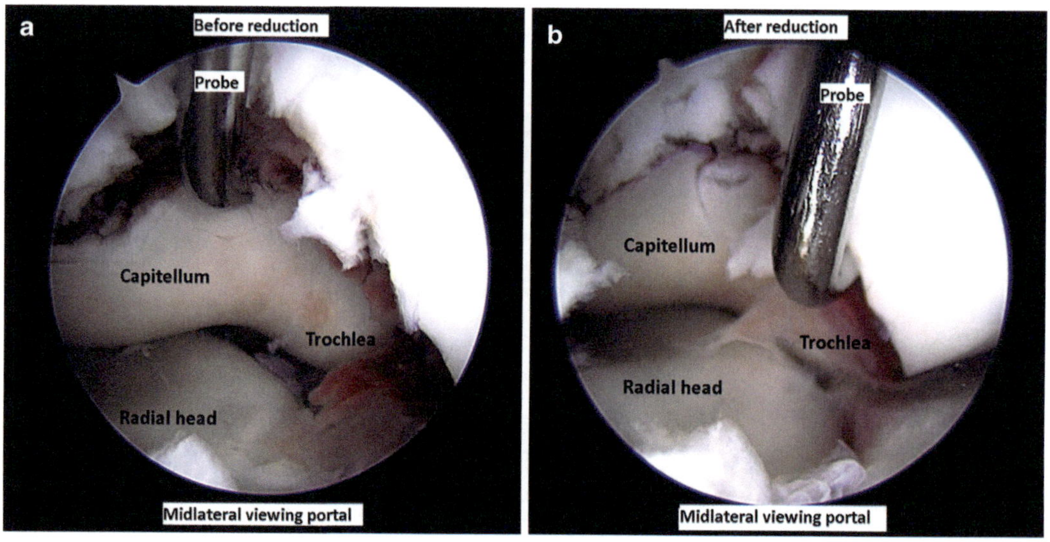

Fig. 9.4 An arthroscopic view of the left elbow in the lateral decubitus position reveals a fragment visible from the mid-lateral portal. A probe was inserted through the posterolateral portal to assist in the reduction, along with a periosteal elevator from the proximal anterolateral portal. (**a**) shows the displaced fragment before reduction, and (**b**) shows the fragment after successful reduction

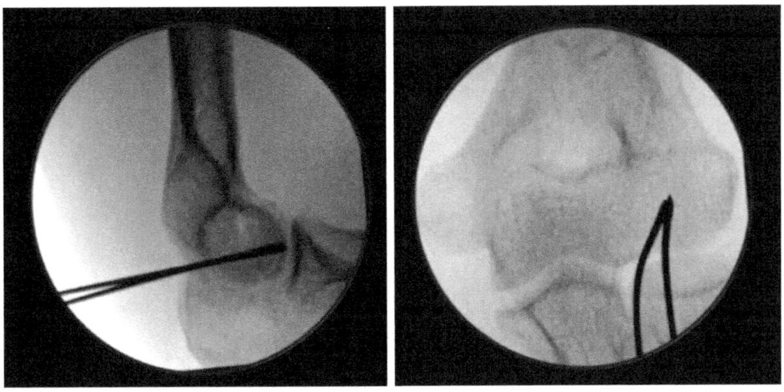

Fig. 9.5 K-wires (size 1.2 mm) were used to maintain reduction and confirmed by image intensifier

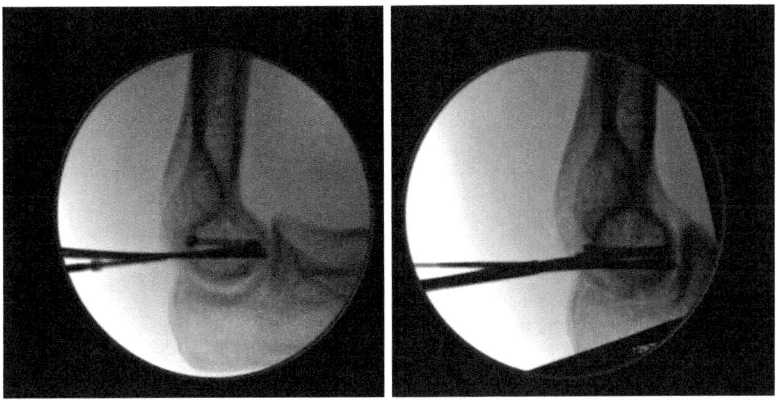

Fig. 9.6 Fracture fixation of the left elbow is performed using headless compression screws under image intensifier guidance. Each screw is positioned over a preplaced wire

The reduction is checked using a probe during full elbow motion and forearm rotation. A thorough arthroscopic examination is conducted to rule out associated lesions. Finally, anteroposterior and lateral plain radiographs of the elbow are taken to confirm fixation (Fig. 9.7; Table 9.1).

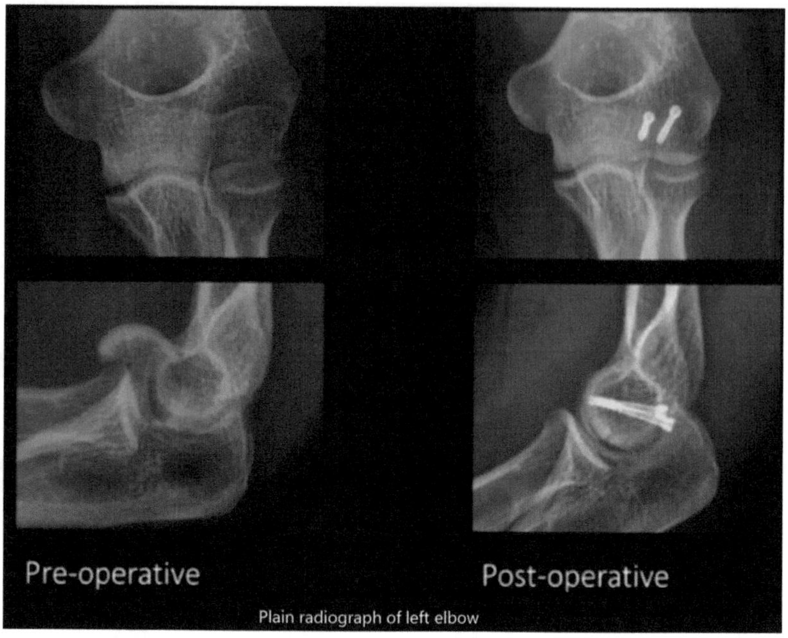

Fig. 9.7 Postoperative radiographs of coronal shear of distal humerus fracture fixation show correct alignment of the left elbow and articular congruency

Table 9.1 Advantages and limitations of arthroscopic assisted capitellum fracture fixation

Advantages	Limitations
Minimally invasive procedure that preserves maximal blood supply Provides enhanced control over reduction and stability of fixation Allows diagnosis and treatment of intra-articular pathology, including removal of loose bodies and drainage of hematomas Ensures precise articular reduction while enabling the removal of small fragments from recesses Does not eliminate the option for conversion to open surgery if necessary	Requires advanced knowledge of elbow anatomy, arthroscopy skills, and trauma expertise Risks to neurovascular structures Limited availability of specialized instruments (aiming devices, cannulated drills) Patient repositioning may be necessary for open surgery conversion (collateral ligament injury)

4 Pearls and Pitfalls (Table 9.2)

Table 9.2 Pearls and pitfalls of arthroscopic assisted capitellum fracture fixation

Pearls	Pitfalls
Carefully selecting patients is essential for achieving successful treatment outcomes The posterolateral portal provides better visualization of the capitellum fracture line, especially when it is not clearly visible through the anterior portal Reduction is performed using manipulative techniques, including distraction and the application of varus force A combination of a probe and a periosteal elevator is used to assist in fragment reduction A K-wire is inserted into the fragment and serves as a joystick for both reduction and provisional fixation across the fracture line	Incorrect portal placement can limit visualization and complicate instrumentation in the narrow working area Inadequate blood removal from the fracture site may hinder visualization and fragment reduction

5 Clinical Outcomes

Arthroscopic techniques for the management of distal humeral coronal shear fractures have evolved over the years, offering minimally invasive alternatives with varying levels of complexity and success. Early efforts, such as Feldmann's 1997 report, demonstrated the feasibility of arthroscopic excision for Type II fractures (Regan and Morrey), utilizing anteromedial and anterolateral portals in cases without joint instability [9]. In 2002, Hardy et al. advanced the approach with arthroscopic reduction and fixation of a Type I Hahn-Steinthal fracture, emphasizing the need for precise screw angulation to avoid radial nerve injury [7]. Mitani et al. (2009) contributed practical refinements by employing two simple portals to achieve reduction with a probe and securing fixation using posteroanteriorly placed screws [8].

Kuriyama et al. (2010) expanded the technique's scope to more complex fractures (Type IIIA, Dubberley), using anterolateral and midlateral portals [6]. Despite success in one case, a conversion to open surgery was required in another, highlighting the challenges of arthroscopic management for highly comminuted fractures.

These cases underscore the growing sophistication of arthroscopic methods, demonstrating their potential for reduced soft tissue trauma and improved visualization while emphasizing the technical challenges and limitations, particularly in more severe fracture types.

In conclusion, while arthroscopy-assisted reduction and cannulated screw fixation for coronal shear fractures of the distal humerus present significant challenges, advancements in elbow arthroscopy techniques have greatly improved the precision and reproducibility of this approach. By offering enhanced visualization of fracture patterns and minimizing the risk of iatrogenic injury to surrounding structures, this evolving technique provides a promising and effective solution for managing these complex injuries, contributing to better surgical outcomes and patient recovery.

References

1. Puloski S, Kemp K, Sheps D, et al. Closed reduction and early mobilization in fractures of the humeral capitellum. J Orthop Trauma; 26. Epub ahead of print 2012. https://doi.org/10.1097/BOT.0b013e318214ded1.
2. Dubberley JH, Faber KI, MacDermid JC, et al. Outcome after open reduction and internal fixation of capitellar and trochlear fractures. J Bone Joint Surg 88. Epub ahead of print 2006. https://doi.org/10.2106/JBJS.D.02954.
3. Mighell M, Virani NA, Shannon R, et al. Large coronal shear fractures of the capitellum and trochlea treated with headless compression screws. J Shoulder Elbow Surg; 19. Epub ahead of print 2010. https://doi.org/10.1016/j.jse.2009.05.012.
4. Ring D. Open reduction and internal fixation of an apparent capitellar fracture using an extended lateral exposure. J Hand Surg 34. Epub ahead of print 2009. https://doi.org/10.1016/j.jhsa.2009.01.026.
5. Watson JJ, Bellringer S, Phadnis J. Coronal shear fractures of the distal humerus: Current concepts and surgical techniques. Shoulder and Elbow; 12. Epub ahead of print 2020. https://doi.org/10.1177/1758573219826529.
6. Kuriyama K, Kawanishi Y, Yamamoto K. Arthroscopic-assisted reduction and percutaneous fixation for coronal shear fractures of the distal humerus: Report of two cases. J Hand Surg 35. Epub ahead of print 2010. https://doi.org/10.1016/j.jhsa.2010.05.021.
7. Hardy P, Menguy F, Guillot S. Arthroscopic treatment of capitellum fracture of the humerus. Arthroscopy; 18. Epub ahead of print 2002. https://doi.org/10.1053/jars.2002.32238.
8. Mitani M, Nabeshima Y, Ozaki A, et al. Arthroscopic reduction and percutaneous cannulated screw fixation of a capitellar fracture of the humerus: a case report. J Shoulder Elbow Surg; 18. Epub ahead of print 2009. https://doi.org/10.1016/j.jse.2008.07.007.
9. Feldman MD. Arthroscopic excision of type II capitellar fractures. Arthroscopy; 13. Epub ahead of print 1997. https://doi.org/10.1016/S0749-8063(97)90011-6.

10 Arthroscopic-Assisted Fixation of Coronoid Fracture

Yun-Rak Choi

1 Background

A coronoid fracture is a break in the coronoid process of the ulna, which is a triangular-shaped bony prominence on the anterior aspect of the ulna. This projection plays a crucial role in stabilizing the elbow joint by providing attachment points for ligaments and muscles [1–4]. Fractures of the coronoid process can affect the congruence of the elbow joint, reducing its inherent stability.

Coronoid fractures are commonly classified into three types as delineated on the lateral radiographic views of the elbow based on the Regan-Morrey classification system:

Type I: Fracture involves a small tip of the coronoid process. This type of fracture is generally stable and often occurs in conjunction with an elbow dislocation.

Type II: Fracture involves a larger portion of the coronoid process but less than 50% of the height of the process. It represents a more significant injury and may be associated with elbow instability.

Type III: Fracture involves more than 50% of the coronoid process. This type is usually associated with significant elbow instability and often accompanies complex elbow injuries, such as dislocation or ligament damage.

Another classification system proposed by O'Driscoll focuses on the location of the fracture on the coronoid process on computed tomographic images and its implications for elbow stability [5]. It is more detailed and includes anteromedial fractures, which are particularly significant for elbow stability due to their impact on the joint's medial compartment.

- Tip fractures: Small fractures from the tip of the coronoid process.
- Anteromedial facet fractures: Fractures involving the anteromedial portion of the coronoid process, which is critical for maintaining the stability of the elbow against varus and posteromedial rotational forces. This type of coronoid fracture is often associated with lateral collateral ligament (LCL) injuries, which contribute to posteromedial rotatory instability (PMRI) of the elbow.
- Basal fractures: Fractures involving the base of the coronoid process, often extending into the trochlear notch and associated with significant instability.

Supplementary Information The online version contains supplementary material available at https://doi.org/10.1007/978-981-95-3732-7_10.

Y.-R. Choi (✉)
Department of Orthopaedic Surgery, Severance Hospital, Yonsei University Health System, Seoul, South Korea
e-mail: yrchoi@yuhs.ac

I.-H. Jeon et al. (eds.), *Elbow Arthroscopy*, https://doi.org/10.1007/978-981-95-3732-7_10

Treatment depends on the type and severity of the fracture. For small tip coronoid fractures, conservative treatment with immobilization in a sling or splint [6], followed by physical therapy, may be sufficient. For Regan-Morrey or O'Driscoll Type II fractures with significant instability or basal coronoid fractures, operative treatment is usually necessary [1]. Surgical options may include open reduction and internal fixation (ORIF) with screws or plates to stabilize the fracture and repair any associated ligament injuries. In severe cases, external fixation may be required to maintain joint stability during healing [7–9].

Most coronoid fractures are not amenable to arthroscopic-assisted fixation because they occur in the setting of a combined injury to the elbow [10]. The indications of arthroscopically assisted reduction and fixation of coronoid fractures are acute (less than 2 weeks after injury) and meaningfully sized fractures inducing incongruency of the ulnohumeral joints [11, 12]. Contraindications are (1) delayed operation >2 weeks, (2) combined olecranon fracture (O'Driscoll type III2), (3) anteromedial facet of the coronoid fracture involving the sublime tubercle (O'Driscoll type II3) deemed unapproachable by arthroscopic methods and requiring anatomic reconstruction by open surgery, (4) replacement for radial head fracture (Mason type III), allowing coronoid fixation by a simultaneous lateral approach, and (5) involvement of more than three columns of the elbow (described by Jupiter) necessitating additional medial collateral ligament repair or external fixation.

2 Indications and Contraindications for Arthroscopically Assisted Reduction and Fixation of Coronoid Fractures

Indications	Relative contraindications
Acute (less than 2 weeks after injury) Meaningfully sized fractures inducing incongruency of the ulnohumeral joints	Delayed operation >2 weeks Combined olecranon fracture (O'Driscoll type III2) Anteromedial facet of the coronoid fracture involving the sublime tubercle (O'Driscoll type II3) Replacement for radial head fracture (Mason type III) Involvement of more than three columns of the elbow (described by Jupiter)

3 Step-by-Step Procedure

3.1 Position, Portal Placement, and Fracture Reduction

The patient is placed in the prone position, with the proximal upper arm supported on an arm positioner to place the arm in 90° of elbow flexion and 90° of shoulder abduction and internal rotation. Important anatomical landmarks include the medial and lateral epicondyles of the humerus, the olecranon, the radial head, and the ulnar nerve. Proper palpation of these landmarks is crucial to avoid neurovascular structures. A sterile rubber tourniquet is applied high on the upper arm after limb exsanguination. A posterior transarticular portal, as described by

Kim et al., is initially established as an entry portal, because attenuated capsular injury on the anterior and lateral columns of the elbow can interrupt the placement of anterior portals. The entry point for the transarticular approach is at the intersection of a horizontal line drawn from the radiocapitellar joint to the olecranon, with a sagittal line drawn just lateral to the olecranon (Video 10.1 [13]). The elbow joint was expanded by injecting sterile saline (20 mL) through an 18 G needle inserted in the transarticular portal and created the portal. Next, a 2.7 mm blunt trocar and sheath are inserted through the transarticular portal, and intra-articular fluid containing hematoma is washed out several times to obtain a better arthroscopic view. Then, a proximal anteromedial and a proximal anterolateral portal are made using an outside-in technique sequentially. And then, a 4.0 mm arthroscope is then introduced through a proximal anterolateral portal, and a probe is inserted through a proximal anteromedial portal, which is used to reduce the displaced coronoid fragment under direct arthroscopic view. After reduction of the coronoid fragment by handling the probe tip from the anteromedial portal, another probe is inserted through a posterior transarticular portal to stabilize the reduced coronoid fragment together with the probe from the proximal anteromedial portal (Fig. 10.1).

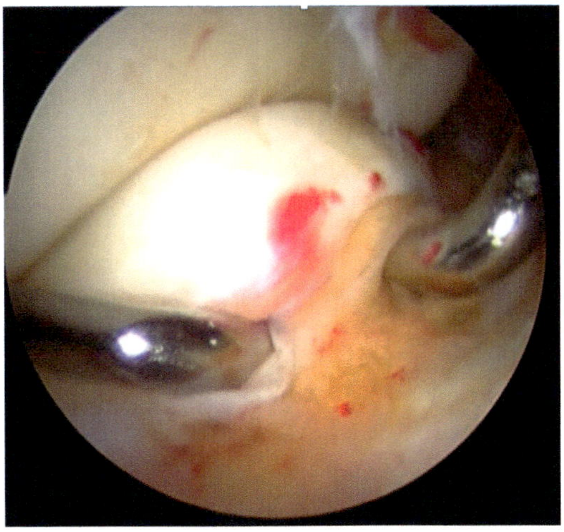

Fig. 10.1 Reduction of coronoid fracture using two probes from the proximal anteromedial portal and the transarticular portal

3.2 Placement of Kirschner Wires for Temporary or Definite Fracture Fixation

After the reduction, 1 or 2 temporary Kirschner (K) wires are inserted from the posterior proximal ulna at the level of the coronoid tip to fix the fracture fragment percutaneously under fluoroscopic guidance (a free hand technique). When coronoid fragments are large enough, 1 or 2 headless compression screws (2.2 or 3.0 mm) are used to fix the fracture fragment over the temporary K-wires (Fig. 10.2). For multifragmented or small coronoid fractures, temporary K-wires are left as the final fixation.

3.3 Management of the Associated Injuries

Displaced radial head fractures associated with a coronoid fracture were reduced and fixed with headless compression screws or a plate and screws using another lateral elbow approach splitting the extensor digitorum communis. The lateral ulnar collateral ligament was repaired using either a metal or a bioabsorbable suture anchor.

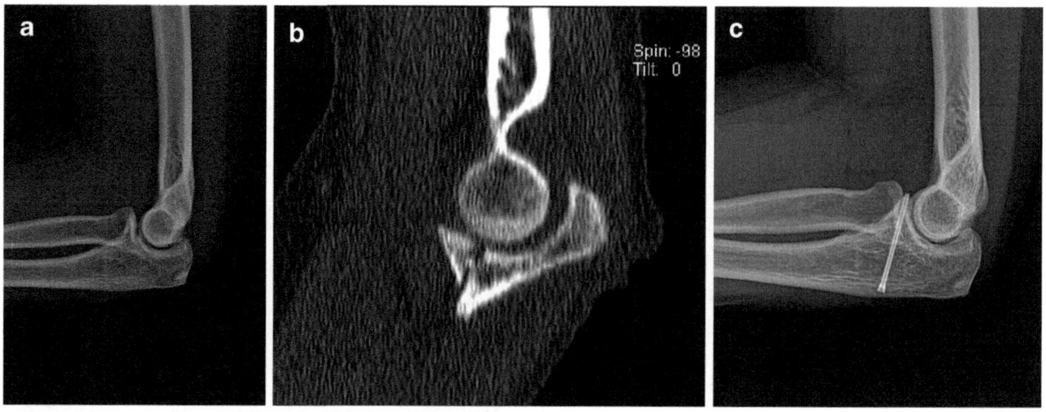

Fig. 10.2 Preoperative radiograph (**a**) and computed tomography (**b**) of a type II coronoid fracture in the Regan-Morrey classification system and postoperative radiograph (**c**) after placement of a headless compression screw to fix the coronoid fragment

4 Pitfalls of the Procedure

Arthroscopic coronoid fixation is a minimally invasive surgical technique used to address fractures of the coronoid process of the ulna. While this approach offers several advantages, such as reduced soft tissue disruption, less postoperative pain, and quicker recovery, it also has several pitfalls and challenges. Understanding these pitfalls is crucial for orthopedic surgeons to avoid complications and ensure optimal outcomes for patients.

4.1 Limited Visualization and Access, Particularly in Complex Fractures

Inadequate visualization may lead to incomplete reduction or improper fixation of the fracture, which can compromise stability and healing. Surgeons must be highly skilled in elbow arthroscopy and may need to use fluoroscopic guidance or consider conversion to open surgery if visualization is inadequate.

4.2 Difficulty in Managing Complex Fractures

Arthroscopy-assisted coronoid fixation may not be suitable for complex fractures, such as comminuted fractures (multiple fragments), fractures involving the base of the coronoid, or fractures associated with extensive soft tissue damage. Attempting to fix complex fractures arthroscopically can lead to inadequate stabilization, residual instability, or failure of fixation. Proper patient selection is critical. Surgeons should consider open techniques for complex fractures that require direct visualization and manipulation.

5 Key Procedure

Video 10.2 Arthroscopy-assisted reduction and fixation of the coronoid fracture

References

1. Beingessner DM, Stacpoole RA, Dunning CE, Johnson JA, King GJ. The effect of suture fixation of type I coronoid fractures on the kinematics and stability of the elbow with and without medial collateral ligament repair. J Shoulder Elb Surg. 2007;16(2):213–7. https://doi.org/10.1016/j.jse.2006.06.015.
2. Closkey RF, Goode JR, Kirschenbaum D, Cody RP. The role of the coronoid process in elbow stability. A biomechanical analysis of axial loading. J Bone Joint Surg Am. 2000;82(12):1749–53. https://doi.org/10.2106/00004623-200012000-00009.
3. Doornberg JN, Ring D. Coronoid fracture patterns. J Hand Surg Am. 2006;31(1):45–52. https://doi.org/10.1016/j.jhsa.2005.08.014.
4. Ring D, Jupiter JB. Fracture-dislocation of the elbow. J Bone Joint Surg Am. 1998;80(4):566–80.
5. Sanchez-Sotelo J, O'Driscoll SW, Morrey BF. Anteromedial fracture of the coronoid process of the ulna. J Shoulder Elb Surg. 2006;15(5):e5–8. https://doi.org/10.1016/j.jse.2005.05.009.
6. Chan K, MacDermid JC, Faber KJ, King GJ, Athwal GS. Can we treat select terrible triad injuries nonoperatively? Clin Orthop Relat Res. 2014;472(7):2092–9. https://doi.org/10.1007/s11999-014-3518-9.
7. Papatheodorou LK, Rubright JH, Heim KA, Weiser RW, Sotereanos DG. Terrible triad injuries of the elbow: does the coronoid always need to be fixed? Clin Orthop Relat Res. 2014;472(7):2084–91. https://doi.org/10.1007/s11999-014-3471-7.
8. Pugh DM, Wild LM, Schemitsch EH, King GJ, McKee MD. Standard surgical protocol to treat elbow dislocations with radial head and coronoid fractures. J Bone Joint Surg Am. 2004;86(6):1122–30. https://doi.org/10.2106/00004623-200406000-00002.
9. Zeiders GJ, Patel MK. Management of unstable elbows following complex fracture-dislocations--the "terrible triad" injury. J Bone Joint Surg Am. 2008;90(Suppl 4):75–84. https://doi.org/10.2106/JBJS.H.00893.
10. Adams JE, Merten SM, Steinmann SP. Arthroscopic-assisted treatment of coronoid fractures. Arthroscopy. 2007;23(10):1060–5. https://doi.org/10.1016/j.arthro.2007.05.017.
11. Lee JM, Yi Y, Kim JW. Arthroscopically assisted surgery for coronoid fractures. Orthopedics. 2015;38(12):742–6. https://doi.org/10.3928/01477447-20151119-04.
12. Oh WT, Do WS, Oh JC, Koh IH, Kang HJ, Choi YR. Comparison of arthroscopy-assisted vs. open reduction and fixation of coronoid fractures of the ulna. J Shoulder Elb Surg. 2021;30(3):469–78. https://doi.org/10.1016/j.jse.2020.06.037.
13. Kim SJ, Jeong JH. Transarticular approach for elbow arthroscopy. Arthroscopy. 2003;19(4):E37. https://doi.org/10.1053/jars.2003.50126.

11 Arthroscopic-Assisted Coronoid Fixation with Lateral Collateral Ligament Repair

Guo Jia, Erica Kholinne, and In-Ho Jeon

1 Background

The coronoid contributes to elbow stability as the primary static stabilizer of the elbow. Isolated coronoid fracture is less commonly found than coronoid fractures associated with elbow dislocations, which can lead to recurrent instability. The loss of coronoid process height of more than 50% will cause elbow instability [1]. Traditionally, fixation of coronoid fracture was performed with open manners utilizing medial, lateral, posterior, and anterior approaches [2]. The main concerns of the open approach are the proximity to the neurovascular structure and difficulty in exposure. Arthroscopic-assisted coronoid fixation allows direct intra-articular observation and excellent visualization of the fracture, hence facilitating the repair of coronoid fracture, especially when the fragment is small. Arthroscopy manner also enables anatomic repair with minimal surgical dissection due to preservation of soft tissue attachments [3].

This chapter describes the arthroscopic management of coronoid fractures, demonstrating its feasibility and effectiveness in treating them with fragment fixation under arthroscopic control.

2 Indications for Arthroscopic-Assisted Coronoid Fixation Surgery

The generally accepted indications for arthroscopic-assisted coronoid fracture fixation are as follows [4]:

1. Patient with Regan and Morrey Type I or II coronoid fracture.
2. Patient with O'Driscoll anteromedial facet fractures.

The contraindications for arthroscopic-assisted coronoid fracture fixation are the presence of concomitant injuries, such as complex elbow dislocations or fractures of the radial head.

Supplementary Information The online version contains supplementary material available at https://doi.org/10.1007/978-981-95-3732-7_11.

G. Jia · I.-H. Jeon
Department of Orthopaedic Surgery, Asan Medical Center University of Ulsan, College of Medicine, Seoul, Republic of Korea

E. Kholinne (✉)
Faculty of Medicine, Universitas Trisakti, Jakarta, Indonesia
e-mail: erica@trisakti.ac.id

I.-H. Jeon et al. (eds.), *Elbow Arthroscopy*, https://doi.org/10.1007/978-981-95-3732-7_11

3 Surgical Technique

3.1 Preoperative Imaging

The patient should have preoperative CT of the elbow, which is essential to define the fracture morphology and identify the severity of the fracture, especially when the fracture involves sublime tubercle, which is unapproachable by arthroscopic methods, hence requiring anatomical reconstruction in open manner [5, 6] (Fig. 11.1).

3.2 Patient Setup and Preparation

The patient is positioned on the operating table in a lateral decubitus position under general anesthesia. The arm is fastened to a padded bolster, with the shoulder raised to 90 degrees and the elbow bent at 90°, allowing the hand to hang freely. Once the skin is prepared and draped, a sterile tourniquet is applied and inflated to 250 mm Hg after the limb has been exsanguinated. The water pump is adjusted to 30 mm Hg. The degree of elbow instability was checked manually under fluoroscopy before the procedure. This is important to rule out cases that are inappropriate for arthroscopic manner. The affected elbow is tested for posteromedial rotatory instability condition with a varus stress test followed by external rotation (Fig. 11.2).

3.3 Portal Establishment and Assessment

Perform diagnostic arthroscopy of the elbow with a 4.5 mm, 30° arthroscope starting from the proximal anteromedial portal. An arthroscopic shaver removes the hematoma, enhancing the visualization of the fracture fragment (Fig. 11.3). After evaluating the fracture fragment, change the viewing portal to proximal anterolateral portal for better visualization. Because visualization from the proximal anteromedial portal is often inadequate, the proximal anterolateral portal is established to compensate for this (Fig. 11.4).

Afterward, a probe or periosteal elevator is inserted through the proximal anteromedial portal to assist the reduction (Fig. 11.5).

While compressing the fragment with the periosteal elevator, the transarticular spinal needle is inserted from the posterior site as a reference trajectory for the screw fixation (Fig. 11.6).

Afterward, the fragment is temporarily fixed with two 1.2 mm retrograde Kirschner wires. An image intensifier confirms anatomic reduction (Fig. 11.7).

A percutaneous guide pins for a 2.4 mm headless compression screw are inserted retrogradely under the direct control of both the image intensifier and the arthroscopic view. A bone curette can protect the neurovascular structure when drilling the guide pins (Figs. 11.8 and 11.9).

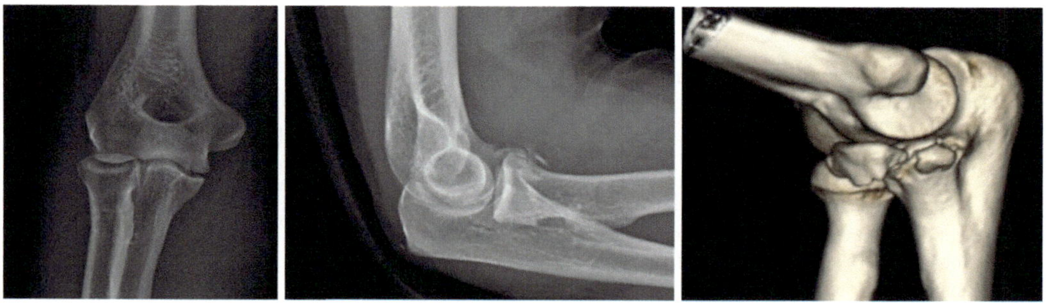

Fig. 11.1 X-ray and CT scan illustrating a type II anteromedial fracture without the insult of sublime tubercle

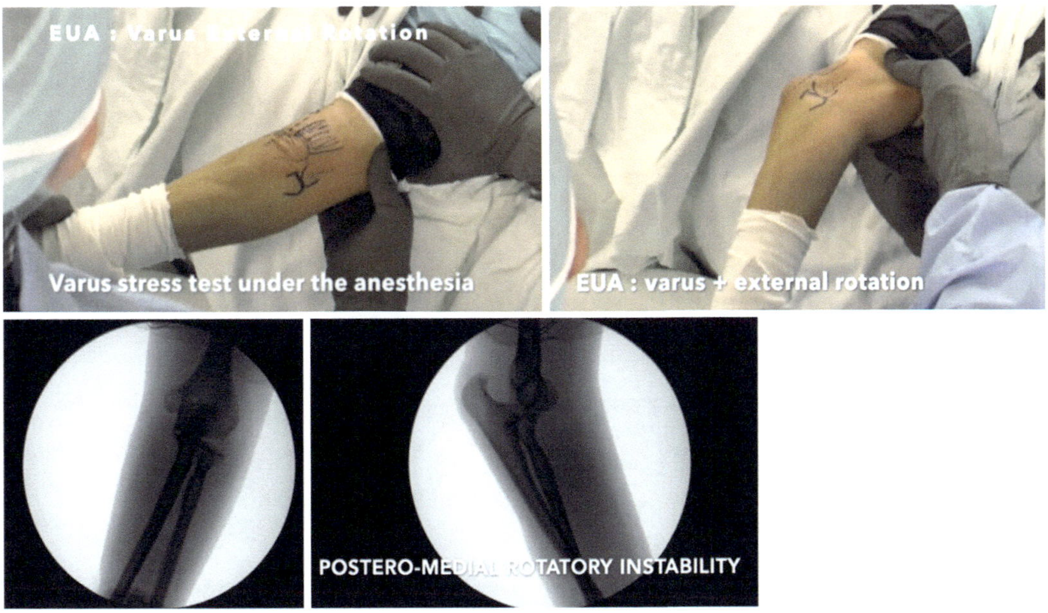

Fig. 11.2 The elbow was tested for posteromedial rotatory instability condition with a varus stress test and external rotation subsequently. The varus stress test resulted in lateral joint opening, and the additional external rotation marked the posteromedial rotatory instability

Fig. 11.3 The hematoma is debrided using an arthroscopic shaver to gain visualization of the fracture site

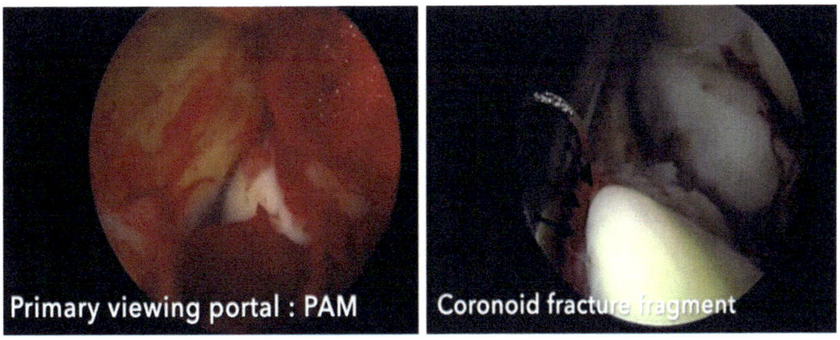

Fig. 11.4 The proximal anterolateral portal provides a better view to visualize the coronoid fracture

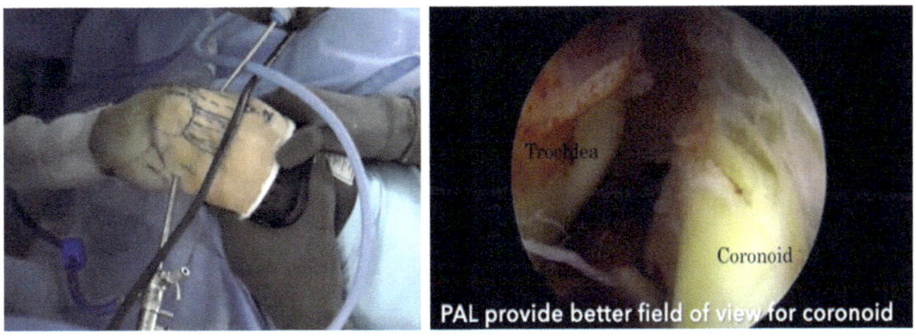

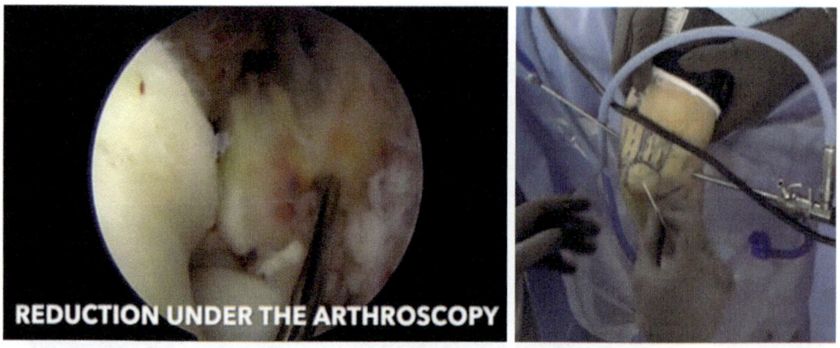

Fig. 11.5 With the arthroscope viewing from the proximal anterolateral portal, a probe was inserted through the proximal anteromedial portal to assist in the reduction

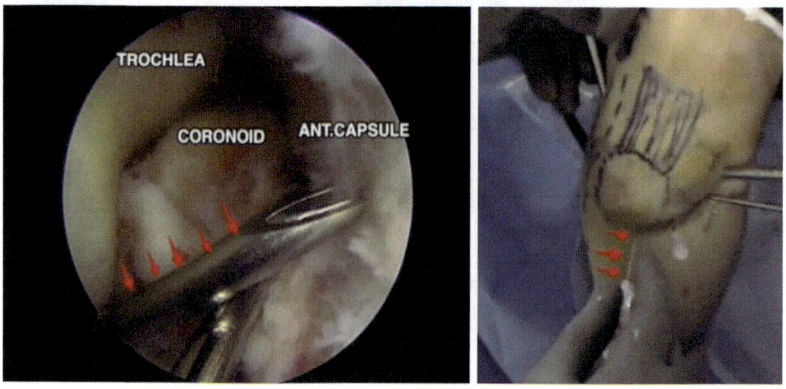

Fig. 11.6 A spinal needle is inserted from the posterior site in transarticular manner as a reference point for the screw fixation

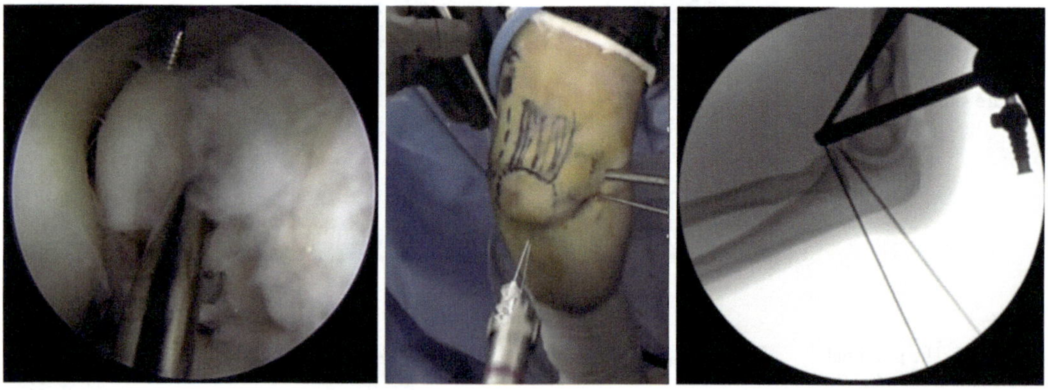

Fig. 11.7 K-wires (size 1.2 mm) were used to maintain reduction, which was confirmed by an image intensifier

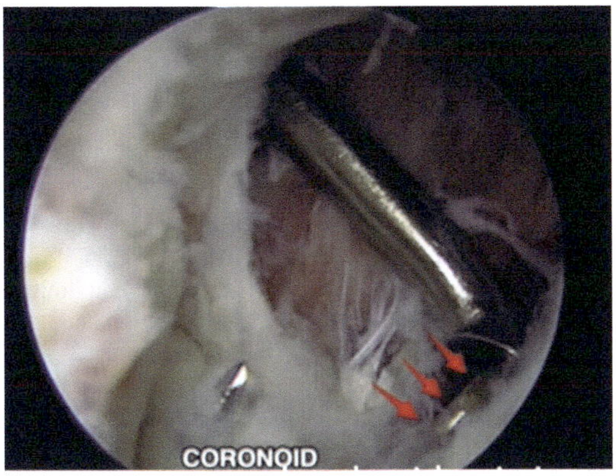

Fig. 11.8 Curette to protect cannulated guide pin insertion

The reduction is checked using a probe during full elbow and forearm rotation. A thorough arthroscopic examination is conducted to rule out associated lesions.

After the procedure, the elbow is immobilized in a long arm splint at 90° of flexion and neutral rotation for 2 weeks. The patient is gradually mobilized to an active range of motion over a 1-month period as tolerated by the pain. Active pronation supination is allowed. Strengthening exercise is allowed when bony healing occurs (Table 11.1).

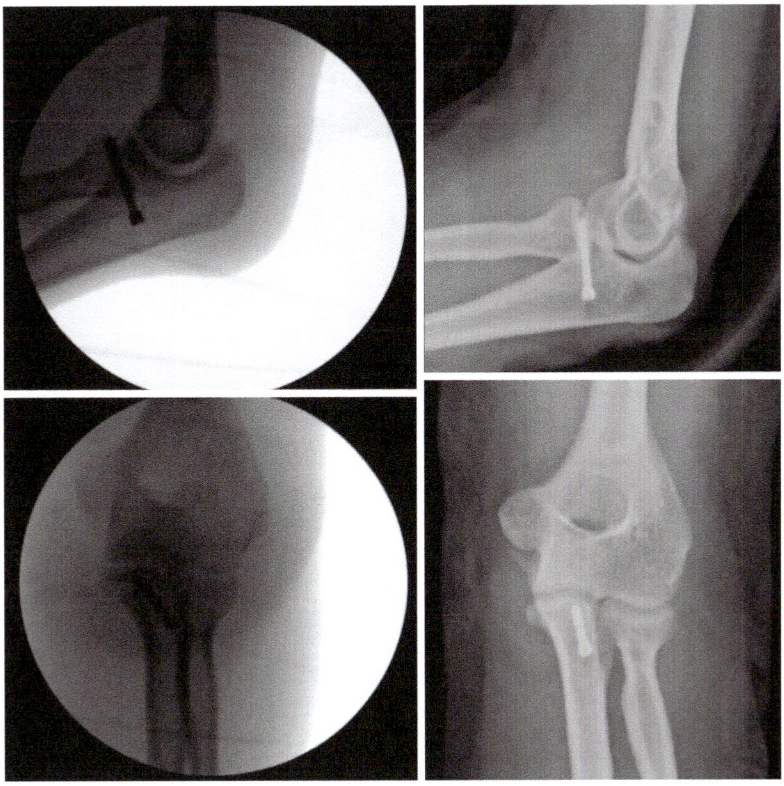

Fig. 11.9 Fracture fixation of coronoid is performed using a headless compression screw under image intensifier guidance

Table 11.1 Advantages and limitations of arthroscopic-assisted coronoid fracture fixation

Advantages	Limitations
Minimally invasive procedure that preserves maximal blood supply Provides enhanced control over reduction and stability of fixation Allows diagnosis and treatment of intra-articular pathology, including removal of loose bodies and drainage of hematomas Ensures precise articular reduction while enabling the removal of small fragments from recesses Does not eliminate the option for conversion to open surgery if necessary	Not suitable for all coronoid fractures Requires advanced knowledge of elbow anatomy, arthroscopy skills, and trauma expertise Risks to neurovascular structures Limited availability of specialized instruments (aiming devices, cannulated drills) Patient repositioning may be necessary for open surgery conversion (collateral ligament injury)

4 Pearls and Pitfalls (Table 11.2)

Table 11.2 Pearls and pitfalls of arthroscopic-assisted coronoid fracture fixation

Pearls	Pitfalls
Carefully selecting patients is essential for achieving successful treatment outcomes The proximal anterolateral portal provides better visualization of the coronoid fracture line A combination of a probe and a periosteal elevator is used to assist in fragment reduction A bone curette is used to protect the guide wire insertion before screw fixation	Incorrect portal placement can limit visualization and complicate instrumentation in the narrow working area Inadequate blood removal from the fracture site may hinder visualization and fragment reduction

5 Clinical Outcomes

The meta-analysis performed by Kholinne et al. demonstrates that ARIF leads to better surgical outcomes than ORIF for coronoid fractures, including greater postoperative range of motion, superior functional scores, and fewer complications [4]. Surgical fixation is essential for fractures causing ulnohumeral instability to enable early motion and prevent stiffness. While ORIF has shown favorable outcomes, ARIF offers superior intra-articular visualization with less soft tissue dissection, reducing complications.

Fracture union time was notably shorter in the ORIF group than in the ARIF group (11.9 vs. 19.7 months), with no cases of nonunion in either group. In this study, ORIF primarily involved plate and screw fixation, while ARIF utilized cannulated screws and Kirschner wire with suture augmentation. The primary objectives of coronoid fixation surgery are achieving anatomic reduction and stable fixation. The use of rigid fixation methods, such as plate and screw in ORIF, may explain the shorter healing time. However, multiple factors influence fracture healing, including patient-specific variables such as age, comorbidities, and lifestyle, as well as injury-related factors like severity, fracture type, and timing of intervention.

The return-to-activity rate showed no significant difference between ORIF (97.2%) and ARIF (94.3%). However, data on the duration of return to activities were limited, as not all studies reported this information. Surgeons typically determine return-to-activity timelines based on surgical type, functional recovery, and radiological findings. The faster union time in the ORIF group may contribute to an earlier return to activities. Given the comparable radiological results between open and arthroscopic approaches, the arthroscopic technique offers benefits such as fewer complications and faster recovery. In contrast, the open technique may be preferable for more complex fractures or cases involving additional elbow joint injuries that require extra-articular reconstruction.

It is also important to acknowledge that arthroscopic surgery is more technically demanding and requires a highly skilled and experienced surgeon to achieve optimal outcomes while minimizing procedure-related complications.

References

1. Hartzler RU, Morrey BF. Coronoid fractures. In: Morrey BF, Sanchez-Sotelo J, editors. Morrey's the elbow and its disorders. Philadelphia, PA: Elsevier; 2018. p. 428–39.
2. Chen HW, Teng XF. A comparative study on the validity and reliability of anterior, medial, and posterior approaches for internal fixation in the repair of fractures of the coronoid process of the ulna. Eur J Med Res. 2018;23(1):40. https://doi.org/10.1186/s40001-018-0336-7.
3. Oh WT, Do WS, Oh JC, Koh IH, Kang HJ, Choi YR. Comparison of arthroscopy-assisted vs. open reduction and fixation of coronoid fractures of the ulna. J Shoulder Elb Surg. 2021;30(3):469–78. https://doi.org/10.1016/j.jse.2020.06.037.
4. Kholinne E, Liu H, Singjie LC, Anastasia M, Kwak JM, Jeon IH. Surgical outcomes and complication rates of arthroscopic-assisted fixation versus open fixation for coronoid fractures: a systematic review and meta-analysis. Shoulder Elbow. 2025;17(1):86–95. https://doi.org/10.1177/17585732241229636.
5. Adams JE, Merten SM, Steinmann SP. Arthroscopic-assisted treatment of coronoid fractures. Arthroscopy. 2007;23(10):1060–5. https://doi.org/10.1016/j.arthro.2007.05.017.
6. Shimura H, Nimura A, Nasu H, Fujishiro H, Imatani J, Okawa A, et al. Joint capsule attachment to the coronoid process of the ulna: an anatomic study with implications regarding the type 1 fractures of the coronoid process of the O'Driscoll classification. J Shoulder Elb Surg. 2016;25(9):1517–22. https://doi.org/10.1016/j.jse.2016.01.024.

Arthroscopic Assessment of Acute Elbow Instability

12

Jae-Man Kwak, Erica Kholinne, and In-Ho Jeon

1 Background

Arthroscopic assessment of ligament instability has emerged as a cornerstone in modern orthopedic practice, particularly for diagnosing and managing subtle and complex joint instabilities [1–3]. These instabilities often escape detection through traditional physical examination and imaging techniques, underscoring the value of arthroscopy. By allowing direct visualization of ligament integrity, dynamic joint mechanics, and associated intra-articular pathology, arthroscopy has become indispensable in the comprehensive evaluation of joint function [4–6].

The elbow joint, a complex hinge-pivot joint, relies on its osseous configuration, capsuloligamentous structures, and dynamic stabilizers for stability. Key stabilizing structures include the medial collateral ligament (MCL), lateral ulnar collateral ligament (LUCL), radial collateral ligament (RCL), and the annular ligament [7–9]. The LUCL, in particular, is the primary stabilizer against posterolateral rotary instability [10]. Damage to these structures, often resulting from trauma or overuse, can lead to symptomatic instability requiring detailed evaluation. Advanced imaging modalities, such as magnetic resonance imaging (MRI), offer valuable insights; however, they lack the dynamic component necessary for a complete assessment, which only arthroscopy can provide [5, 11].

Understanding the biomechanics of ligament function is equally critical. The elbow joint is subject to significant forces during activities such as throwing, weightlifting, and repetitive overhead motions, making it vulnerable to ligament injuries [12, 13]. Athletes, especially baseball pitchers and tennis players, are at high risk. Arthroscopy not only facilitates the diagnosis of these injuries but also helps correlate biomechanical stresses with observed pathology, guiding tailored treatment strategies. Furthermore, advancements in arthroscopic equipment and techniques have expanded the scope of diagnostic and therapeutic capabilities, making it possible to address complex conditions that were previously deemed inoperable [2, 3, 7, 14–16].

As the indications for arthroscopic procedures in trauma cases, such as fractures, continue to expand, the demand for arthroscopic evaluation of both acute and chronic ligament injuries is also

Supplementary Information The online version contains supplementary material available at https://doi.org/10.1007/978-981-95-3732-7_12.

J.-M. Kwak (✉)
Department of Orthopedic Surgery, Uijeongbu Eulji Medical Center, College of Medicine, Eulji University, Uijeongbu, Republic of Korea

E. Kholinne
Faculty of Medicine, Universitas Trisakti, Jakarta, Indonesia

I.-H. Jeon
Department of Orthopedic Surgery, Asan Medical Center, University of Ulsan College of Medicine, Seoul, Republic of Korea

I.-H. Jeon et al. (eds.), *Elbow Arthroscopy*, https://doi.org/10.1007/978-981-95-3732-7_12

increasing. In response to this trend, this presentation aims to introduce methods that have been validated through the author's experimental research, as well as findings and techniques that have been documented in the literature.

2 Indications and Contraindications

2.1 Indications

- *Suspected ligament instability:* Clinical scenarios where ligament laxity or rupture is suspected, such as after acute trauma or repetitive stress injuries. Arthroscopy is particularly useful in cases where imaging findings are inconclusive.
- *Chronic joint pain:* Pain unresponsive to conservative treatments, often linked to ligament insufficiency or secondary degenerative changes. Arthroscopy allows for precise identification and targeted intervention.
- *Recurrent dislocations or subluxations:* Patients with a history of elbow dislocations or subluxations often present with ongoing instability episodes that significantly impact their joint function and daily activities. Arthroscopy provides a dynamic and detailed evaluation of the joint structures, enabling the surgeon to assess the extent of damage to critical stabilizing elements such as the lateral collateral ligament complex, medial collateral ligament, and the joint capsule. Recurrent instability may be caused by ligament insufficiency, cartilage defects, or even subtle biomechanical imbalances that are difficult to detect through noninvasive imaging modalities. Arthroscopic evaluation not only helps confirm the diagnosis but also provides real-time feedback on joint stability under stress, allowing for precise identification of the underlying pathology and guiding tailored treatment approaches, including ligament repair, reconstruction, or debridement of associated intra-articular pathology.
- *Failure of conservative management:* Persistent symptoms despite interventions such as physical therapy, bracing, or injections. In cases of advanced lateral epicondylitis, prolonged use of steroid injections may contribute to ligament insufficiency, which can lead to instability. Arthroscopy can be instrumental in assessing such subclinical instability and determining the appropriate course of action.
- *Assessment of associated intra-articular pathology:* Arthroscopy allows for a comprehensive evaluation of conditions that may coexist with or contribute to joint instability. These include osteochondral lesions, which can cause mechanical symptoms and pain due to cartilage and subchondral bone damage, synovitis, characterized by inflammation of the synovial membrane that may lead to joint swelling and discomfort, and loose bodies, which are fragments of cartilage or bone that can become trapped in the joint, causing locking, catching, or additional instability. By directly visualizing these intra-articular pathologies, arthroscopy provides critical insights into the underlying causes of instability and guides appropriate treatment strategies.

2.2 Contraindications

- *Severe joint stiffness:* Markedly restricted range of motion (ROM) can pose significant challenges for performing arthroscopic procedures. Joint stiffness, often resulting from post-traumatic adhesions, capsular contractures, or chronic inflammation, limits the ability to manipulate the joint and properly position arthroscopic instruments. This can compromise both the accuracy of diagnostic evaluations and the safety of the procedure by increasing the risk of iatrogenic damage to surrounding structures, such as cartilage or neurovascular tissues. In cases of severe joint stiffness, limited arthroscopic access may prevent thorough visualization of intra-articular structures, including ligaments, cartilage, and synovium, thereby reducing the efficacy of the procedure.

- *Active infection:* Joint infections pose a significant risk of spreading pathogens through arthroscopic portals, leading to severe complications.
- *Extensive soft tissue damage:* In cases where concomitant soft tissue injuries, such as severe ligament tears, extensive capsular disruption, or muscle damage, obstruct visualization or hinder proper instrument manipulation, the utility of arthroscopy may be limited. Additionally, if physical examination and imaging studies have already confirmed severe joint instability or extensive soft tissue compromise, performing arthroscopy may not be necessary in all cases. Instead, open surgical approaches or alternative methods may be more appropriate for directly addressing the identified pathology, particularly when the instability or damage is already well-documented and does not require further diagnostic confirmation. Arthroscopy should be reserved for situations where it provides additional diagnostic or therapeutic value beyond what has already been determined through clinical and imaging evaluations.

3 Step-by-Step Procedure (Kwak and Jeon Test)

3.1 Portals Placement

- Anatomical landmarks, including the medial and lateral epicondyles, radial head, and olecranon, are meticulously marked preoperatively. The ulnar nerve's course is also identified to minimize the risk of iatrogenic injury.
- Adequate fluid management is critical. The use of pressurized saline systems ensures joint distension, enhances visualization, and reduces the risk of extravasation into surrounding soft tissues.
- The procedure begins with the placement of standard arthroscopic portals, tailored to the specific joint pathology and anatomical considerations. The diagnostic portal (posterolateral portal) is critical to be placed for comprehensive visualization in ulnohumeral joint and radiocapitellar joint (Fig. 12.1).

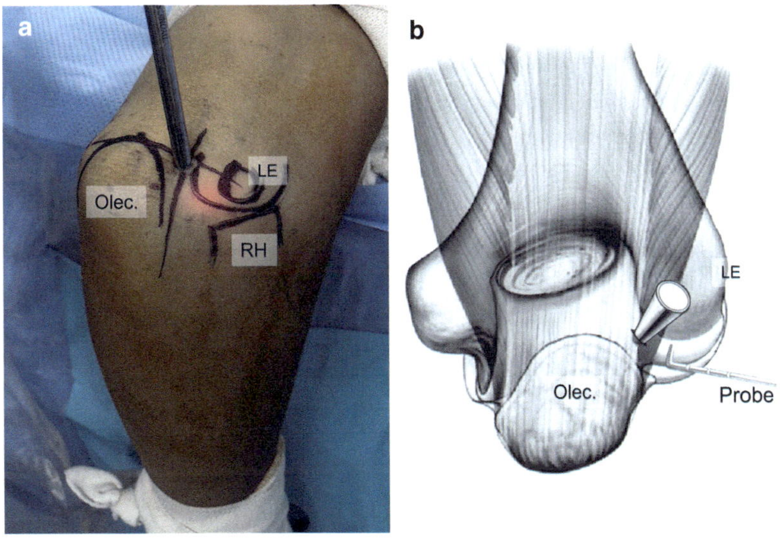

Fig. 12.1 The images show the placement of posterolateral portal which give the comprehensive visualization in posterior radiocapitellar joint. Figure (**a**) shows specific anatomical landmarks. Figure (**b**) is an anatomical diagram of the elbow joint, highlighting the placement of the posterolateral portal.

3.2 Clearance of Synovium

- To ensure clear visualization of the target areas, including the radiocapitellar space and the ulnohumeral joint, it is essential to perform adequate clearance of the synovium and surrounding soft tissues around the posterolateral portal. This allows for unobstructed access and precise evaluation of the joint structures during arthroscopy.

3.3 Dynamic Stress Testing

- Dynamic arthroscopic stress tests serve as the cornerstone for evaluating ligament instability, providing real-time assessment of joint behavior under stress. Specifically, for the evaluation of posterolateral instability, a posterolateral stress test should be performed with the elbow positioned at 30° of flexion and in full supination, which is the most provocative position for eliciting posterolateral instability [6, 17]. This positioning places the lateral ligament complex under tension, allowing for the detection of any subluxation, gapping, or abnormal joint motion during arthroscopic visualization. By replicating the instability mechanism dynamically, this test provides crucial diagnostic information for confirming ligament insufficiency and guiding treatment decisions.
- Real-time visualization allows the surgeon to document ligament gapping, excessive joint translation, and associated pathologies, providing a comprehensive assessment.

3.4 Direct Visualization

- During the stress test, if the radiocapitellar joint widens to the extent that the anterior margin of the radial head becomes visible, this indicates advanced instability, likely due to a complete tear of the lateral collateral ligament complex. This finding is referred to as the "drive-through sign" of the radiocapitellar joint (Fig. 12.2a, Video 12.1).
- Similarly, during the stress test, if the ulnohumeral joint widens to the extent that the medial trochlea becomes visible, this also suggests severe instability, likely caused by a complete tear of the lateral collateral ligament complex. This finding is termed the "medial trochlea sign" of the ulnohumeral joint (Fig. 12.2b, Video 12.2).
- In our experiments, both the drive-through sign of the radiocapitellar joint and the medial trochlea sign of the ulnohumeral joint were observed in cases of advanced ligament injuries that required surgical intervention for ligament reconstruction or repair.

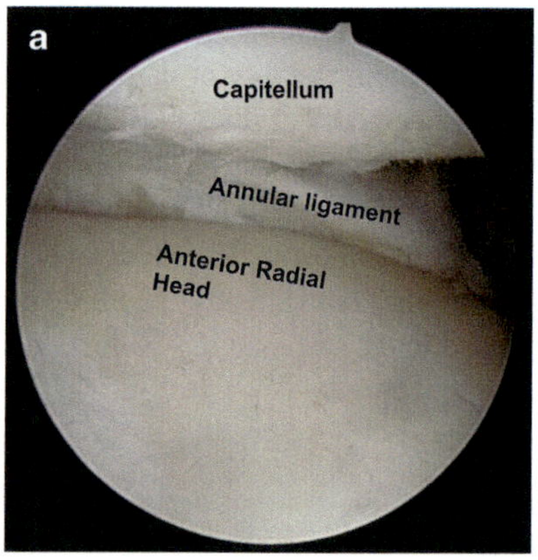

Fig. 12.2a The "drive-through sign" of the radiocapitellar joint

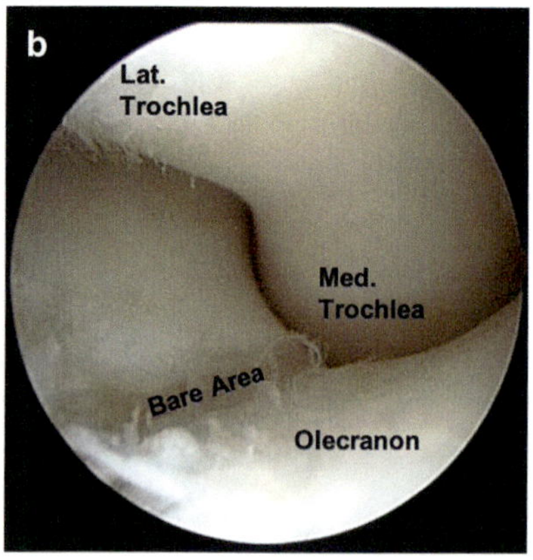

Fig. 12.2b The "medial trochlea sign" of the ulnohumeral joint

4 Other Arthroscopic Evaluation Methods

4.1 Annular Drive-Through Test (Arrigoni Test) [18]

- *Procedure:* The radial head is gently pushed anteriorly by the examiner's thumb while passing a 4.2 mm shaver posteriorly between the radial head and annular ligament. This test evaluates the tension and integrity of the LUCL.
- *Key findings:* Successful passage of the shaver indicates ligament disruption, whereas resistance suggests an intact LUCL. Gap measurements of 4.5 mm or more confirm ligamentous laxity.
- *Tips:* Maintain a steady hand while pushing the radial head to avoid excessive force, which could obscure subtle findings.

4.2 Proximal Radioulnar Joint Instrumentation (Kniesel Test) [19]

- *Procedure:* An instrument, such as a switching stick, is inserted into the proximal radioulnar joint between the radial head and coronoid process. The degree of joint widening is measured to evaluate ligament stability.
- *Key findings:* Measurements of 3–6 mm indicate mild instability, whereas gaps exceeding 6 mm suggest severe ligament compromise.
- *Tips:* Ensure precise placement of the instrument to obtain accurate measurements. Avoid overdistending the joint, which may lead to false positives.

4.3 Loose Collar Sign [20]

- *Observation:* This visual indicator involves sagging of the annular ligament around the radial head, exposing the radial neck. It is a hallmark of advanced ligament instability.
- *Tips:* Use a 30° scope to improve visualization of this subtle sign, particularly in the lateral compartment.

4.4 Other Supplemental Maneuvers [20]

- *Posterior supination test:* Performed by extending and supinating the elbow under direct arthroscopic visualization. Excessive gapping between the trochlea and olecranon indicates posterior instability.
- *Axial pull test:* Downward traction is applied to the forearm with the elbow flexed at 90°. Varus tilting at the radiocapitellar joint confirms instability.
- *Tips:* Combine these maneuvers with dynamic stress testing for a comprehensive assessment.

Each of these methods provides unique insights and complements the primary arthroscopic evaluation, ensuring a comprehensive assessment of ligament instability. Detailed technique and consistent practice are essential to achieving reliable results.

5 Caution Points

- *Portal placement:* Accurate portal placement is essential to avoid neurovascular injury. Preoperative imaging and anatomical markings are invaluable in achieving this goal.
- *Joint distension:* Overdistension can obscure visualization and compromise the procedure. Optimal intra-articular pressure must be maintained throughout.
- *Patient-specific factors:* Prior surgeries, anatomical variations, and comorbid conditions must be considered to tailor the procedure to individual needs.

6 Key Procedure Highlight

- *Dynamic arthroscopic testing.*
  - This technique involves the application of stress maneuvers under direct arthroscopic visualization, providing unparalleled insights into ligament integrity.
  - Dynamic testing also aids in determining the need for surgical repair or reconstruction, particularly in borderline cases.

References

1. Hsu JW, Gould JL, Fonseca-Sabune H, Hausman MH. The emerging role of elbow arthroscopy in chronic use injuries and fracture care. Hand Clin. 2009;25:305–21. https://doi.org/10.1016/j.hcl.2009.05.009.
2. Kim JW, Yi Y, Kim TK, Kang HJ, Kim JY, Lee JM, Bae KH, Joo MS. Arthroscopic lateral collateral ligament repair. J Bone Joint Surg Am. 2016;98:1268–76. https://doi.org/10.2106/jbjs.15.00811.
3. Moskal MJ, Savoie FH 3rd, Field LD. Elbow arthroscopy in trauma and reconstruction. Orthop Clin North Am. 1999;30:163–77. https://doi.org/10.1016/s0030-5898(05)70069-9.
4. Kholinne E, Liu H, Kim H, Kwak JM, Koh KH, Jeon IH. Systematic review of elbow instability in association with refractory lateral epicondylitis: myth or fact? Am J Sports Med. 2021;49:2542–50. https://doi.org/10.1177/0363546520980133.
5. Kirschbaum S, Plachel F, Kerschbaum M, Gerhard C, Thiele K. Does sonography allow an objective and reproducible distinction between stable, hypermobile, and unstable elbow joints? J Shoulder Elb Surg. 2021;30:1142–51. https://doi.org/10.1016/j.jse.2020.11.023.
6. Kwak JM, Rotman D, Lievano JR, Fitzsimmons JS, O'Driscoll SW. Ultrasonographic measurement of elbow Varus laxity with a sequential injury model of the lateral collateral ligament-capsular complex. Orthop J Sports Med. 2021;9:23259671211048941. https://doi.org/10.1177/23259671211048941.
7. Camp CL, Smith J, O'Driscoll SW. Posterolateral rotatory instability of the elbow: part II. Supplementary examination and dynamic imaging techniques. Arthrosc Tech. 2017;6:e407–11. https://doi.org/10.1016/j.eats.2016.10.012.
8. De Giorgi S, Vicenti G, Bizzoca D, Carrozzo M, Baglioni M, Virgilio A, Moretti L, Moretti B. Lateral collateral ulnar ligament reconstruction techniques in posterolateral rotatory instability of the elbow: a systematic review. Injury. 2020; https://doi.org/10.1016/j.injury.2020.11.010.
9. Bernholt DL, Rosenberg SI, Brady AW, Storaci HW, Viola RW, Hackett TR. Quantitative and qualitative analyses of the lateral ligamentous complex and extensor tendon origins of the elbow: An anatomic study. Orthop J Sports Med. 2020;8:2325967120961373. https://doi.org/10.1177/2325967120961373.
10. Morrey BF, An KN. Articular and ligamentous contributions to the stability of the elbow joint. Am J Sports Med. 1983;11:315–9. https://doi.org/10.1177/036354658301100506.
11. Gilotra MN, Fridman J, Enobun B, Kuntz AF, Glaser DL, Huffman GR. Risk factors associated with atraumatic posterolateral rotatory instability. JSES Int. 2021;5:827–33. https://doi.org/10.1016/j.jseint.2021.02.008.
12. Dunning CE, Zarzour ZD, Patterson SD, Johnson JA, King GJ. Ligamentous stabilizers against posterolateral rotatory instability of the elbow. J Bone Joint Surg Am. 2001;83:1823–8. https://doi.org/10.2106/00004623-200112000-00009.
13. Seo JB, Yi HS, Kim KB, Yoo JS. Clinical outcomes of arthroscopic lateral ulnar collateral ligament repair with or without intra-articular fracture. J Orthop Surg (Hong Kong). 2020;28:2309499020908348. https://doi.org/10.1177/2309499020908348.
14. Shim JW, Yoo SH, Park MJ. Surgical management of lateral epicondylitis combined with ligament insufficiency. J Shoulder Elb Surg. 2018;27:1907–12. https://doi.org/10.1016/j.jse.2018.06.011.
15. van Riet RP. Assessment and decision making in the unstable elbow: management of simple dislocations. Shoulder Elbow. 2017;9:136–43. https://doi.org/10.1177/1758573216686533.
16. Van Tongel A, Macdonald P, Van Riet R, Dubberley J. Elbow arthroscopy in acute injuries. Knee Surg Sports Traumatol Arthrosc. 2012;20:2542–8. https://doi.org/10.1007/s00167-012-1904-y.
17. O'Driscoll SW, Bell DF, Morrey BF. Posterolateral rotatory instability of the elbow. J Bone Joint Surg Am. 1991;73:440–6.
18. Arrigoni P, Cucchi D, D'Ambrosi R, Butt U, Safran MR, Denard P, Randelli P. Intra-articular findings in symptomatic minor instability of the lateral elbow (SMILE). Knee Surg Sports Traumatol Arthrosc. 2017;25:2255–63. https://doi.org/10.1007/s00167-017-4530-x.
19. Kniesel B, Huth J, Bauer G, Mauch F. Systematic diagnosis and therapy of lateral elbow pain with emphasis on elbow instability. Arch Orthop Trauma Surg. 2014;134:1641–7. https://doi.org/10.1007/s00402-014-2087-4.
20. Koso R, Logli A, Mirvish A, Baratz M. Arthroscopic evaluation for posterolateral rotatory instability of the elbow. Shoulder Elbow. 2024:17585732241293326. https://doi.org/10.1177/17585732241293326.

13 Acute Elbow Instability: Arthroscopic Repair or Augmentation of the Lateral Collateral Ligament Complex

Cholawish Chanlalit

1 Background

Elbow is a joint with the most common dislocation second to the shoulder. The dislocation usually occurs during adolescence and early adulthood. Types of elbow dislocation depend on mechanisms of injury. The most common type is the posterior dislocation, which occurs up to 90% of elbow dislocations. Most of the time, it is usually presents as a simple elbow dislocation with no associated fracture. Elbow dislocation with associated fractures, including fractures of the radial head or coronoid is called a complex fracture dislocation, which will not be discussed in this chapter. The second most common type is anterior dislocation. The rarest type is divergent type which is an ulnohumeral joint dislocation with radioulnar joint separation [1, 2].

The common mechanism of injury is falling on the outstretching hand (FOOSH). Falling with elbow extended, the force contributed from the body weight continuously rotates the forearm externally relative to the humerus. This results in a tear starting from lateral collateral ligament (LCL) to anterior and posterior capsules. If the force continues to proceed, the injury will extend to medial collateral ligament (MCL). Once the MCL is torn, the elbow can easily dislocate. This mechanism of elbow dislocation is known as Horii's circle.

2 Pathoanatomic Staging

Acute elbow instability is a spectrum from subluxation to dislocation, which goes along with the pathoanatomic stage that demonstrates the capsuloligamentous disruption. O'Driscoll divided the elbow instability into three pathoanatomic stages [3, 4].

Stage 1: Elbow sprain
Lateral ulnar collateral ligament (LUCL) rupture and possible tear of the remaining lateral collateral ligament are resulted from the forearm-rotation event, mentioned previously. This leads to posterolateral rotatory subluxation and then spontaneous relocation. A physical examination of lateral pivot-shift test under adequate pain control can be possibly positive.
Stage 2: Elbow subluxation
Additional tear of anterior and posterior soft tissue (capsule) disruption causes the elbow to subluxate. Plain radiographs will show the appearance of the trochlea riding on the coronoid process or the coronoid process crawling and compressing under the trochlea.
Stage 3: Elbow dislocation
In stage 3, it is divided into 3a, 3b, 3c to indicate the severity of the injury to the surrounding tissues of the injured elbow.

(continued)

Supplementary Information The online version contains supplementary material available at https://doi.org/10.1007/978-981-95-3732-7_13.

C. Chanlalit (✉)
Center of Excellence in Upper Extremity and Sports Medicine, HRH Princess Maha Chakri Sirindhron Medical Center, Faculty of Medicine, Srinakharinwirot University, Nakhon Nayok, Thailand

I.-H. Jeon et al. (eds.), *Elbow Arthroscopy*, https://doi.org/10.1007/978-981-95-3732-7_13

Stage 3a: Anterior band of MCL (aMCL) is intact
With an intact aMCL, the elbow will be stable after the elbow reduction because the aMCL, as the primary stabilizer, is intact and functional. Therefore, after the reduction, the valgus stress test will be stable or gives negative value.
Stage 3b: Anterior band of MCL (aMCL) is ruptured
With a completely torn aMCL, after the reduction, the valgus stress test will be unstable or gives a clear positive value. In this stage, after the elbow reduction, the muscles that cross the joint will play important role in providing stability to the elbow, which are the common extensor and flexor-pronator tendons. Therefore, pronation of forearm will increase the stability of the elbow.
Stage 3c: All soft tissues are stripped off from the distal humerus
With all detached soft tissues, pronation of forearm will no longer help increase the stability of the elbow. At this stage, the elbow is very unstable, especially when the elbow is in extension. It is necessary to flex the elbow (usually more than 40°) to maintain the ulnohumeral joint in place. In addition, the severity in this group is very obvious. Even wearing a cast, loosening of the elbow joint within the cast will be seen on the plain radiograph.

3 Management

Acute elbow dislocation is considered an emergency condition that requires reduction as it is the first priority. There are many techniques on reduction and pain management during the reduction. After reduction, conservative therapy is the mainstay. Regardless of the primary therapy chosen in simple elbow dislocations, early functional follow-up care protocol with early elbow motion is shown to be superior to the immobilization therapy with a duration of more than 2 weeks [5, 6].

4 The Principles of Surgery

The MCL has high potential of self-healing. In stable elbow, MCL can heal and achieve considerable final elbow stability. Meanwhile, in complete loss of primary and secondary soft tissue constraints (pathoanatomic stage 3c), the elbow becomes extremely unstable. This problem can be solved by flex the elbow deeply to maintain the elbow in place. In this situation, the MCL, capsule, and various parts of the elbow can be healed on their own capability, which then later provide elbow stability. However, the prolonged immobilization of elbow in this position will lead to elbow stiffness, especially in flexed position. This can eventually cause disability of the elbow and slow down the recovery of the elbow function [7].

In another approach, LCL is the first structure to be disrupted in elbow dislocation. Since potential self-healing of LCL is not as good as that of MCL, repairing the lateral structures would prevent consequences of chronic posterolateral rotatory instability. Suturing the LCL, tendons, and muscles that cross the joint on the lateral side of elbow can be performed easier and safer from nerve injury complication than suturing the MCL. Repairing these structures can restore a certain degree of stability to the elbow while allowing the MCL to heal itself. Repairing MCL is considered for high demand groups such as overhead athlete or martial art athlete.

In unstable elbow, surgery can avoid prolonged immobilization of elbow in flexed position and allow elbow motion. After the surgery, the elbow may be allowed to move as tolerated or may be motioned within a locked hinged elbow brace with a predetermined range of motion for only a short period of time. Early motion can reduce the problem of elbow joint stiffness and facilitates the recovery of the muscles across the elbow [7].

The entity of the surgery for elbow dislocation provides benefit for patients to gain earlier recovery than conservative treatment and prevents the dissatisfied sequalae. Long term follow-up studies after conservative treatment of elbow dislocation found that many patients reported pain and symptoms or sign of elbow instability, but recurrent dislocations were rarely reported [6–8].

5 Advantage of Arthroscopic Surgery

The advantage of arthroscopic surgery is that it can assess for concomitant injuries such as loose bodies, osteochondral fragments, or chondral fragments, which often cannot be seen on plain film X-ray.

In minimally invasive surgery, many studies have proposed several techniques for suturing the collateral ligament, which may or may not suture the tendon or muscles simultaneously. The LCL repair can recondition the unstable elbow to become stable enough for MCL to gain a properly healed condition. Therefore, arthroscopic surgery is a minimally invasive surgery that can suture both LCL and lateral tendons resulting in adequate elbow stability, as well as treating concomitant injuries at the same time [6, 7, 9–13].

6 Surgical Technique

6.1 Positioning

After the patient is anesthetized, the stability of the elbow can be evaluated again at this time. Then the patient is positioned in a lateral decubitus position with the elbow lying on an arm support, making sure the elbow can be freely flexed and extended. The elbow is draped with wide and convenient space for moving the scope and working instruments around the elbow during arthroscopic surgery (Fig. 13.1a, b). With this setting, the stability can still be checked after surgery and eventually the conversion to open surgery can be performed when necessary.

6.2 Portals for Arthroscopic LCL Suturing

The author usually starts the arthroscopic examination in the volar compartment. A proximal anteromedial portal is initially established for a viewing portal for insertion of an arthroscopic lens with a diameter of 4.0 mm as a routine. After that, anterolateral portal is created using an outside-in technique under direct visualization via arthroscopic camera. The skin landmark for this portal is just anterior to radiocapitellar joint line (Fig. 13.1c, d). When done, the elbow can be inspected for the torn ligament and capsule, as well as concomitant lesions, in volar compartment (Fig. 13.2a).

Probe, shaver, and grasper can be used in the volar compartment area. Most often, chondral fragments are found at the tip of coronoid. In such cases, the fragment can be removed in the same setting, using proximal anteromedial as viewing portal and anterolateral portal as working portal (Fig. 13.2b).

In cases where the volar compartment has a lot of scar tissue (usually not found in acute cases) or the capsule is torn into strips, creation of a proximal anterolateral portal (Fig. 13.1d) for inserting a retractor can provide more working space in the joint without the necessity to increase the water pressure. Especially in a relatively new elbow injury, limiting the water pressure can reduce the chance of swelling from fluid leakage.

When entering the dorsal compartment, it is usually started by looking through the direct posterior portal. The posterolateral portal will be used as the working portal (Fig. 13.1e).

Pearl and Pitfall for Selecting the Posterolateral Portal as the Working Portal

- Care does not injure the ulnar nerve, by avoid to putting the portal too medialized
- Easy for insert the instrument to reach the centre of lateral facet of the lateral epicondyle.

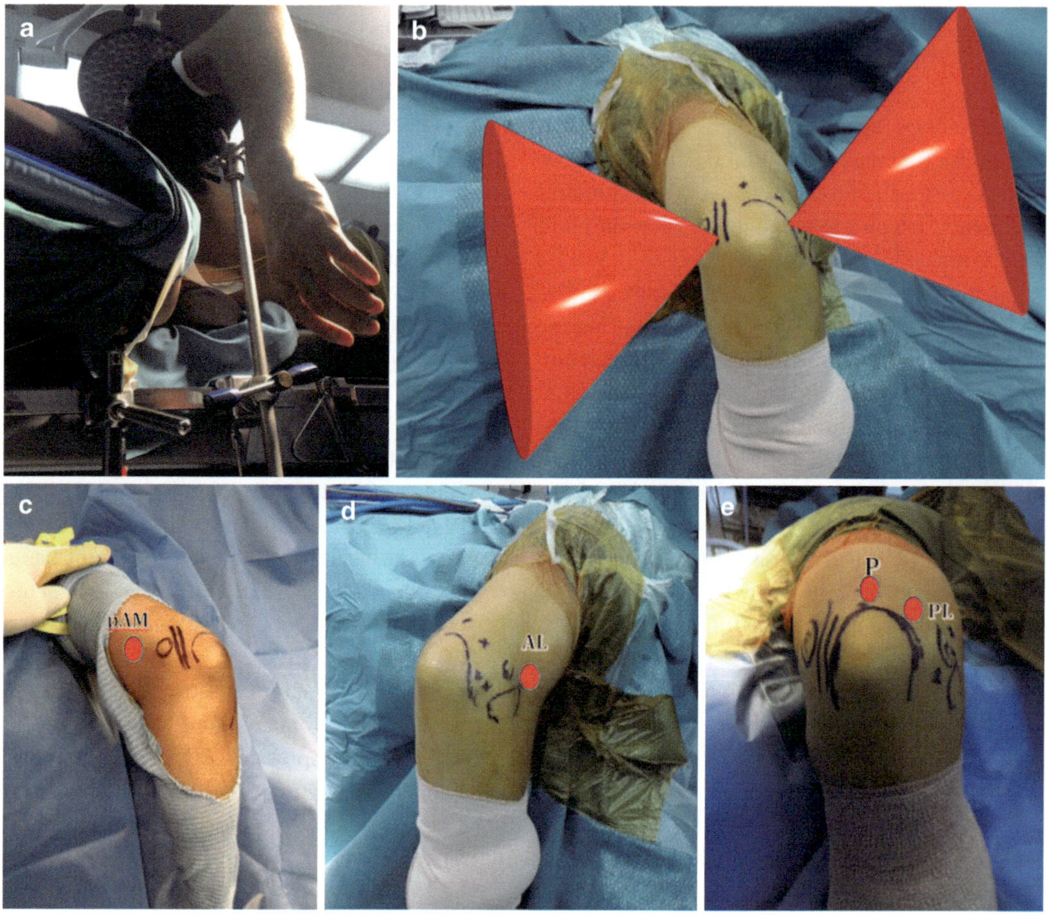

Fig. 13.1 (**a**) Lateral decubitus with arm support. (**b**) The red cone shape represents the space for arthroscopic instrument movement. (**c**) Proximal anteromedial (pAM) portal. (**d**) Anterolateral portal (AL) and the proximal anterolateral portal (pAL). (**e**) P Posterior portal, PL posterolateral portal

Pearl and Pitfall for Reducing the Chance of Misorientation During Arthroscopic Surgery in the Dorsal Compartment of the Elbow

- At the starting, make sure that the tip of the scope and instrument are in the olecranon fossa.
- Create and extend the working space by using a shaver or radiofrequency cautery. Be aware and make sure the instruments are in the joint. For example, the posterior capsule can be removed. However, if the muscle is seen while debriding the capsule, it means that the instruments are at the area that is too superficial and enter the triceps muscle plane.
- Identified olecranon by flexing and extending the elbow, the olecranon will move, but the olecranon fossa in distal humerus will not move.
- Then extend to posteromedial and posterolateral space or gutter.

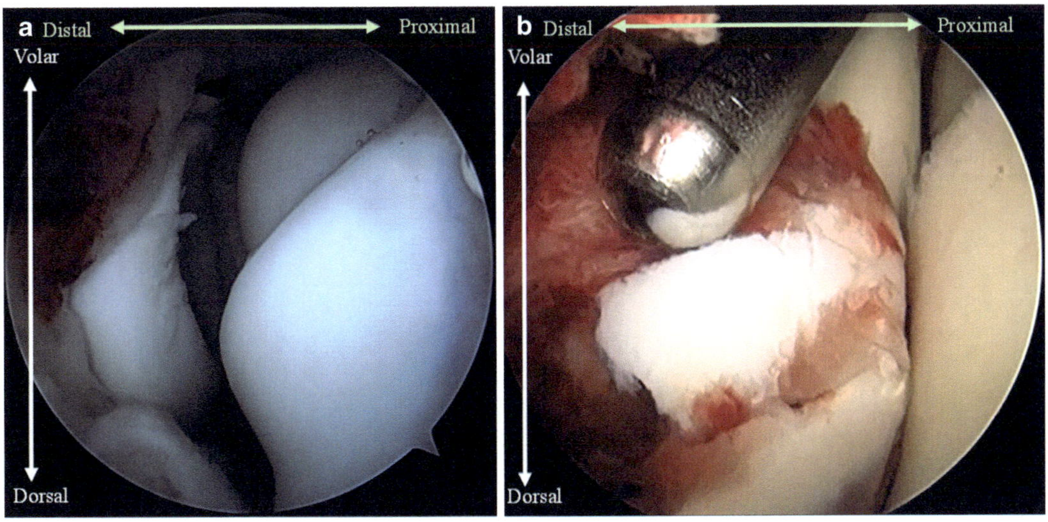

Fig. 13.2 Examination in volar compartment (**a**) Viewing from proximal anteromedial portal, capsular tear and widening of radiocapitellum and ulnohumeral joint widening are shown. (**b**) Chondral fragment on tip of coronoid is demonstrated (R radius, Ca capitellum, T trochlea, Co coronoid)

After achieving the working and viewing portals, you must clearly determine the step in of elbow arthroscopy, basically determine where you are within the joint.

Once the arthroscopic viewing and working portals are established at the dorsal compartment of the elbow, in the initial unstable elbow dislocation, the following characteristics are often found (Fig. 13.3):

- *Positive drive-through sign*
- *Widening of ulnohumeral joint*. Looking at ulnohumeral gap from the posterior portal, an assistant stabilizes the humerus while the surgeon extends the elbow and rotates the forearm to supination. At this moment, the ulnohumeral joint opening becomes very large.
- *Naked lateral facet of lateral condyle* confirms that the lateral collateral complex is torn from the humeral side. In some cases, peeling of free avulsed fragments, capsule, and collateral complex may be found as free-floating structure in the joint.

6.3 Steps in Repair LCL Complex (Video 13.1)

Prepare the footprint of the LCL insertion at the lateral facet of lateral condyle with a shaver through the posterolateral portal (Fig. 13.4a). In the posterolateral portal area, use a half-pipe as the guide to the elbow, followed by a curved aiming guide for a 1.8 mm soft anchor (Y-Knot®flex, Conmed) with double-loaded sutures (Fig. 13.4b).

The reason why the author prefers to use the soft suture anchor is that it is small and does not damage much bone tissue. It also offers a curved aiming guide that can be tilted to adjust the angle to be able to reach the area of the LCL attachment at the lateral facet of the lateral condyle as much as possible. The soft suture anchor can be applied through the posterolateral portal without creating another incision, which is usually required when using a rigid suture anchor.

After that, the soft suture anchor is inserted into the bone. Figure 13.5a shows both pairs (four limbs) of the sutures coming out from the elbow joint through the posterolateral portal. A

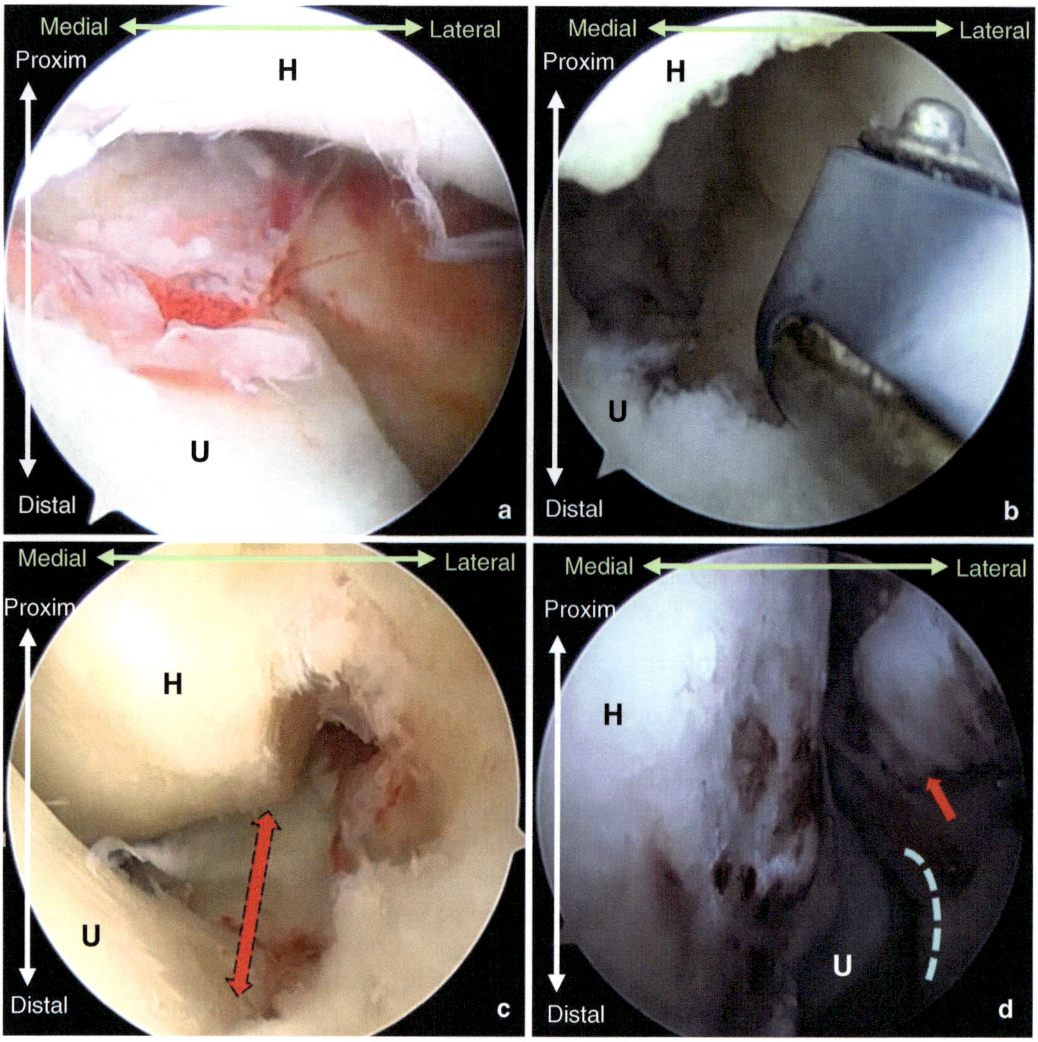

Fig. 13.3 (**a**, **b**) Drive through sign: viewing from the posterior portal with the elbow extended, the arthroscope can pass through the lateral gutter or easily visualize the radial head. (**c**) Ulnohumeral joint widening: when the elbow is extended and the forearm is supinated, the two head red arrows demonstrate the widening of ulnohumeral joint. (**d**) Blue strip line was labeling the annular complex, the red arrow indicates the avulsion of the LCL

small skin incision is made over the lateral side of the elbow, which is usually distal to the soft spot portal (Fig. 13.5d). In cases of dislocated elbows, it is quite difficult to clearly identify the small skin incision site. Usually, it is around the radial head. Identifying the incision site can be facilitated by using a needle for percutaneous piercing from skin through various structures that can be gathered and repaired back to the lateral facet of the lateral condyle site under arthroscopic view. Then, a small skin incision is created for introducing the suture lasso (suture passer). The author prefers to use an 18- or a 20-gauge needle with polydioxanone suture (PDS) inserted in a loop pattern. It is pierced through the created small skin incision and let the tip of the needle grasp the lateral collateral complex and capsule sites which are then sutured together to the origin of LCL humeral attachment (Fig. 13.5b, c).

Through the posterolateral portal, a suture retriever is used to grab the loop of the PDS and one limb of the four sutures. Both PDS and the

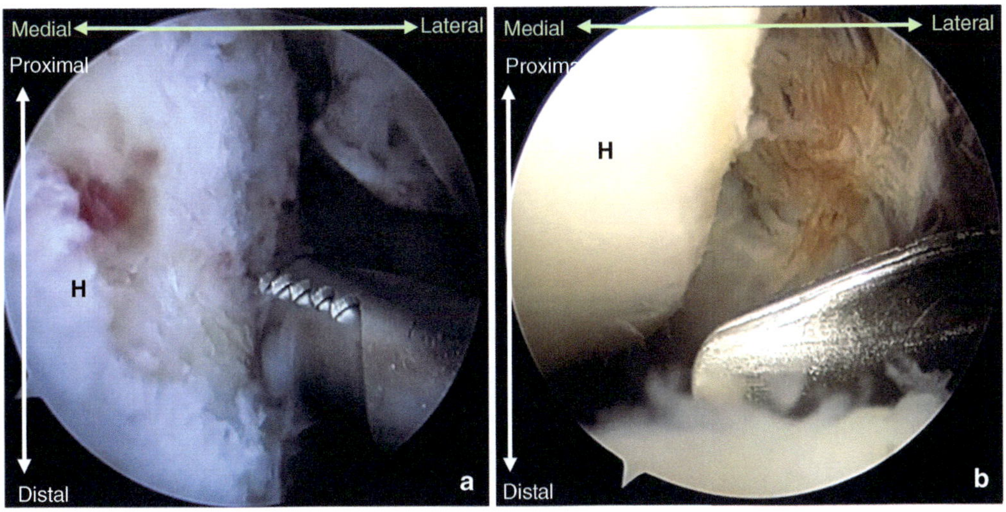

Fig. 13.4 (**a**) Looking from the posterior portal, a shaver is introduced through the posterolateral portal to prepare the humeral footprint for LCL repair. (**b**) A half-pipe instrument is used, as the author's arthroscopic surgery never uses a cannular (H humerus)

suture must be pulled out from the joint at the same time to avoid soft tissue obstruction which is when the suture gets stuck in the portal while shuttling suture limb to exit from the small skin incision (Fig. 13.6a). Next, the steps for shuttling are similarly repeated on a limb of the other pair of sutures. However, the lasso is pierced on a different area to grasp more of the lateral collateral complex. The pierce is made through the same one small skin incision or another incision where the surgeon think that would obtain a maximal grab area of collateral complex ligament. In the end, each limb of each suture was left exiting the joint through the posterolateral portal, and the other limb through the small skin incision as demonstrated in the arthroscopic view (Fig. 13.6b, c) and outside view in (Fig. 13.7b, c).

Create the soft tissue tunnel by using a clamp to dilate subcutaneous tissue from the small skin incision to the posterolateral portal (Fig. 13.7a). Then retrieve the two limbs of sutures from the posterolateral portal through the percutaneous skin incision area (Fig. 13.7b, c). Now both limbs of each suture come out at the skin incision area.

While putting the patient's elbow in approximately 40°–45° degrees flexion and forearm in neutral rotation, each pair of sutures are tied for surgical knots. During the tying, the appropriate suture tension can be adjusted. At the same time, the arthroscopic view of the joint can monitor the closing of the lateral ulnohumeral gap and can see all structures that are previously grasped being tightened back to the lateral epicondyle area (Fig. 13.8).

6.4 Postoperative Rehabilitation

The compression dressing was applied in cooperation with a slab to control the elbow posture in slight extension to help reduce the swelling. The arm sling was applied after removing the compression dressing and after the swelling had subsided. Two to three sessions of passive-assisted range of motion exercise were initiated as early as tolerated. The range of motion could be improved with progressive active-controlled range of motion exercises as tolerated during this period.

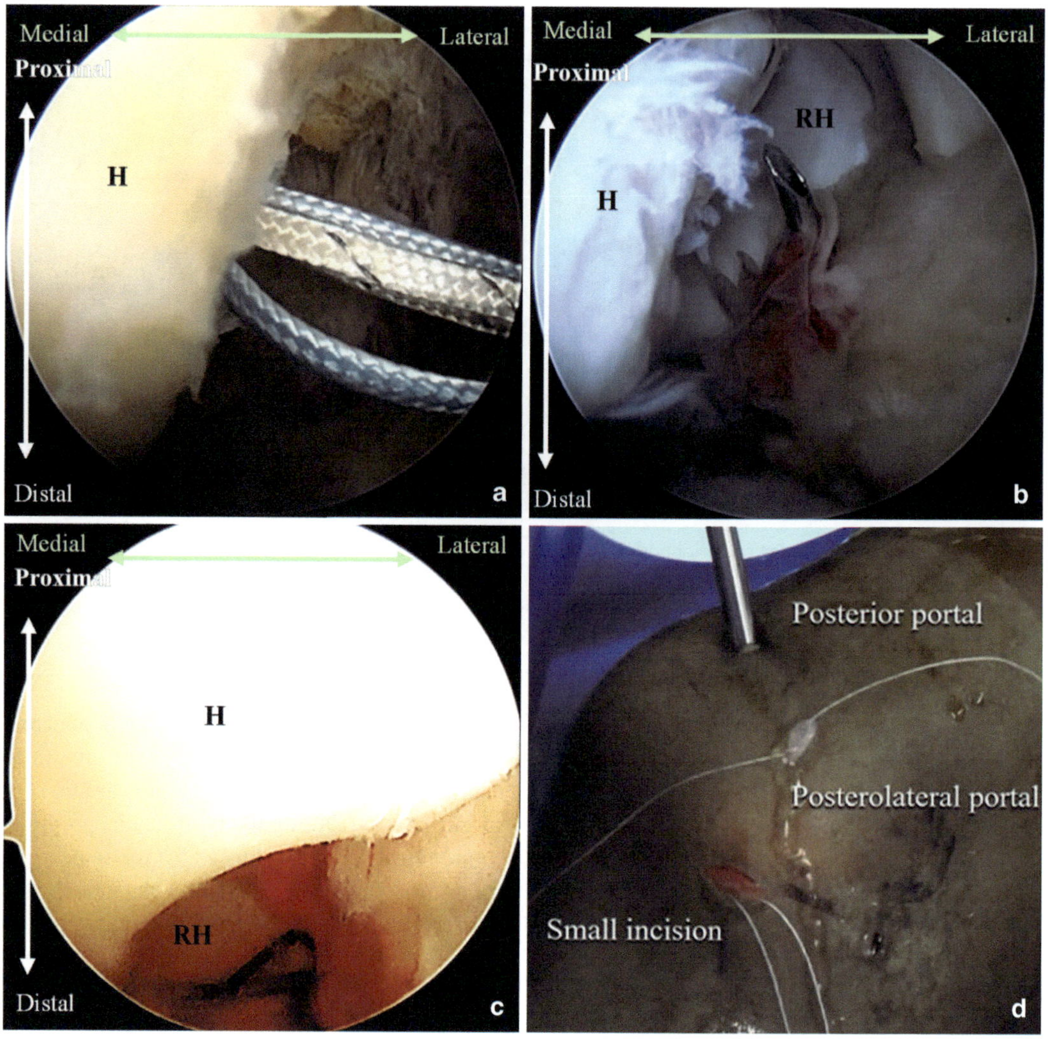

Fig. 13.5 (**a**) Demonstrates the four limbs of suture from soft anchor. (**b**) The commercial lasso was introduced through a small skin incision to catch the annular ligament in the joint. (**c**) Alternative for commercial lasso be polydioxanone suture (PDS) lasso with an 18-gauge needle can also grasp the structures in the joint as effectively as the commercial lasso. (**d**) Portals and small skin incision for the LCL repair (H humerus, RH radial head)

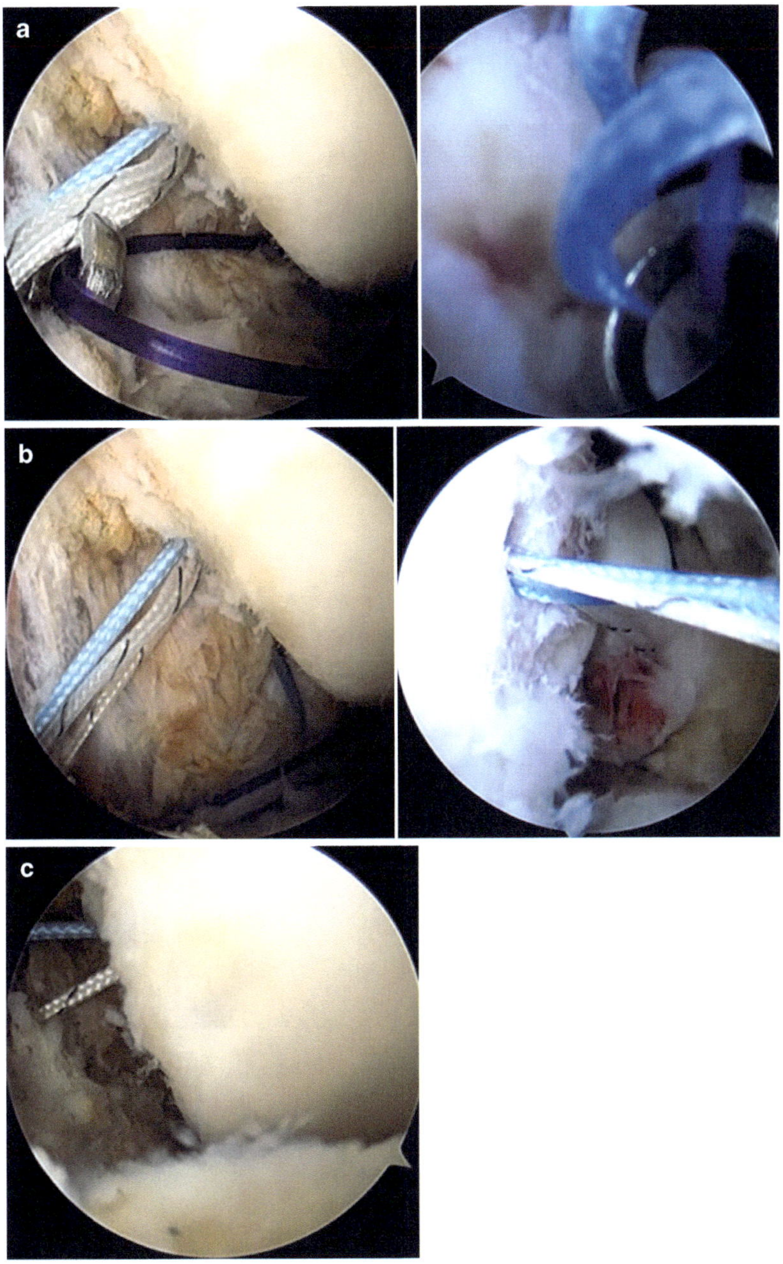

Fig. 13.6 (**a**) Lasso loop and one limb of the suture were taken out from the posterolateral portal in one time to prevent the soft tissue interpose while shutting the suture. (**b**) Each tail of the two pairs of sutures is shuttled through the small skin incision. (**c**) Arthroscopic view demonstrates each tail of each two sutures were out from joint through the posterolateral portal

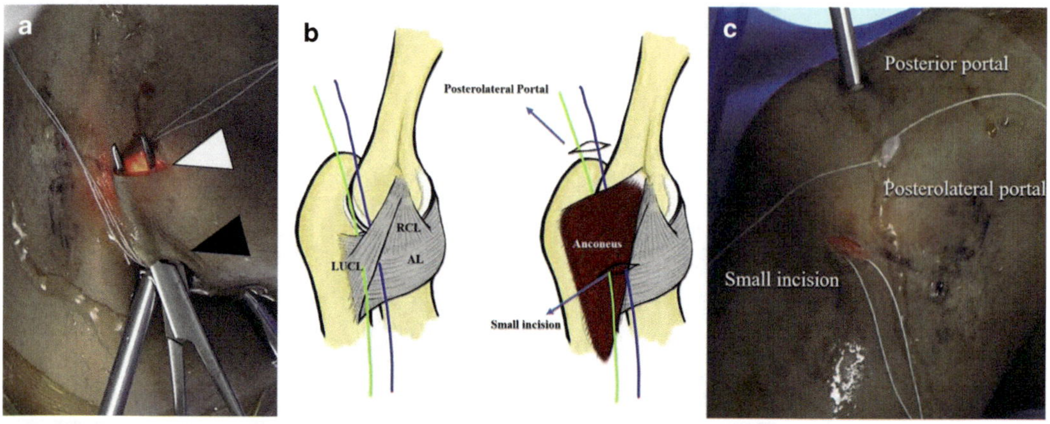

Fig. 13.7 (**a**) The subcutaneous tunnel was created with the small straight clamp. (**b**) The diagram demonstrates that the sutures are passed through the ligament and capsule, and on top of the muscle layer. (**c**) On the external view, each limb of each suture exits from the joint in different area (posterolateral portal and small skin incision)

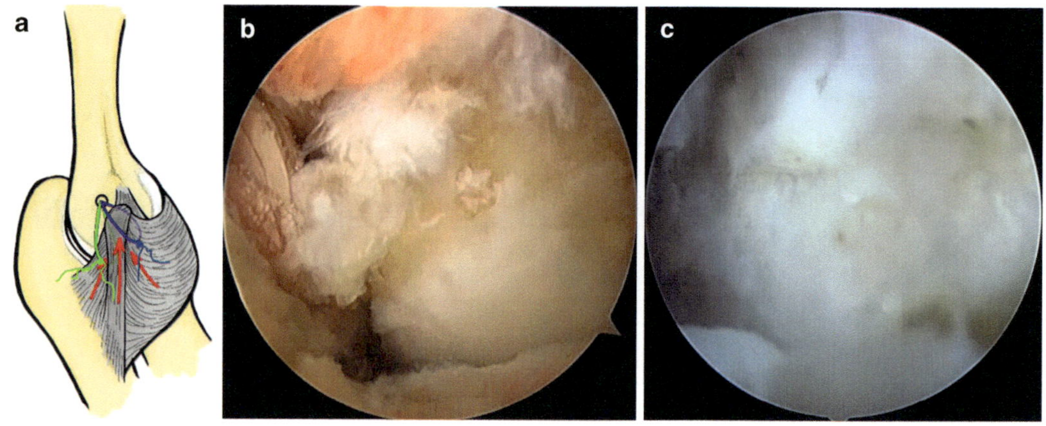

Fig. 13.8 (**a**) The diagram demonstrates that the LCL complex was tied with two suture knots. (**b, c**) The ulnohumeral gap from left and right elbow were closed even when forceful forearm supination was applied after repair the LCL

References

1. Josefsson PO, Nilsson BE. Incidence of elbow dislocation. Acta Orthop Scand. 1986;57(6):537–8. https://doi.org/10.3109/17453678609014788.
2. Dizdarevic I, Low S, Currie DW, Comstock RD, Hammoud S, Atanda A Jr. Epidemiology of elbow dislocations in high school athletes. Am J Sports Med. 2016;44(1):202–8. https://doi.org/10.1177/0363546515610527.
3. O'Driscoll SW. Elbow instability. Acta Orthop Belg. 1999;65(4):404–15.
4. O'Driscoll SW, Morrey BF, Korinek S, An KN. Elbow subluxation and dislocation. A spectrum of instability. Clin Orthop Relat Res. 1992;280:186–97. https://doi.org/10.1097/00003086-199207000-00024.
5. Schubert I, Strohm PC, Maier D, Zwingmann J. Simple traumatic elbow dislocations; benefit from early functional rehabilitation: a systematic review with meta-analysis including PRISMA criteria. Medicine (Baltimore). 2021;100(44):e27168. https://doi.org/10.1097/MD.0000000000027168.
6. Calderazzi F, Garzia A, Leigheb M, Menozzi M, Nosenzo A, Ceccarelli F, et al. Simple and stable elbow dislocations: results after conservative treatment. Acta Biomed. 2020;91(4-S):224–31. https://doi.org/10.23750/abm.v91i4-S.9637.
7. Jauffrit D, Heraudet P, Tibbo M, Erbland A, Carlier Y, Mansat P, et al. Simple acute postero-lateral

elbow dislocation: a historical perspective. Injury. 2024;55(3):111353. https://doi.org/10.1016/j.injury.2024.111353.

8. Geyer S, Lacheta L, Seilern Und Aspang J, Willinger L, Lutz PM, Lappen S, et al. Patient satisfaction, joint stability and return to sports following simple elbow dislocations: surgical versus non-surgical treatment. Arch Orthop Trauma Surg. 2023;143(3):1481–9. https://doi.org/10.1007/s00402-022-04383-8.
9. Kim JW, Lee SH, Kim SJ, Park JS. Surgical technique for arthroscopic lateral collateral ligament repair. JBJS Essent Surg Tech. 2016;6(3):e33. https://doi.org/10.2106/JBJS.ST.16.00030.
10. Heo YM, Yi JW, Lee JB, Lee DH, Park WK, Kim SJ. Unstable simple elbow dislocation treated with the repair of lateral collateral ligament complex. Clin Orthop Surg. 2015;7(2):241–7. https://doi.org/10.4055/cios.2015.7.2.241.
11. Mahasupachai N, Premsiri A, Chanlalit C. Arthroscopic lateral collateral ligament repair for the acute elbow dislocation in primary lateral sclerosis patient: a case report. Orthop Rev (Pavia). 2022;14(1):32287. https://doi.org/10.52965/001c.32287.
12. Ek ET, Wang KK. Arthroscopic repair of the lateral ulnar collateral ligament of the elbow using a knotless suture anchor. Arthrosc Tech. 2018;7(2):e77–81. https://doi.org/10.1016/j.eats.2017.08.057.
13. Martinez FM, Martinez Garcia C, Lopez AG, Leon-Munoz VJ, Medina FS. Acute dislocation of the elbow: an all-arthroscopic repair of the lateral ligament complex. Arthrosc Tech. 2023;12(10):e1827–e36. https://doi.org/10.1016/j.eats.2023.06.014.

Chronic Elbow Instability: Arthroscopic Imbrication of the Lateral Collateral Ligament

14

Pieter Caekebeke, Flynn van Riet, and Roger van Riet

1 Background

There are several advantages of an all-arthroscopic technique to restore lateral stability of the elbow versus open techniques using a graft [1]. Arthroscopy allows the surgeon to evaluate the entire elbow, and associated pathology, such as loose bodies or cartilage lesions, can be treated arthroscopically in many cases. Arthroscopic imbrication of the lateral collateral ligament has been shown to yield excellent results with a minimal chance of complications. It has therefore become one of the standard options to treat lateral instability for surgeons trained in elbow arthroscopy [2]. The basics of elbow arthroscopy will be discussed in other chapters. In this chapter, we will focus on the arthroscopic imbrication of the lateral collateral ligament (LCL) complex.

Supplementary Information The online version contains supplementary material available at https://doi.org/10.1007/978-981-95-3732-7_14.

P. Caekebeke
Orthopaedic Surgery, Ziekenhuis Oost-Limburg, Genk, Belgium

University of Hasselt, Hasselt, Belgium

University of Antwerp, Antwerp, Belgium

F. van Riet
University of Antwerp, Antwerp, Belgium

R. van Riet (✉)
University of Antwerp, Antwerp, Belgium

Orthopaedic Surgery, University Hospital Antwerp, Antwerp, Belgium

AZ Monica, Orthoca, Antwerp, Belgium

2 Indications and Contraindications for Arthroscopic LCL Imbrication

Arthroscopic LCL imbrication is indicated for patients with Grade 1 or 2 posterolateral rotatory instability (PLRI) according to O'Driscoll [3]. This technique is especially beneficial in cases where concomitant pathologies such as loose bodies or cartilage lesions can be addressed arthroscopically. This procedure is contraindicated in patients with Grade 3 PLRI (severe recurrent instability), collagen diseases such as Ehlers-Danlos, or any contraindications to elbow arthroscopy or general anesthesia (Table 14.1).

Table 14.1 Indications and contraindications to arthroscopic

Indications	Contraindications
Grade 1–2 [4] PLRI[a]	Severe recurrent instability (Gr 3) [4]
	Collagen disease (e.g., Ehler-Danlos)
	Contraindications for elbow arthroscopy
	Contraindications for anesthesia

[a]*PLRI* posterolateral rotatory instability [3]

I.-H. Jeon et al. (eds.), *Elbow Arthroscopy*, https://doi.org/10.1007/978-981-95-3732-7_14

3 Step-by-Step Surgical Procedure

The surgical technique has been published previously [2, 5], and a schematic overview can be found in Fig. 14.1. In our practice, arthroscopic procedures of the elbow are performed under general anesthesia, with patients placed in the lateral decubitus position (Fig. 14.2). The arm is carefully positioned on a support to avoid any compression on the antecubital space, as this could compromise the arthroscopic view and push neurovascular structures closer to the instruments. A tourniquet is applied after exsanguination, and a useful technique is to rest the tourniquet on the support, adding stability and preventing antecubital compression.

Before any incisions are made, a thorough clinical examination of the elbow is conducted, including tests for lateral instability. Anatomical landmarks such as the ulnar nerve, olecranon, and radial head are marked on the skin to aid in identifying the origin and insertion of the lateral ulnar collateral ligament (LUCL) later in the procedure. The elbow joint is then insufflated with approximately 30 ml of saline to optimize the arthroscopic view, especially since the capsule is usually loose and requires a relatively high volume for proper distension (Fig. 14.3).

The procedure begins with the creation of a standard anteromedial portal, positioned 2 cm proximal and 1 cm anterior to the medial epicondyle. A blunt trocar is used to enter the joint, gliding over the anterior surface of the humerus toward the radial head. Using a 4.5 mm, 30° scope, the anterior compartment is systematically inspected, starting with the radial head (Fig. 14.4) and moving to the coronoid, coronoid fossa, radial fossa, and anterior capsule. If necessary, a lateral working portal is made under direct visualization, guided by a needle (Fig. 14.5).

Other procedures like synovectomy, loose body, or osteophyte removal are performed now.

To continue the inspection, a posterolateral portal is made at the lateral tip of the olecranon (Fig. 14.6), and the scope is directed toward the olecranon fossa. The scope is then guided into the ulnar gutter, where valgus stress is applied to test the integrity of the medial collateral ligament (MCL). If necessary, a central posterior portal can be used to address any identified pathology. The inspection proceeds by directing the scope to

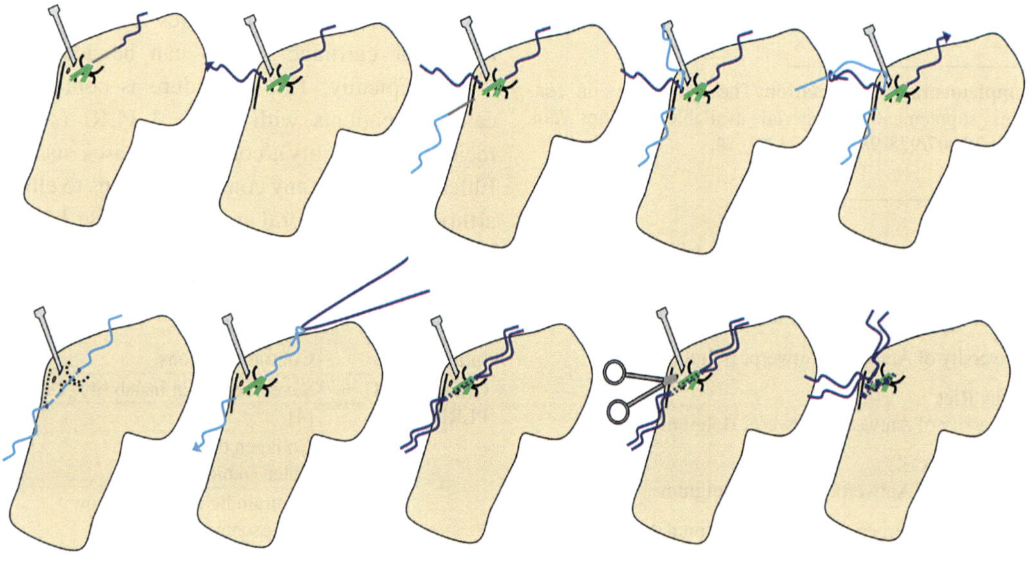

Fig. 14.1 Lateral outside view of the elbow. Subcutaneous border of the ulna, radial head and capitellum are drawn in black. LCL and LUCL are drawn in green. Reproduced with permission ©MoRe Foundation 2026. All Rights Reserved

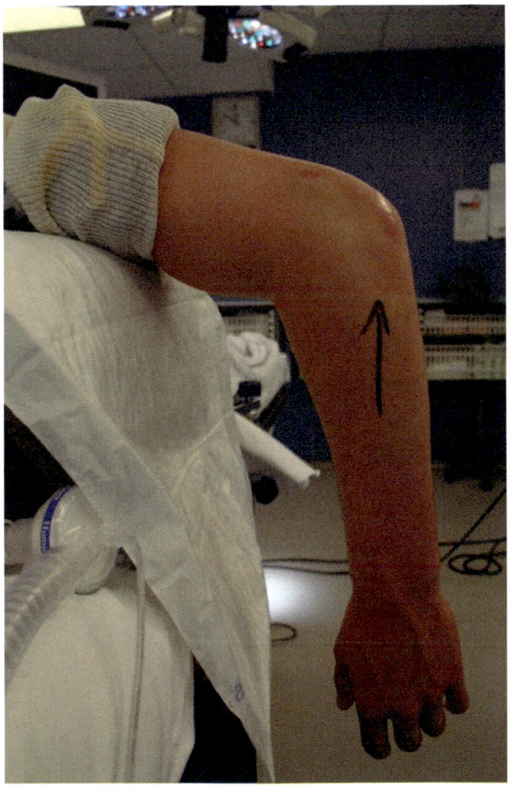

Fig. 14.2 The patient is positioned in lateral decubitus. The tourniquet is resting on a holder leaving the antecubital joint area free. Reproduced with permission ©MoRe Foundation 2026. All Rights Reserved

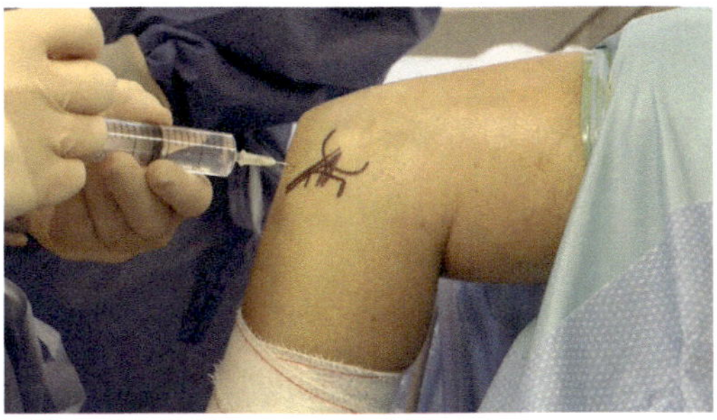

Fig. 14.3 The joint is insufflated from the soft-spot portal with approximately 30 ml saline. Reproduced with permission ©MoRe Foundation 2026. All Rights Reserved

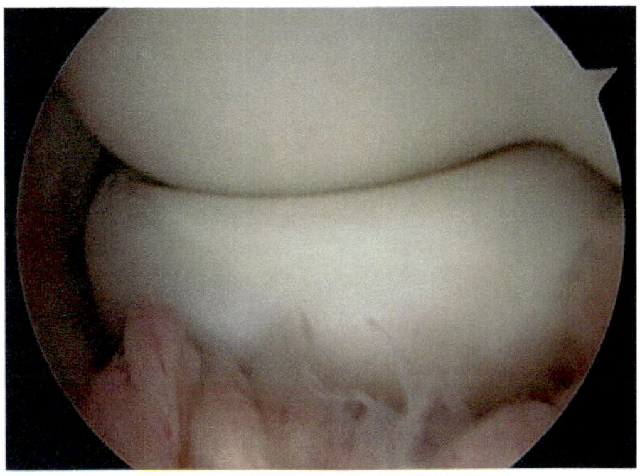

Fig. 14.4 Anterior view of the radial head with mild synovitis and sagging of the annular ligament. Reproduced with permission ©MoRe Foundation 2026. All Rights Reserved

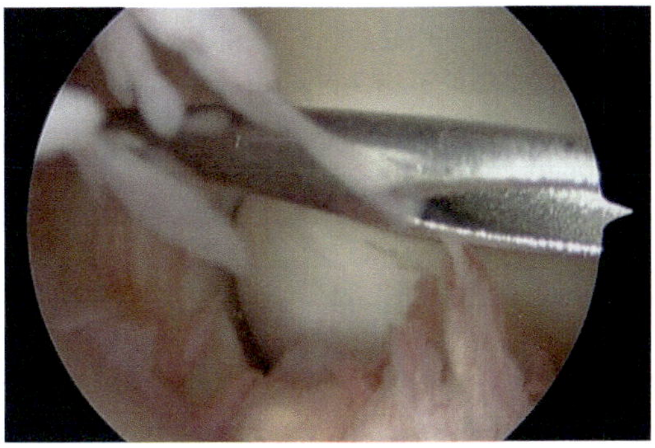

Fig. 14.5 A needle is used to determine the optimal position of the lateral portal under direct arthroscopic view. Reproduced with permission ©MoRe Foundation 2026. All Rights Reserved

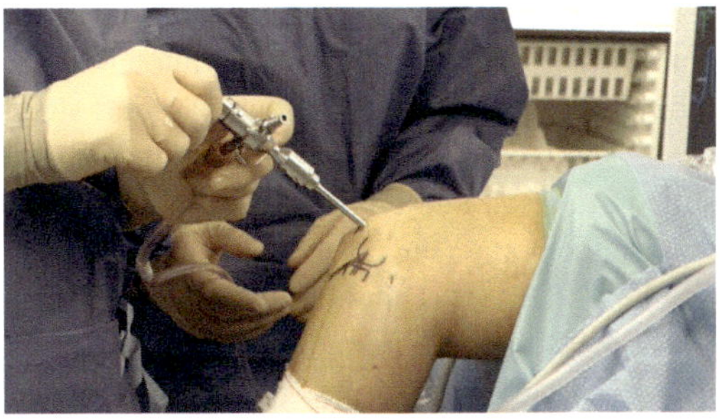

Fig. 14.6 The posterolateral portal is made on the proximal lateral tip of the olecranon, and the tip of the trocar is directed toward the olecranon fossa. Reproduced with permission ©MoRe Foundation 2026. All Rights Reserved

the radial gutter, with the elbow extended to 30°. Rotation of the cannula away from the olecranon facilitates entry into the radial gutter.

Once in the radial gutter, a synovial fold or synovitis often obstructs the view of the radial head, but this can be cleared using a soft tissue shaver (Fig. 14.7). At this stage, the arthroscopic rotatory instability (ARI) test is performed [5]. With axial traction and varus stress applied to the

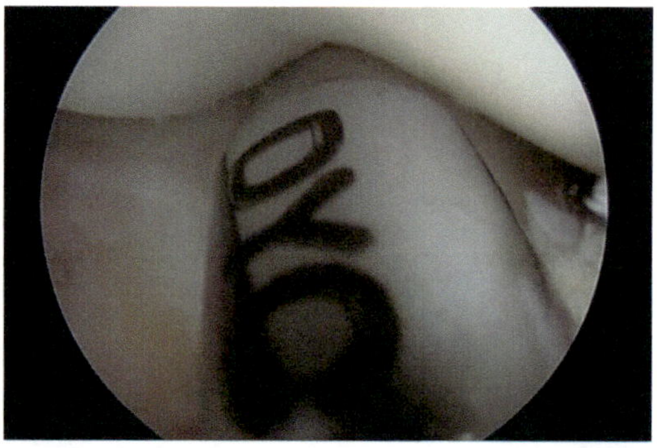

Fig. 14.7 The posterolateral synovial fringe and plica are removed to obtain a good view on the posterior radiocapitellar joint. Reproduced with permission ©MoRe Foundation 2026. All Rights Reserved

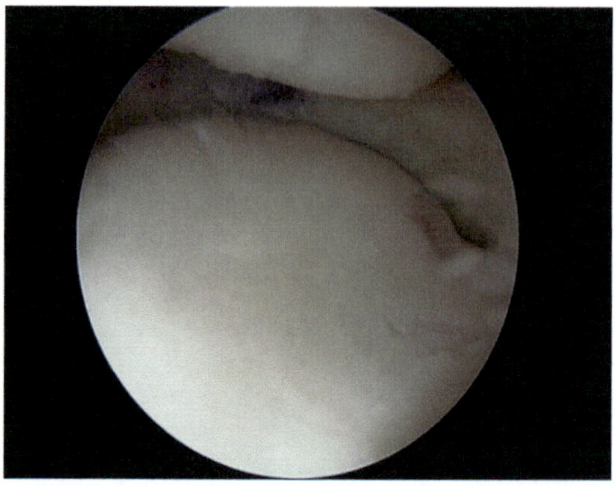

Fig. 14.8 With axial traction, varus stress, and forearm supination, observe the posterior translation of the radial head, indicating instability. Reproduced with permission ©MoRe Foundation 2026. All Rights Reserved

elbow, the radial head may translate posteriorly when the forearm is fully supinated, indicating instability (Fig. 14.8).

For the imbrication procedure, a 14G needle loaded with a polydioxanone suture (PDS II, Ethicon, J&J Medical, USA) cut in half (Fig. 14.9) is inserted into the center of the lateral epicondyle and directed toward the radial gutter (Fig. 14.10). Once the needle tip is visible, the suture is shuttled into the joint and retrieved through the soft-spot portal with a grasper (Fig. 14.11). The needle is then reloaded with the other half of the suture and inserted along the subcutaneous border of the ulna, directed over the LUCL insertion into the radial gutter (Fig. 14.12). Care is taken to stay close to the bone, which enhances the imbrication and minimizes the risk of damaging neurovascular structures. The suture is again retrieved through the soft-spot portal, and both ends are tied together outside the portal (Fig. 14.13).

The PDS is now fully intra-articular (Fig. 14.14), running from the lateral epicondyle, over the LUCL insertion at the supinator crest, and exiting distally at the subcutaneous border of the ulna. A loop is tied in the proximal end (Fig. 14.15), and a second PDS is pulled halfway through it, creating a doubled suture (Fig. 14.16). The double strand is cut at its end, so now we

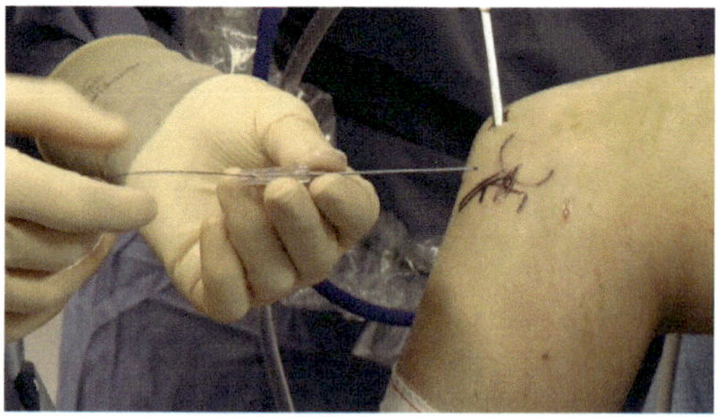

Fig. 14.9 A 14 G needle is loaded with a PDS. Reproduced with permission ©MoRe Foundation 2026. All Rights Reserved

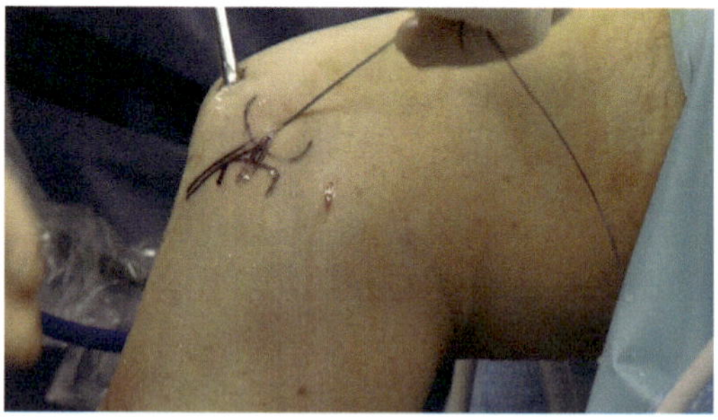

Fig. 14.10 The needle is inserted at the insertion of the LCL complex at the center of the lateral epicondyle and directed toward to posterior part of the radiohumeral joint. Reproduced with permission ©MoRe Foundation 2026. All Rights Reserved

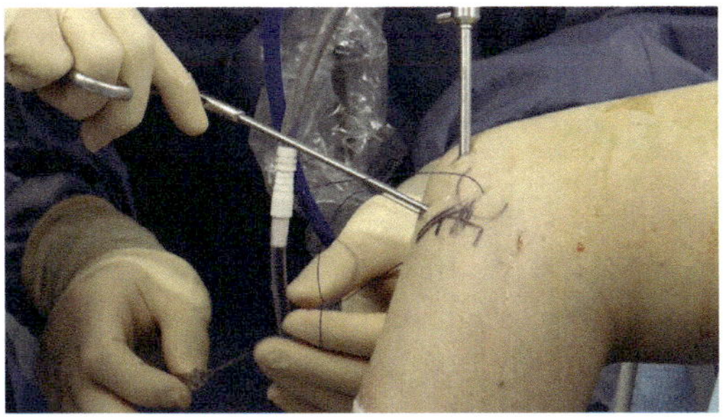

Fig. 14.11 The distal end of the suture is retrieved from the soft-spot portal. Reproduced with permission ©MoRe Foundation 2026. All Rights Reserved

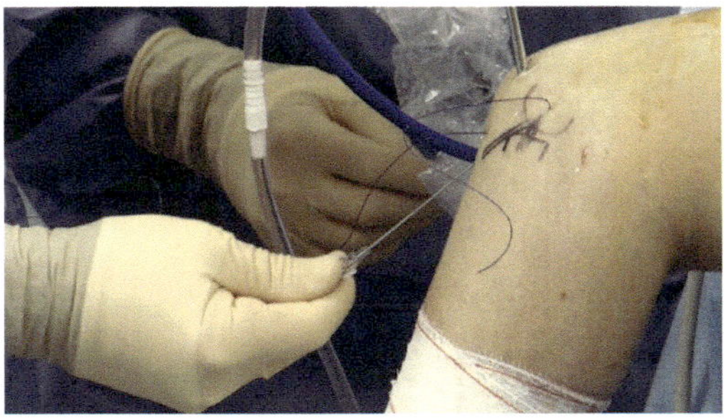

Fig. 14.12 The reloaded needle is inserted at the subcutaneous border of the ulna, directed over the LUCL insertion into the radial gutter. Reproduced with permission ©MoRe Foundation 2026. All Rights Reserved

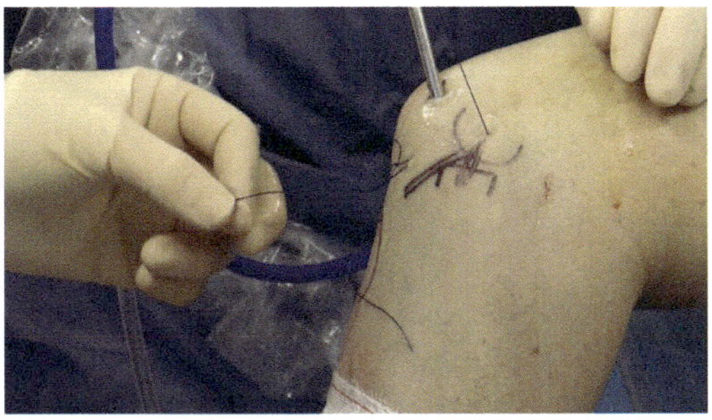

Fig. 14.13 Both sutures are tied outside the soft spot and pulled proximally. This creates one continuous suture strand running intra-articularly from insertion to origin of the LCL. Reproduced with permission ©MoRe Foundation 2026. All Rights Reserved

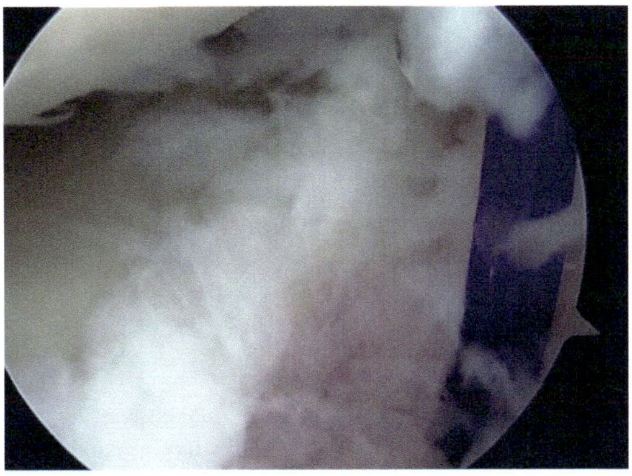

Fig. 14.14 Arthroscopic view from the posterolateral portal showing the intra-articular portion of the PDS suture. Reproduced with permission ©MoRe Foundation 2026. All Rights Reserved

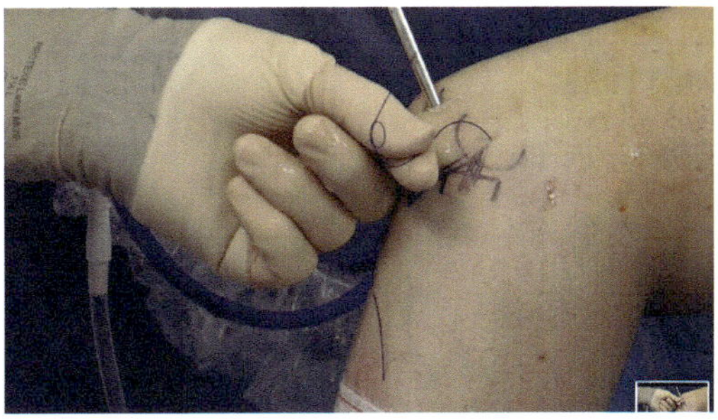

Fig. 14.15 A loop is tied in the proximal part of the suture. Reproduced with permission ©MoRe Foundation 2026. All Rights Reserved

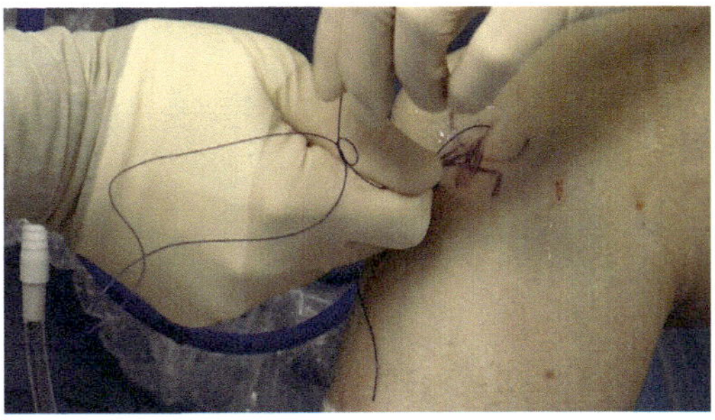

Fig. 14.16 A second PDS is brought hallway in the loop of the first suture. This creates a doubled PDS that is then pulled distally to create two strands. Reproduced with permission ©MoRe Foundation 2026. All Rights Reserved

have two sutures running as discussed above. These strands are then subcutaneously routed out of the soft-spot portal from the insertion and origin, respectively (Fig. 14.17). We now have a loop over both the insertion and origin. LCL complex, posterolateral capsule, and anconeus are included in the loop. Stability testing is repeated with the sutures both relaxed and tightened, ensuring adequate stability when tightened (Fig. 14.18). The scope is then removed, and the

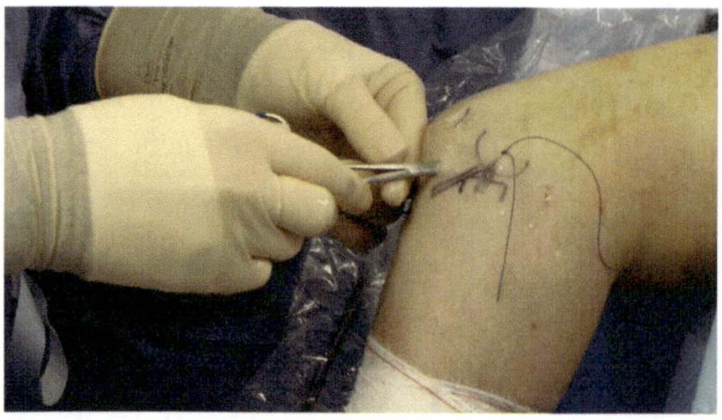

Fig. 14.17 Both the distal and proximal ends of the two sutures are shuttled subcutaneously from origin and insertion out of the soft spot. Reproduced with permission ©MoRe Foundation 2026. All Rights Reserved

sutures are tied separately with precise tension, effectively imbricating the LUCL, posterolateral capsule, and anconeus. Finally, all portals are closed, and the elbow is protected in a removable splint (eXo Elbow, Jakedesign, Belgium) and is removed on the first postoperative day, after which a dynamic brace can be used. Full flexion is permitted immediately while extension is gradually increased over the following weeks. For the first 2 weeks, extension is allowed up to 60°, followed by 30° for another 2 weeks. Full range of motion in the brace is allowed from week 4.

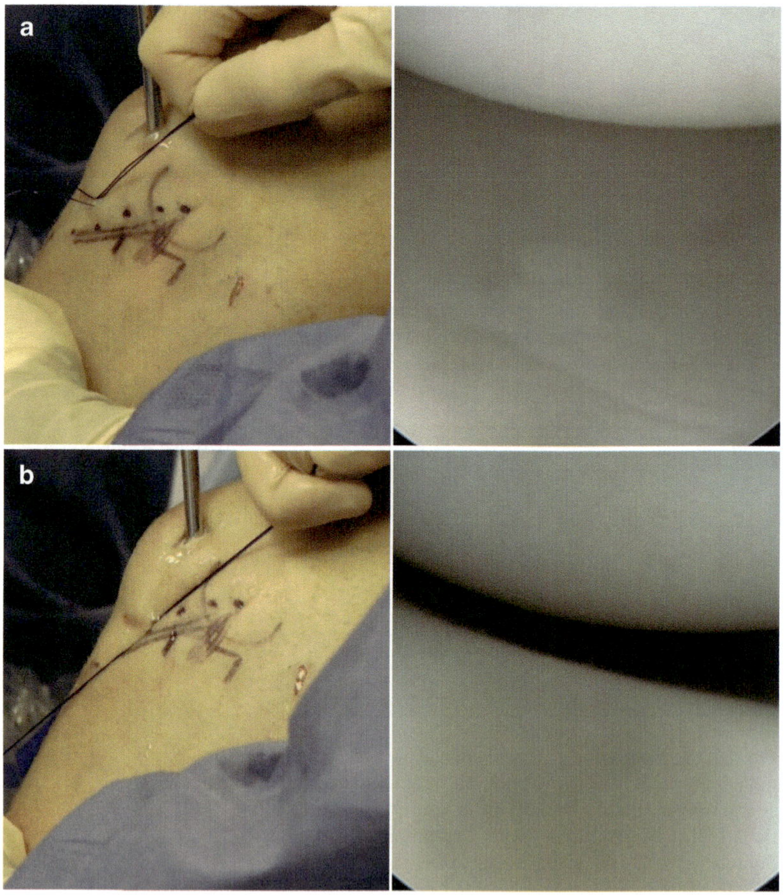

Fig. 14.18 (**a**) The ARI test shows a subluxation of the joint with the sutures loose. (**b**) The ARI test is negative with both sutures tightened, verifying the stabilizing effect of the imbrication. Reproduced with permission ©MoRe Foundation 2026. All Rights Reserved

4 Break Down the Procedure into Clear, Sequential Steps (Fig. 14.1)

4.1 Pre-procedure Setup

- *Anesthesia*: General anesthesia.
- *Patient positioning*: Lateral decubitus position with the arm supported, ensuring no compression on the antecubital space.
- *Tourniquet application*: Apply a tourniquet at 250 mm Hg after exsanguination and position it on the support for added stability (Fig. 14.2).
- *Landmark identification*: Identify and mark key anatomical landmarks, including the ulnar nerve, olecranon, lateral epicondyle, and radial head.
- *Joint insufflation*: Insufflate the elbow joint with approximately 30 ml of saline (Fig. 14.3).

4.2 Initial Diagnostic Arthroscopy

- *Anteromedial portal creation*: Create a portal 2 cm proximal and 1 cm anterior to the medial epicondyle using a No. 15 blade.
- *Joint entry*: Insert a blunt trocar, guiding it over the anterior humerus surface toward the radial head.
- *Anterior compartment inspection*: Use a 4.5 mm, 30° scope to systematically inspect the radial head, coronoid, coronoid fossa, radial fossa, and anterior capsule (Fig. 14.4).
- *Lateral portal creation (if needed):* Under direct visualization, create a lateral working portal with outside-in needle guidance (Fig. 14.5).
- *Concomitant procedures:* Synovectomy and removal of osteophytes or loose bodies can be performed now.

4.3 Posterior Compartment Inspection

- *Posterolateral portal creation*: Create a portal at the lateral tip of the olecranon, directing the trocar toward the olecranon fossa (Fig. 14.6).
- *Medial collateral ligament (MCL) testing*: Apply valgus stress to the elbow while inspecting the ulnar gutter and the integrity of the MCL.
- *Central posterior portal creation*: A central posterior portal can be made if there is a need for a working portal in the posterior compartment.
- *Lateral gutter inspection:* Extend the elbow to 30° and guide the scope into the radial gutter. Rotate the cannula to ease entry.
- *Synovial fold resection*: Use a soft tissue shaver to clear the synovial fold and improve visibility of the radial head (Fig. 14.7).

4.4 Arthroscopic Rotatory Instability (ARI) Test

Perform the ARI test: With axial traction, varus stress, and forearm supination, observe the posterior translation of the radial head, indicating instability (Fig. 14.8).

4.5 LCL Complex Imbrication—Suture Placement

- *Needle insertion (lateral epicondyle):* Load a 14G needle with PDS II suture (Fig. 14.9) and insert it into the lateral epicondyle, directing it toward the radial gutter (Fig. 14.10).
- *Suture retrieval:* Shuttle the suture into the joint and retrieve it through the soft-spot portal using a grasper (Fig. 14.11).

- *Needle insertion (subcutaneous border of ulna)*: Reload the needle with the other half of the suture and insert it along the subcutaneous border of the ulna, directed over the LUCL insertion into the radial gutter (Fig. 14.12).
- *Second suture retrieval:* Retrieve the second suture through the soft-spot portal.

4.6 LCL Complex Imbrication—Suture Preparation and Tightening

- *Create one suture strand:* Tie the suture ends together and pull proximally so it creates a single strand in line with the LUCL (Fig. 14.13). It can be inspected intra-articularly with the scope in the posterolateral portal (Fig. 14.14).
- *Double-strand creation:* Tie a loop in the proximal end of the first suture (Fig. 14.15), pull a new strand through the loop to create a doubled strand (Fig. 14.16), and route the ends out of the soft-spot portal (Fig. 14.17).
- *Stability testing:* Perform stability tests under direct arthroscopic view with sutures tightened and relaxed to confirm improved stability (Fig. 14.18).
- *Knot tightening:* Once confirmed, tighten the sutures with the correct tension and bury the knots away from the portal.

4.7 Portal Closure and Postoperative Protocol

- *Portal closure:* Close all arthroscopic portals.
- *Postoperative splinting:* A removable resting splint is used with the elbow in 70° of flexion (eXo elbow, JakeDesign, Belgium).
- *Brace application:* On the first postoperative day, remove the splint and apply a brace. Full flexion is allowed immediately. For the first 2 weeks, extension is allowed up to 60°, followed by 30° for another 2 weeks. Full range of motion is allowed from week 4.

5 Important Points to Watch Out for During the Surgery

Pearls

1. *Landmark identification*:
    - Mark anatomical landmarks (e.g., ulnar nerve, lateral epicondyle).
2. *Systematic joint inspection*:
    - Perform a thorough and systematic inspection of the joint compartments, addressing any concomitant pathologies that contribute to instability.
3. *Stability testing*:
    - Use the arthroscopic rotatory instability (ARI) test to assess lateral ligament integrity and instability under direct view.
4. *Portal creation*:
    - Create a distal posterolateral portal to enhance the view in the radial gutter, facilitating better access and visualization.
5. *Needle insertion*:
    - Insert the needle close to the bone, especially when passing near the radial head and LUCL insertion, to strengthen the imbrication and reduce the risk of neurovascular injury.
6. *Suture management*:
    - Carefully shuttle and retrieve sutures through the soft-spot portal to maintain a controlled environment and ensure accurate suture placement. Remove the scope before tightening sutures to achieve complete reduction.
7. *Knot tightening*:
    - Tie the sutures separately and bury them away from the portal to prevent knot irritation.

Pitfalls

1. *Suture breakage*:
    - The PDS suture may break when overtightened, compromising the stability of the repair. If it is noted during the procedure, it should simply be repeated.
2. *Severe instability*:
    - Although it may potentially be used for cases of severe instability, this method has

not been proven to be effective, and alternative approaches may be necessary.

3. *Missed pathologies*:
   - Focusing solely on the primary instability may lead to missing other associated conditions, such as synovitis, osteoarthritis, fractures, or nonunion, which could compromise overall surgical success.

6 Key Procedure Highlight (Video 14.1: Courtesy of MoRe Foundation)

- *Indications*: Arthroscopic LCL imbrication is indicated for patients with Grade 1 or 2 posterolateral rotatory instability (PLRI) according to O'Driscoll. Arthroscopy is especially beneficial in cases where concomitant pathologies such as loose bodies or cartilage lesions can be addressed arthroscopically.
- *Contraindications*: This procedure is contraindicated in patients with Grade 3 PLRI (severe recurrent instability), collagen disease like Ehler-Danlos, or any contraindications to elbow arthroscopy or general anesthesia.
- *Stability testing*: Use the arthroscopic rotatory instability (ARI) test to assess ligament integrity and instability under direct view. This is crucial for confirming the presence of lateral ligamentous complex injury.
- *Sequential suture placement:* Insert PDS II sutures from the lateral epicondyle and subcutaneous border of the ulna towards the joint. Retrieve them through the posterolateral portal, tie the suture ends together, and pull proximally so the knot exits the skin creating a single strand in line with the LUCL. Create a double strand, confirm improved stability.
- *Knot tightening:* Tighten the sutures separately with the correct tension.

References

1. Conti Mica M, Caekebeke P, van Riet R. Lateral collateral ligament injuries of the elbow – chronic posterolateral rotatory instability (PLRI). EFORT Open Rev. 2016;1(12):461–8. https://doi.org/10.1302/2058-5241.160033.
2. Kohlprath R, Vuylsteke K, van Riet R. Arthroscopic lateral collateral ligament imbrication of the elbow: short-term clinical results. J Shoulder Elb Surg. 2022;31(11):2316–21. https://doi.org/10.1016/j.jse.2022.06.001.
3. O'Driscoll SW, Bell DF, Morrey BF. Posterolateral rotatory instability of the elbow. J Bone Joint Surg Am. 1991;73(3):440–6. https://doi.org/10.2106/00004623-199173030-00017.
4. O'Driscoll SW, Morrey BF, Korinek S, An KN. Elbow subluxation and dislocation. A spectrum of instability. Clin Orthop Relat Res. 1992;280:186–97. https://doi.org/10.1097/00003086-199207000-00024.
5. Vandenberghe M, van Riet R. The unstable elbow: from open ligamentoplasty to arthroscopic techniques. In: Barco R, Sanchez-Sotelo J, editors. Essential techniques in elbow surgery. Cham: Springer International Publishing; 2016. p. 133–9.

Chronic Posterolateral Rotatory Instability: Arthroscopic Lateral Ulnar Collateral Ligament Reconstruction

15

Jia Guo, Erica Kholinne, and In-Ho Jeon

1 Background

Posterolateral rotatory instability (PLRI) is regarded as the most common pattern of elbow joint instability, typically resulting from a deficiency in the lateral collateral ligament (LCL) complex. In particular, the lateral ulnar collateral ligament (LUCL) functions as a key stabilizer against external rotation forces and varus stress at the ulnohumeral joint [1]. Surgical repair of the LUCL is generally indicated for acute injuries, while recurrent symptomatic chronic PLRI often requires LUCL reconstruction [2, 3].

Various open surgical techniques for LUCL reconstruction have been described, with the "docking technique" being the most widely accepted approach. Recent advancements in elbow arthroscopy have contributed to significant progress in arthroscopic-assisted LUCL reconstruction [4]. It offers several benefits, including reduced tissue disruption, a lower risk of injury to surrounding stabilizing structures, enhanced assessment of instability severity to inform surgical decision-making, and the ability to address concomitant intra-articular pathologies [5]. This chapter provides a step-by-step guide to the surgical technique for arthroscopic-assisted lateral ulnar collateral ligament reconstruction.

2 Indications and Contraindications

2.1 Indications

Arthroscopic LUCL reconstruction is indicated in patients with chronic symptomatic posterolateral rotatory instability (PLRI) of the elbow resulting from LUCL deficiency. Chronic symptomatic PLRI is defined by the following criteria:

1. Symptom duration exceeding 3 months with persistent lateral elbow pain, locking, or recurrent instability.
2. Failure of conservative treatment, that is, recurrent elbow dislocation, persistent subluxation, or dislocation despite bracing.
3. Inability to maintain joint reduction beyond 30° of elbow flexion.

Supplementary Information The online version contains supplementary material available at https://doi.org/10.1007/978-981-95-3732-7_15.

J. Guo (✉) · I.-H. Jeon
Department of Orthopaedic Surgery, Asan Medical Center, University of Ulsan, College of Medicine, Seoul, Republic of Korea

E. Kholinne
Faculty of Medicine, Universitas Trisakti, Jakarta, Indonesia

I.-H. Jeon et al. (eds.), *Elbow Arthroscopy*, https://doi.org/10.1007/978-981-95-3732-7_15

2.2 Contraindications

2.2.1 Relative Contraindications

1. Severe disruption of native anatomy due to prior trauma or advanced degenerative arthritis.
2. History of ulnar nerve transposition, which may complicate surgical access and graft placement.

2.2.2 Absolute Contraindications

Presence of concomitant radial head or coronoid fractures requiring open reduction and internal fixation (ORIF).

3 Step-by-Step Procedure

3.1 Patient Positioning

With the patient under general anesthesia, a preoperative assessment of elbow instability is performed, including varus laxity and lateral pivot-shift tests. The patient is positioned in the lateral decubitus position, and the arm is secured to a padded support with the shoulder abducted to 90° and the elbow flexed to 90°, allowing the forearm to hang freely. A sterile tourniquet is applied and inflated to 250 mm Hg. A 4.5 mm, 30° arthroscope is used, with the arthroscopic pump pressure set to 30 mm Hg.

3.2 Portal Establishment and Arthroscopic Assessment

Bony and soft-tissue landmarks are identified and marked prior to the procedure. The Soft-spot portal is identified at the center of the triangular interval formed by the olecranon tip, lateral epicondyle, and radial head (Fig. 15.1). To distend the elbow joint for insufflation, a 20 mL saline is injected through an 18-gauge needle inserted into the soft-spot portal.

Arthroscopic diagnosis involves assessing elbow laxity and identifying associated pathologies or injuries using two viewing portals to enable a complete examination. The proximal anteromedial portal is established 2 cm proximal to the medial epicondyle and 1–2 cm anterior to the medial intermuscular septum to visualize the anterior compartment. Through this portal, widening of the radiocapitellar joint space can be observed in an unstable elbow, consistent with findings on preoperative stress radiography (Fig. 15.2).

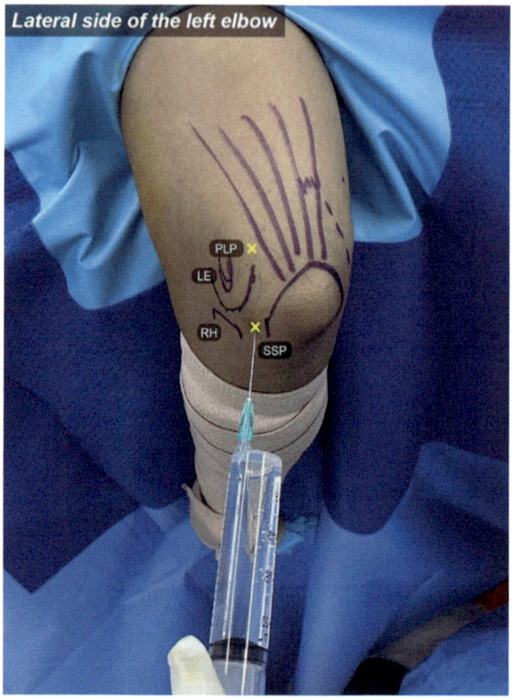

Fig. 15.1 Setup and portals for arthroscopy. The patient is positioned in the lateral decubitus position with the left elbow secured in 90° of flexion. Yellow crosses indicate the portal sites: the soft-spot portal and the posterolateral portal. For joint insufflation, 20 mL of saline is injected through the soft-spot portal. Abbreviations: LE lateral epicondyle, PLP posterolateral portal, RH radial head, SSP soft-spot portal

The proximal posterolateral portal is created 2–3 cm proximal to the olecranon tip, along the lateral edge of the triceps tendon, to allow visualization of the posterolateral compartment. A typical positive "drive-through" sign, defined by the ability to advance the arthroscope through the ulnohumeral joint, may suggest medial collateral ligament (MCL) or LUCL deficiency [6].

To assess the specific pattern and extent of LUCL deficiency, the arthroscopic rotatory

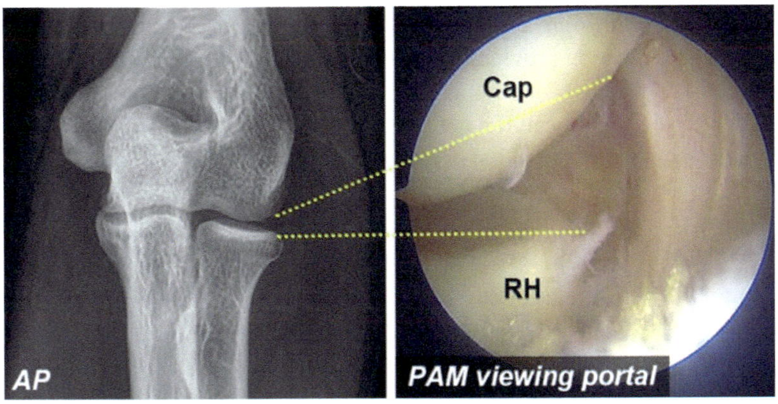

Fig. 15.2 Arthroscopic assessment of elbow joint laxity (left elbow, lateral decubitus position). The viewing portal is established through the proximal anteromedial portal. Widening of the radiocapitellar joint space is observed, consistent with findings from preoperative stress radiography findings. Abbreviations: AP anteroposterior view, Cap capitellum, PAM proximal anteromedial, RH radial head

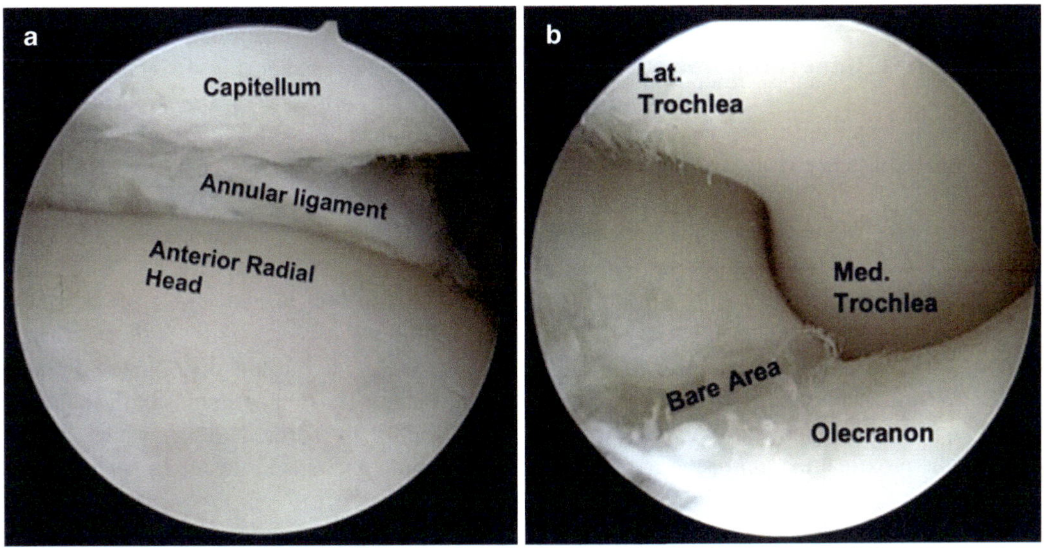

Fig. 15.3 Arthroscopic signs of advanced LCL injury. (**a**) Drive-through sign: In Stage 3 LCL injury, posterolateral subluxation of the radial head allows the anterior border of the radial head to be visualized from the posterolateral viewing portal using a 30° arthroscope. (**b**) Medial trochlea sign: This sign is typically observed in cases of ulnohumeral joint (UHJ) laxity. Because the trochlea is not normally visible unless the UHJ is subluxated, its visualization is considered pathognomonic for end-stage LCL injury. (Adapted from: Kwak JM, Int Orthop. 2024 Jan)

instability test is recommended under posterolateral rotatory stress. Arthroscopic findings indicative of advanced LCL injury include the "medial trochlea" sign, characterized by unusual visibility of the medial trochlea, and the "sunset" sign, characterized by visibility of the anterior rim of the radial head (Fig. 15.3, Video 15.1). [5]

In addition, any concomitant pathologies or injuries, such as synovial plica syndrome and lateral epicondylitis, can be addressed during the arthroscopic examination.

Arthroscopic instability testing is essential to confirm the diagnosis of LUCL deficiency and to determine the necessity for LUCL reconstruction. Furthermore, performing an arthroscopic assessment prior to graft fixation provides a reference joint gap, which can later be compared with the post-reconstruction joint gap to confirm adequate graft tensioning and stabilization [7].

3.3 Graft Harvest and Preparation

An intraoperative assessment confirmed the presence of the ipsilateral palmaris longus tendon. A 1 cm incision is made over the distal wrist crease, and a tendon stripper is used to harvest a 15–20 cm segment of the tendon. The graft is then prepared by the assisting surgeon using whipstitch running sutures with 5-0 ETHIBOND (Ethicon) at both free ends (Fig. 15.4).

3.4 Ulnar Tunnel Preparation

Using the supinator crest as a landmark for the ulnar tunnel, located just distal to the proximal margin of the radial head [8], a 2 cm incision was made over the posterior ulna at the level of the radial neck (Fig. 15.5). A double-strand LUCL reconstruction is performed by drilling two 2.2 mm-diameter bone tunnels with a 1–1.5 cm osseous bridge between them (Fig. 15.6).

The distal tunnel is created first, just proximal to the supinator crest and approximately 15 mm distal to the proximal margin of the radial head, as indicated by previous computer model studies [9]. The second bone tunnel is created proximal and posterior to the first, maintaining a 1–1.5 cm bony bridge between them. A cerclage or looped stiff fiber wire may be used to assist with graft passage, depending on surgeon's preference. In this procedure, a PDS suture is used to facilitate graft shuttling.

3.5 Humeral Tunnel Preparation

After creating the ulnar tunnel, the humeral tunnel is prepared by making a skin incision centered over the lateral epicondyle. The humeral attachment of the graft is positioned at the center of the capitellum to achieve isometric reconstruction, ensuring consistent tension throughout the full range of the flexion-extension arc [8]. The isometric point on the capitellum for suture anchor placement is confirmed using an intraoperative image intensifier (Fig. 15.7).

Following soft-tissue clearance from the subchondral bone of the lateral epicondyle, a 3.0 mm knotless bioabsorbable suture anchor (Smith & Nephew) is inserted at the confirmed isometric point. With the guide positioned at the predetermined location, a 2.4 mm drill hole is created. The suture anchor, loaded with a single-strand No. 2-0 FiberWire repair suture, is then advanced through the guide into the drill hole and seated with a mallet. The double strands of the palmaris longus graft are secured to the suture anchor using a sliding knot (Fig. 15.8).

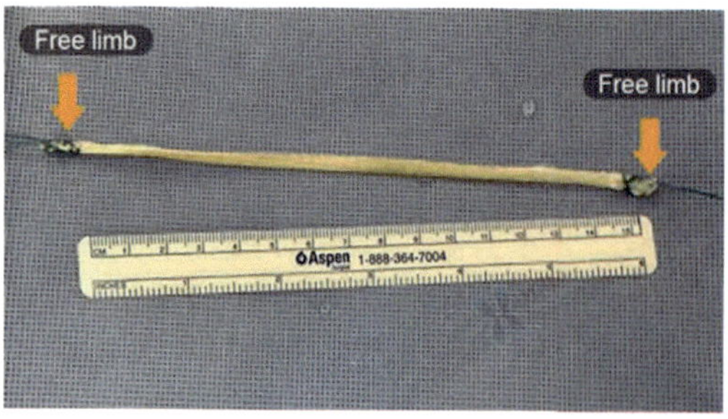

Fig. 15.4 Graft preparation. The ipsilateral palmaris longus tendon is harvested and prepared for use as a graft to facilitate smooth passage through the 2.2 mm ulnar tunnel. Each free end is sutured using a whipstitch running technique with 5-0 ETHIBOND (Ethicon)

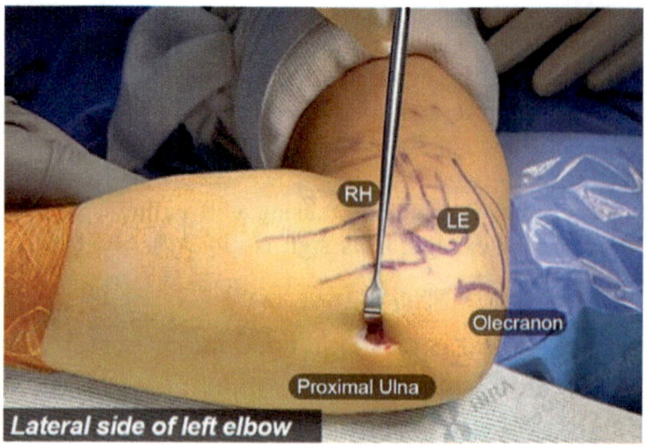

Fig. 15.5 Small incision at the posterior ulna of the left elbow in the lateral decubitus position. A 2 cm incision is made over the posterior ulna at the level of the radial neck prior to creating the ulnar tunnels. Abbreviations: LE lateral epicondyle, RH radial head

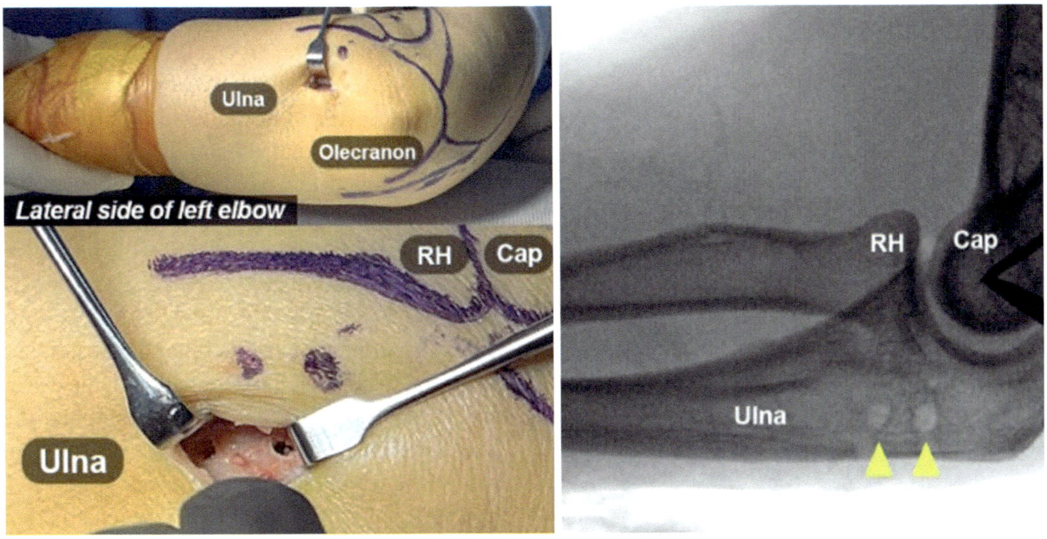

Fig. 15.6 Ulnar tunnel creation on the left elbow in the lateral decubitus position. Two convergent ulnar tunnels, each 2.2 mm in diameter, are created with a 1- to 1.5 cm osseous bridge between them. The intraoperative image intensifier highlights the tunnels and bony bridge, marked by yellow triangles. Abbreviations: Cap capitellum, RH radial head

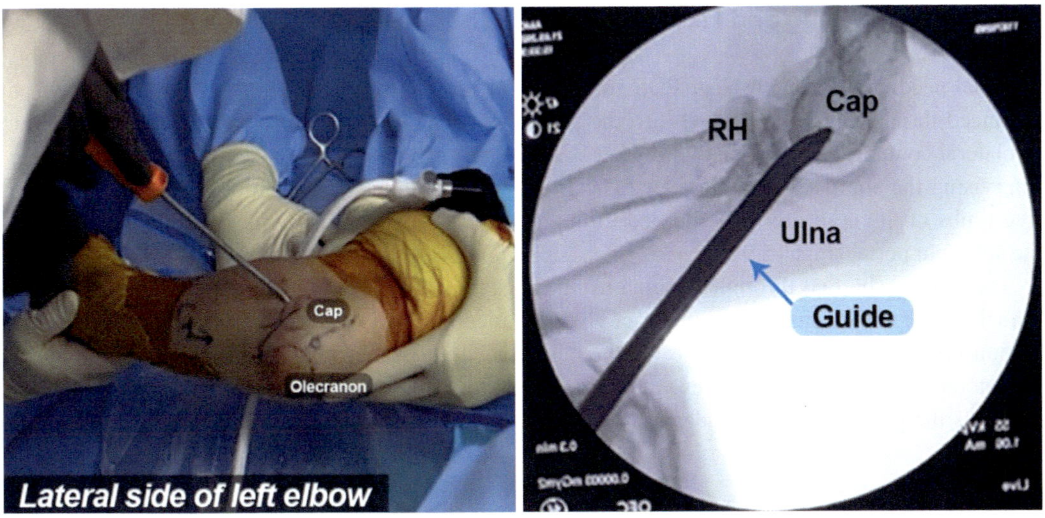

Fig. 15.7 Isometric point on the capitellum of the left elbow in the lateral decubitus position. During humeral tunnel preparation, the isometric point on the capitellum is identified using an intraoperative image intensifier. Abbreviations: Cap capitellum, RH radial head

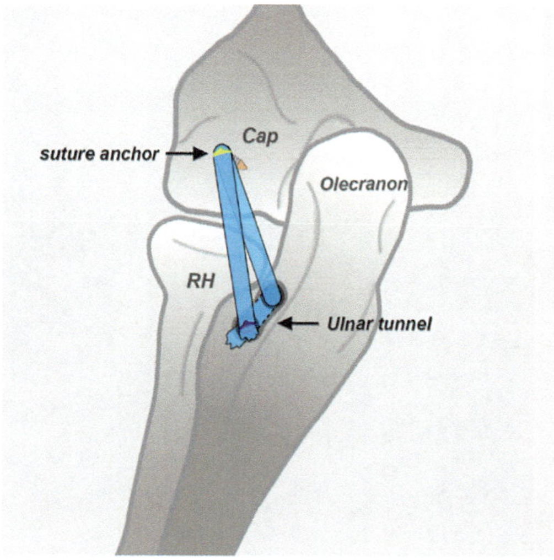

Fig. 15.8 Graft fixation method for the left elbow in the lateral decubitus position. The double-stranded palmaris longus graft is secured to the suture anchor on the humeral side using a sliding knot. On the ulnar side, the two free limbs are sutured together and tied with a knot. Abbreviations: Cap capitellum, RH radial head

3.6 Graft Passing and Fixation

A spinal needle loaded with No.1 PDS suture is advanced through the ulnar tunnel into the posterolateral compartment to assist with graft shuttling using the shuttle relay technique. The two free limbs of the graft are then shuttled through the soft-spot portal (Fig. 15.9).

The graft is shuttled through the ulna using a tunnel shuttle relay technique, with direct visualization provided by the arthroscope via the posterolateral portal. During this step, the surgeon confirms the graft placement under arthroscopy, ensuring that it is properly positioned at the posterior aspect of the radial head (Fig. 15.9). Once the graft is passed, the two free ends are retrieved through the soft-spot portal. One limb is passed to the predrilled ulnar tunnel. The graft is then cycled, tensioned, and fixed with the elbow in 90° of flexion and neutral rotation (Fig. 15.9). For augmentation, the two ends of the graft were sutured together using a 1-0 ETHIBOND (*Ethibond Excel; Ethicon, US LLC*) (Fig. 15.8). The arthroscope is reinserted into the posterolateral portal to confirm the elimination of the drive-through sign, the medial trochlear sign, and the radial head sunset sign following reconstruction. Finally, the wound is closed in layers.

This novel arthroscopic LUCL reconstruction serves as an alternative procedure for managing chronic PLRI and has shown promising outcomes (Fig. 15.10), although further data are needed to validate its efficiency. This technique offers several advantages over the open approach. First, it allows for comprehensive assessment of elbow stability and associated pathologies, facilitating informed surgical decision-making. Notably, arthroscopic evaluation provides strong visual evidence of the severity of LUCL deficiency in cases of PLRI.

Additionally, this minimally invasive technique reduces soft-tissue dissection and minimizes the risk of damaging other elbow stabilizers, such as the anconeus muscle. Precise identification of the humeral attachment site for accurate isometric reconstruction can be achieved through a small incision, aided by an intraoperative image intensifier.

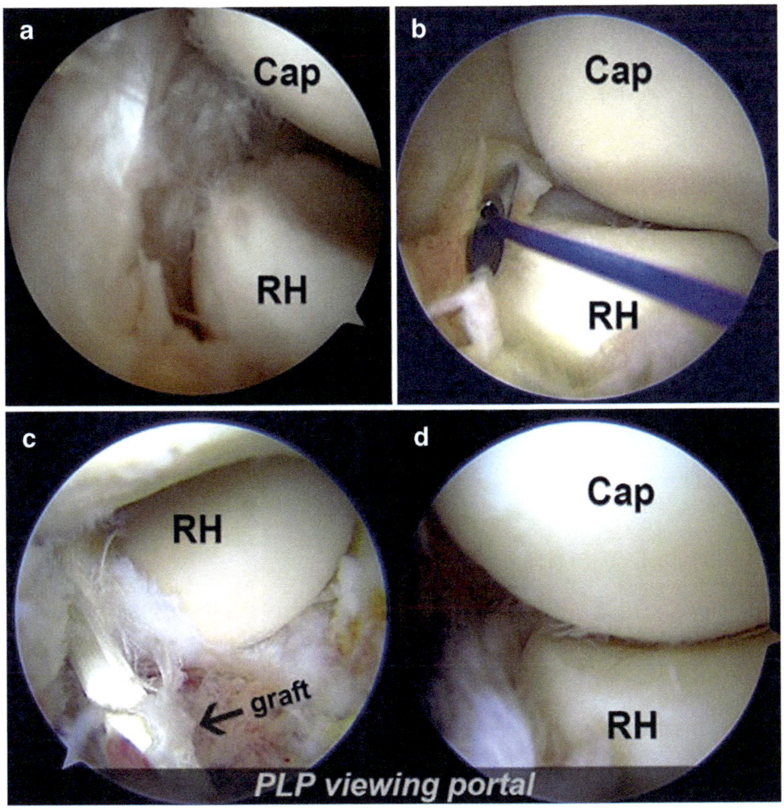

Fig. 15.9 Arthroscopic view of the left elbow in the lateral decubitus position showing graft passage from the posterolateral viewing portal. (**a**) Widening of the radiocapitellar joint gap is visible prior to lateral ulnar collateral ligament (LUCL) reconstruction. (**b**) A spinal needle loaded with No. 1 polydioxanone suture (PDS, Ethicon) is passed through the ulnar tunnel and introduced into the posterolateral compartment. (**c**) The graft is positioned at the posterior aspect of the radial head using the shuttle relay technique. (**d**) After graft passage and fixation, the joint space is reduced by tensioning the graft. Abbreviations: Cap capitellum, PLP posterolateral portal, RH radial head

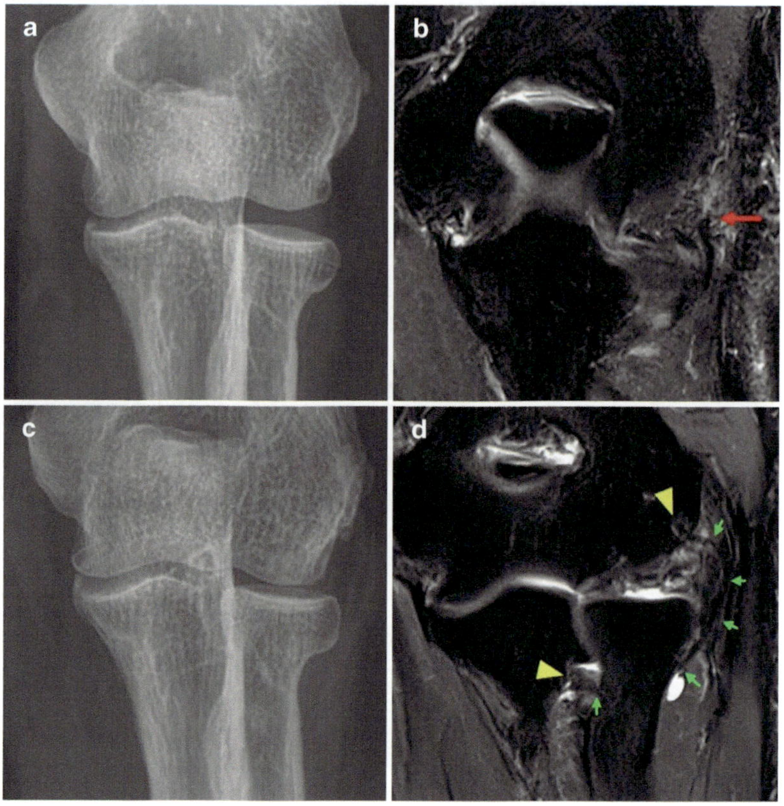

Fig. 15.10 Preoperative and postoperative MRI and X-ray of arthroscopic LUCL reconstruction for LUCL deficiency with concomitant lateral epicondylitis. (**a**) Preoperative stress X-ray shows widening of the radiocapitellar joint space. (**b**) Preoperative MRI reveals LUCL tear at the humeral insertion (red arrow). (**c**) One-year postoperative X-ray demonstrates a reduced radiocapitellar joint space. (**d**) One-year postoperative MRI shows graft integrity at both humeral and ulnar insertions (yellow arrows). The graft appears intact and located along the posterior aspect of the radial head

4 Pitfalls of the Procedure

1	The humeral and ulnar footprints should be identified under image intensification to ensure optimal graft placement.
2	The graft should be positioned on the posterior side of the radial head, with confirmation achieved via arthroscopic visualization through the proximal posterolateral portal.
3	Eliminating the “medial trochlear sign” is essential for effective lateral collateral ligament complex reconstruction, as it confirms proper tightening of the ulnohumeral joint.

References

1. Badhrinarayanan S, Desai A, Watson JJ, White CHR, Phadnis J. Indications, outcomes, and complications of lateral ulnar collateral ligament reconstruction of the elbow for chronic posterolateral rotatory instability: a systematic review. Am J Sports Med. 2021;49(3):830–7. Epub 20200902
2. Nestor BJ, O’Driscoll SW, Morrey BF. Ligamentous reconstruction for posterolateral rotatory instability of the elbow. J Bone Joint Surg Am. 1992;74(8):1235–41.
3. Camp CL, Sanchez-Sotelo J, Shields MN, O’Driscoll SW. Lateral ulnar collateral ligament reconstruction

for posterolateral rotatory instability of the elbow. Arthrosc Tech. 2017;6(4):e1101–e5. Epub 20170724
4. Guo J, Kholinne E, Ben H, Park J, Jeon IH. Arthroscopic-assisted lateral ulnar collateral ligament reconstruction for posterolateral rotatory instability of the elbow: a technical note. Arthrosc Tech. 2024;13(11):103101. Epub 20240725.
5. Kwak JM, Kholinne E, Hwang SJ, Jeon IH. Arthroscopic assessment for lateral collateral ligament complex deficiency of the elbow: a cadaveric study. Int Orthop. 2024;48(1):143–50. Epub 20231213
6. Goodwin D, Dynin M, Macdonnell JR, Kessler MW. The role of arthroscopy in chronic elbow instability. Arthroscopy. 2013;29(12):2029–36. Epub 20131008
7. Geyer S, Heine C, Winkler PW, Lutz PM, Lenich A, Scheiderer B, et al. LUCL reconstruction of the elbow: clinical midterm results based on the underlying pathogenesis. Arch Orthop Trauma Surg. 2022;142(8):1809–16. Epub 20210219
8. Kholinne E, Ha TH, Tan J, Jeon IH. Three-dimensional computed tomography modeling for kinematic analysis of double-strand lateral ulnar collateral ligament reconstruction. J Shoulder Elb Surg. 2019;28(7):1378–86. Epub 20190516
9. Moritomo H, Murase T, Arimitsu S, Oka K, Yoshikawa H, Sugamoto K. The in vivo isometric point of the lateral ligament of the elbow. J Bone Joint Surg Am. 2007;89(9):2011–7.

Part IV

Nerve Disorders

Endoscopic Intra-Articular Cubital Tunnel Release

16

Norimasa Takahashi and Hiroyuki Sugaya

1 Background

Mild to moderate ulnar neuropathy with or without associated elbow osteoarthritis can be successfully treated with nonsurgical management. However, patients who fail nonsurgical treatments often require surgical intervention. Controversy exists over the optimal procedure for decompression of the ulnar nerve. Standard surgical approaches include open in situ decompression, subcutaneous transposition, intramuscular transposition, and submuscular transposition. We have performed subcutaneous anterior transposition of the ulnar nerve in the supine position, followed by arthroscopic arthroplasty in the prone position for cubital tunnel syndrome associated with osteoarthritic elbow joint. Since 2011, we have been performing ulnar nerve decompression using arthroscopy in prone position for cubital tunnel syndrome with osteoarthritis.

Supplementary Information The online version contains supplementary material available at https://doi.org/10.1007/978-981-95-3732-7_16.

N. Takahashi (✉)
Sports Medicine & Joint Center, Funabashi Orthopaedic Hospital, Funabashi, Japan

H. Sugaya
Tokyo Sports & Orthopaedic Clinic, Tokyo, Japan

2 Surgical Indication

The best indication for arthroscopic release is in patients with elbow osteoarthritis with mild to moderate neuropathy. Elbow contracture with or without mild neuropathy is an indication.

Ulnar nerve instability has been empirically considered an indication.

Severe neuropathy including muscle weakness or atrophy is thought to be outside of the indication. Revision surgery for cubital tunnel syndrome is contraindication.

3 Surgical Procedure

Elbow arthroscopy is performed under general anesthesia in the prone position (Fig. 16.1). A standard 4 mm arthroscope, a radiofrequency device (VAPR VUE, Depuy Synthes), and a shaver (DYONICS PLATINUM, Smith & Nephew) are used. An arthroscopic fluid management system (DOUBLEFLO, Smith & Nephew) is used instead of a tourniquet, which is mounted by an 0.9% sodium chloride irrigation 3000 mL (ARTHROMATIC, Baxter) with 1 mg adrenaline. Standard anteromedial portal and anterolateral portal are used for the procedure in anterior joint space. Two portals are established in the soft spot for the procedure in the posterolateral joint space. A standard posterolateral portal (Fig. 16.2), which is a main viewing portal for the procedure in the olecranon

I.-H. Jeon et al. (eds.), *Elbow Arthroscopy*, https://doi.org/10.1007/978-981-95-3732-7_16

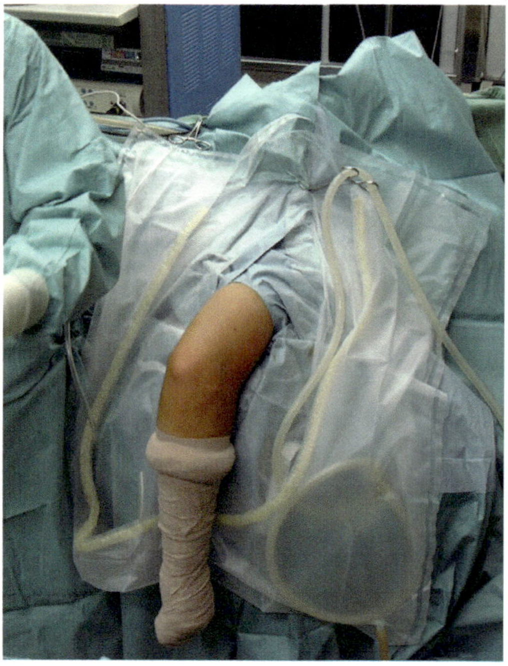

Fig. 16.1 Left elbow. Arthroscopy setting in prone position

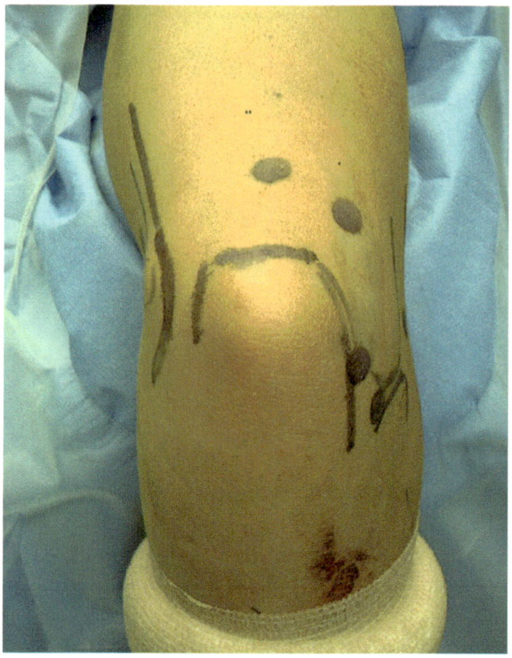

Fig. 16.2 Left elbow. Portals for posterior joint space * posterolateral portal, ** posterior portal

fossa, is established under viewing from the soft spot portal. Then, a posterior portal is established through the triceps (Fig. 16.2). An arthroscopic shaver and a radiofrequency probe are inserted to debride synovium and other tissues through this posterior portal. The initial step of the ulnar nerve release is to clear the olecranon fossa to obtain excellent visualization of the posteromedial capsule and medial gutter. In cases of elbow osteoarthritis, the procedure involves the removal of osteophytes and loose bodies, as well as the resection of osteophytes from the medial gutter. For ulnar nerve decompression, the posteromedial joint capsule is punctured and partially excised using a radiofrequency probe or a biter from the posterior portal (Fig. 16.3a). The radiofrequency probe is mainly used in coagulation mode when close to the nerve. The posteromedial capsule is resected in a proximal to distal direction starting from the medial side of olecranon fossa. Then, the capsule defect is carefully enlarged to identify the ulnar nerve (Fig. 16.3b). After the ulnar nerve is identified, it is retracted dorsally using a rod from the posterior portal. An 18 G needle is inserted into the area of capsular defect (Fig. 16.4a), followed by a knife which is called a suicide portal (Figs. 16.4b and 16.5). The suicide portal is alternatingly used with the posterior portal to distally excise both the joint capsule and Osborne ligament. Decompression is complete when there are no cord-like tissues remaining and the muscle fibers of common flexors are visible (Figs. 16.6, 16.7, and 16.8). After ulnar nerve decompression, we often observe improved blood flow to the nerve (Fig. 16.9).

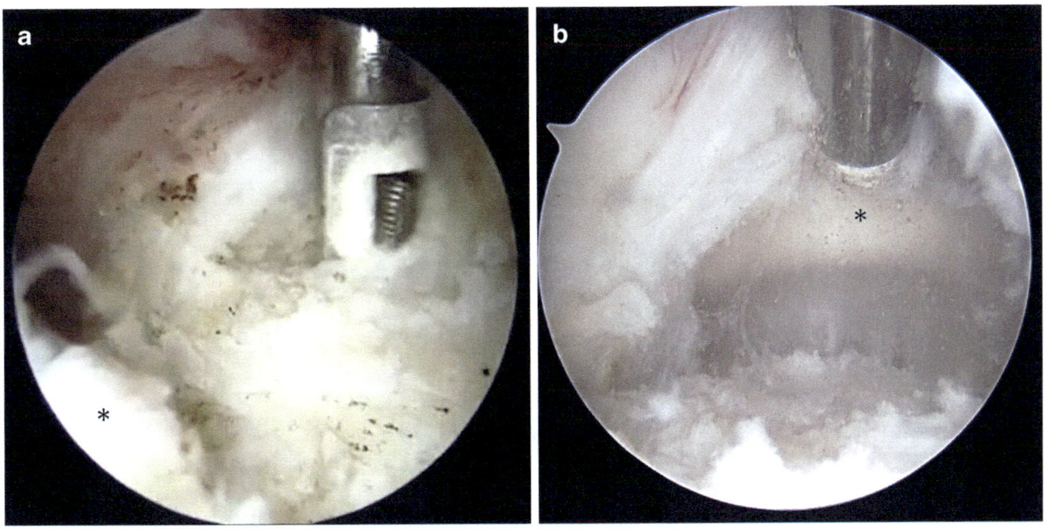

Fig. 16.3 Left elbow. posteromedial capsule resection (**a**) * olecranon, (**b**) *ulnar nerve

Fig. 16.4 Suicide portal (red circle), * medial epicondyle, ** antero-medial portal

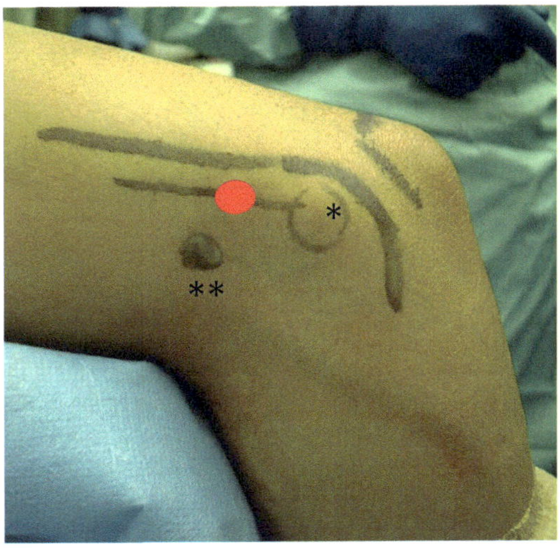

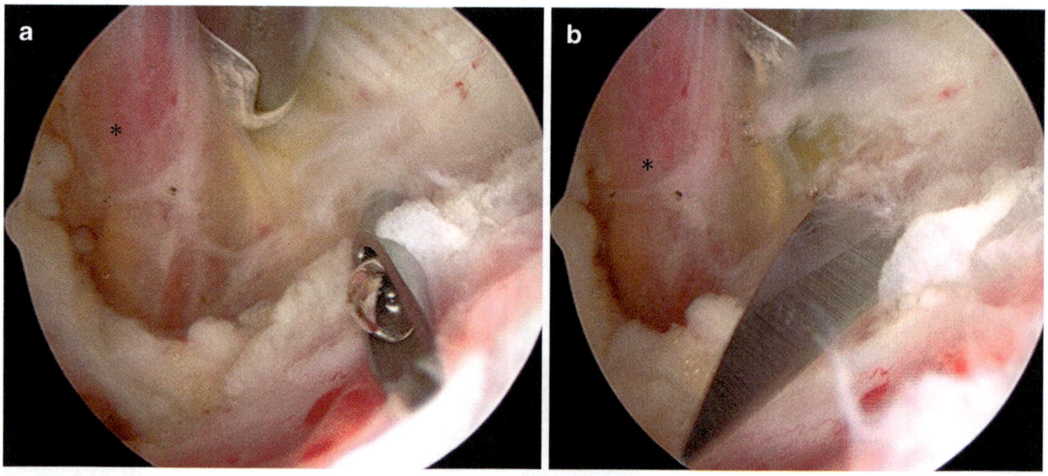

Fig. 16.5 Established suicide portal * ulnar nerve (**a**) 18 G needle penetration, (**b**) incision

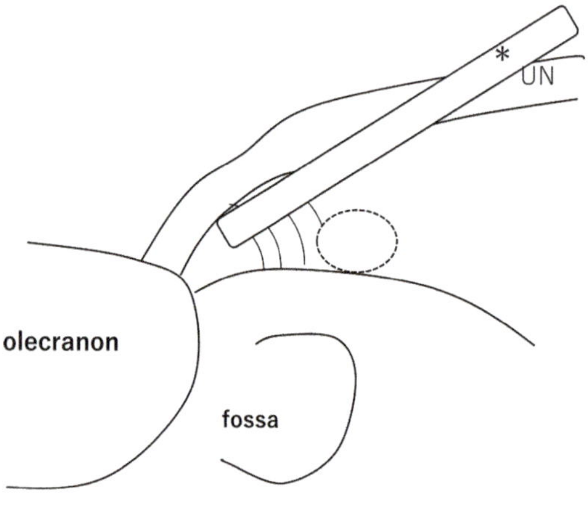

Fig. 16.6 Schema of suicide portal. An ulnar nerve was retracted with rod, when suicide portal was created

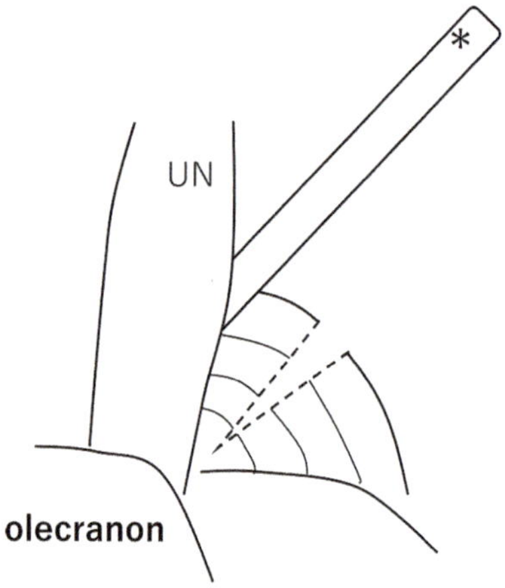

Fig. 16.7 Osborne ligament is released from the suicide portal (fibrous band of the two heads of FCU)

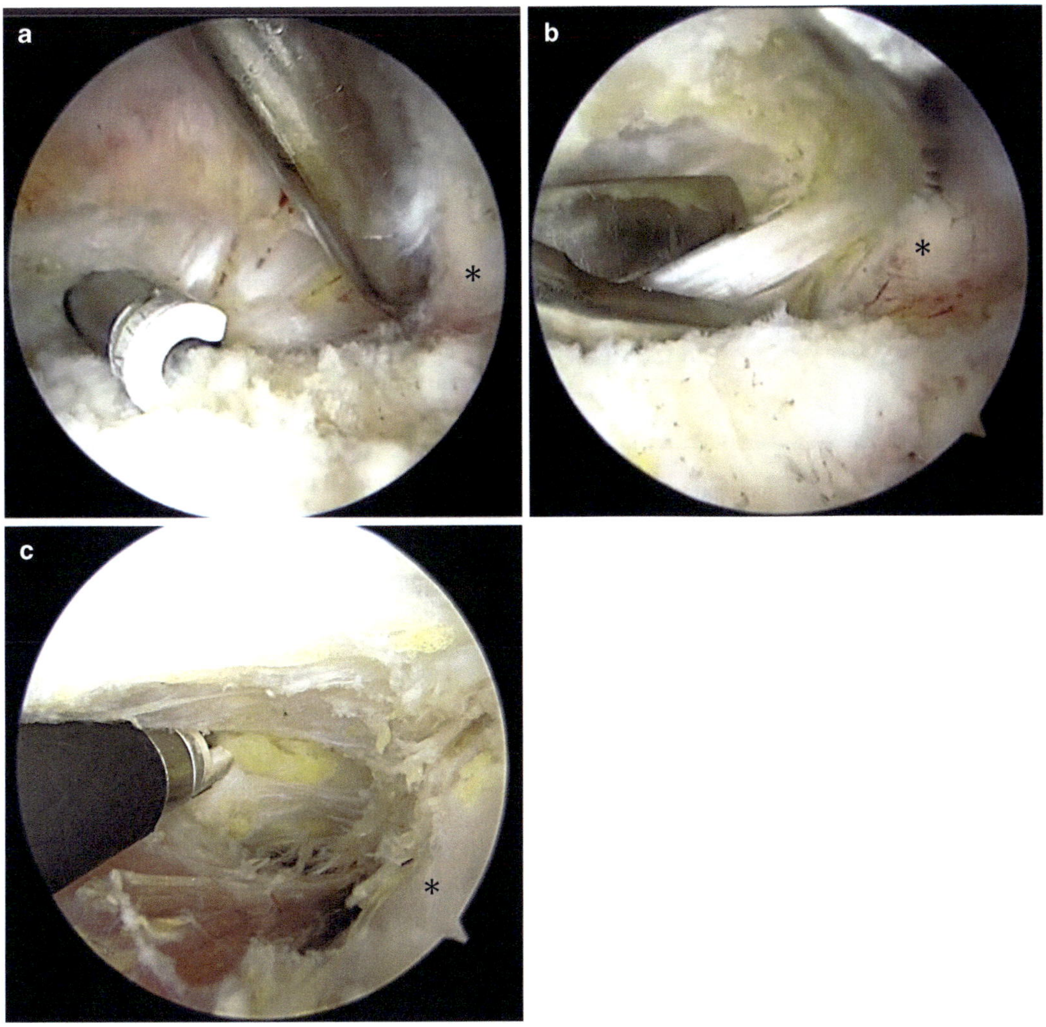

Fig. 16.8 Left elbow. Osborne ligament was released step by step, when ulnar nerve (*) was laterally retracted (**a**, **b**). Muscle fiber of common flexor was observed, when decompression is finished (**c**)

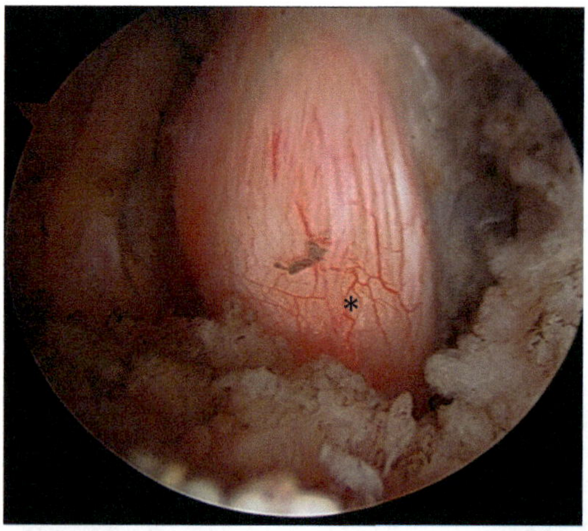

Fig. 16.9 Right elbow. After decompression, blood flow around the ulnar nerve is improved

4 Postop Rehabilitation

The range of motion exercise starts the next day after surgery. No immobilization is necessary.

5 Clinical Outcomes

Between 2011 and 2017, 48 elbows in 48 patients who underwent arthroscopic ulnar nerve release were retrospectively reviewed. These included 40 cases of osteoarthritis, 3 of primary cubital tunnel syndrome, 3 of elbow contracture, 1 of synovial osteochondromatosis, and 1 of ulnar nerve instability. Among them, 39 patients were followed postoperatively. No nerve injury was observed. Mild to moderate numbness remained in 6 patients. Revision surgeries were performed in 4 patients including 3 persistent nerve symptoms and a recurrent nerve symptom.

Case: A 52-year-old female, left-handed wheelchair tennis player

She was referred to our hospital with left elbow pain and numbness of 4th and 5th finger for 6 months. Range of motion were 115 in flexion and −20 in extension. The nerve conduction velocity in the ulnar nerve was 52.9 m/s on the right and 34.6 m/s on the left. Severe elbow osteoarthritis was observed (Figs. 16.10 and 16.11). Arthroscopic debridement was performed with the ulnar nerve decompression (video 16.1). The nerve symptoms improved right after the surgery. The ranges at 3 months were 128 in flexion and −3 in extension (Fig. 16.12). After 4 and a half years, the ranges were 115 in flexion and −15 in extension, with nerve symptoms.

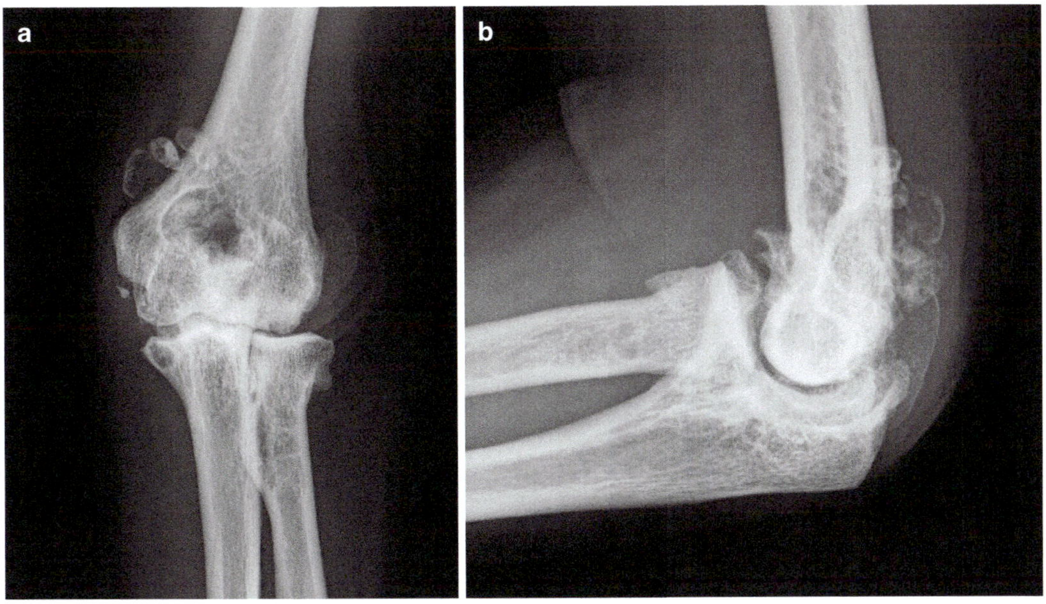

Fig. 16.10 51-year-old female Preop Xray (**a**) AP view (**b**) lateral view

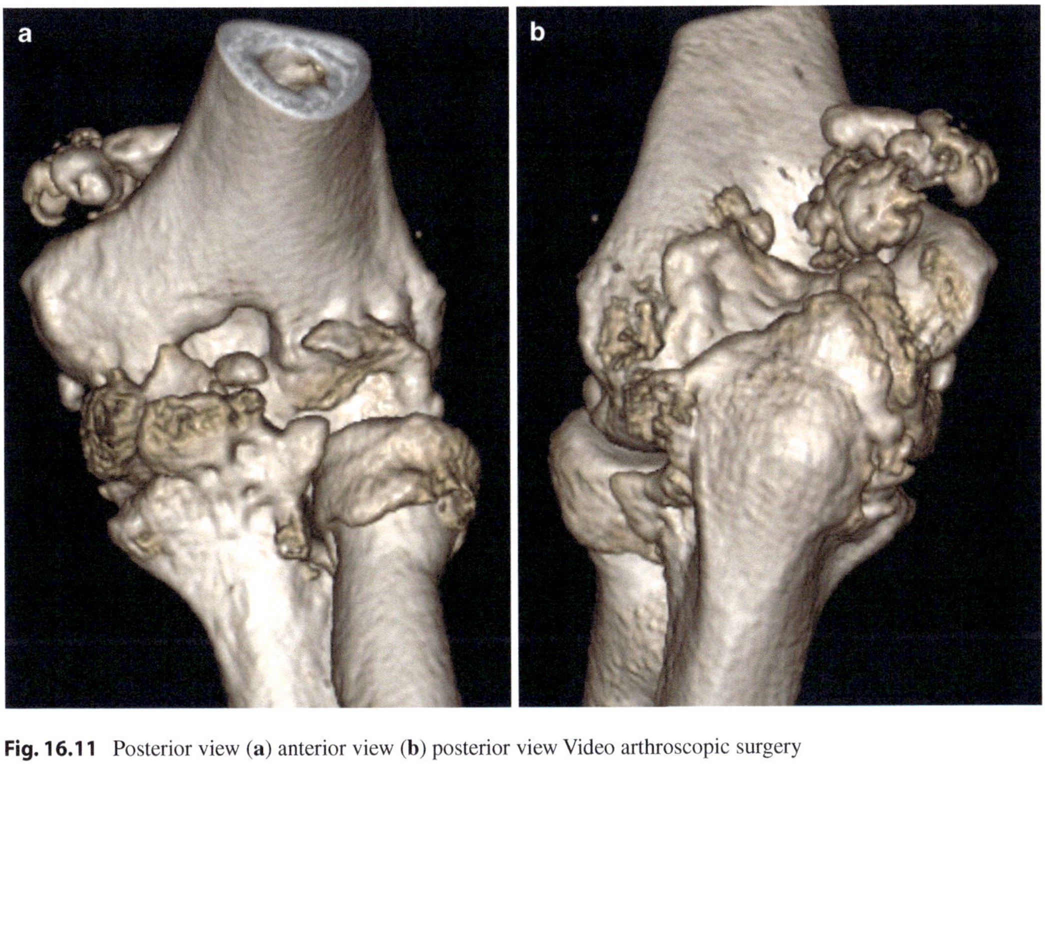

Fig. 16.11 Posterior view (**a**) anterior view (**b**) posterior view Video arthroscopic surgery

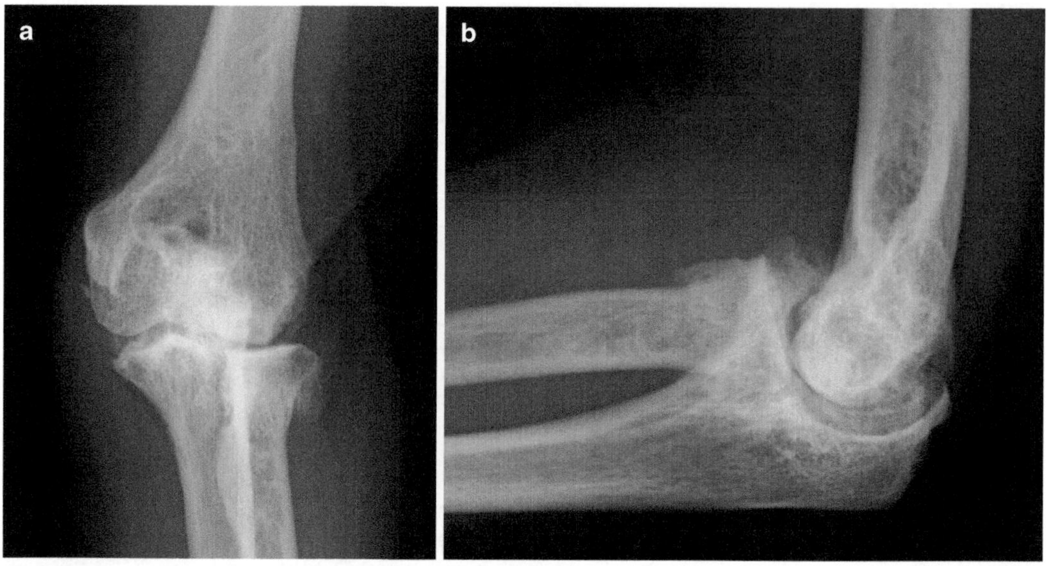

Fig. 16.12 Postop Xray (**a**) ap view (**b**) lateral view

Endoscopic Extra-Articular Cubital Tunnel Release

17

Panai Laohaprasitiporn and Gregory Bain

1 Background

1.1 Overview of Cubital Tunnel Syndrome

Cubital tunnel syndrome is the second most common compressive neuropathy after carpal tunnel syndrome, characterized by compression and traction of the ulnar nerve as it traverses the elbow. Clinical presentation varies, ranging from intermittent numbness in the ring and little fingers to decreased grip strength, and, in advanced cases, claw hand deformity involving the ulnar two fingers and intrinsic muscle wasting.

In the early stages of cubital tunnel syndrome, when symptoms are primarily sensory with minimal grip and pinch weakness, and there is no muscle atrophy, conservative management is preferred. This includes activity modification, physical therapy, and splinting. However, in cases where sensory or motor deficits persist, or symptoms do not improve with conservative treatment, surgical decompression is indicated.

Open decompression of the ulnar nerve, with or without transposition, has long been considered the standard surgical approach for cubital tunnel syndrome. Recently, the utilization of endoscopic techniques for ulnar nerve decompression has gained increasing popularity.

1.2 Anatomy and Its Surgical Relevance

A thorough understanding of the cubital tunnel anatomy is crucial for comprehending both the pathophysiology of cubital tunnel syndrome and the surgical techniques used in its treatment. The ulnar nerve, which arises from the brachial plexus (C8-T1), descends along the arm and traverses several anatomical regions prone to compression. At the level of the elbow, multiple potential sites of ulnar nerve entrapment exist, contributing to the development of cubital tunnel syndrome. These include the arcade of Struthers, the medial intermuscular septum, the cubital tunnel formed by Osborne's ligament, anconeus epitrochlearis muscle, and the fascia of the flexor carpi ulnaris muscle (Fig. 17.1).

Proximally, the arcade of Struthers, a fibrous band between the medial triceps and intermuscu-

Supplementary Information The online version contains supplementary material available at https://doi.org/10.1007/978-981-95-3732-7_17.

P. Laohaprasitiporn
Department of Orthopaedic Surgery, Flinders University and Flinders Medical Centre, Adelaide, SA, Australia

Department of Orthopaedic Surgery, Faculty of Medicine Siriraj Hospital, Mahidol University, Bangkok, Thailand

G. Bain (✉)
Department of Orthopaedic Surgery, Faculty of Medicine Siriraj Hospital, Mahidol University, Bangkok, Thailand
e-mail: greg@gregbain.com.au

I.-H. Jeon et al. (eds.), *Elbow Arthroscopy*, https://doi.org/10.1007/978-981-95-3732-7_17

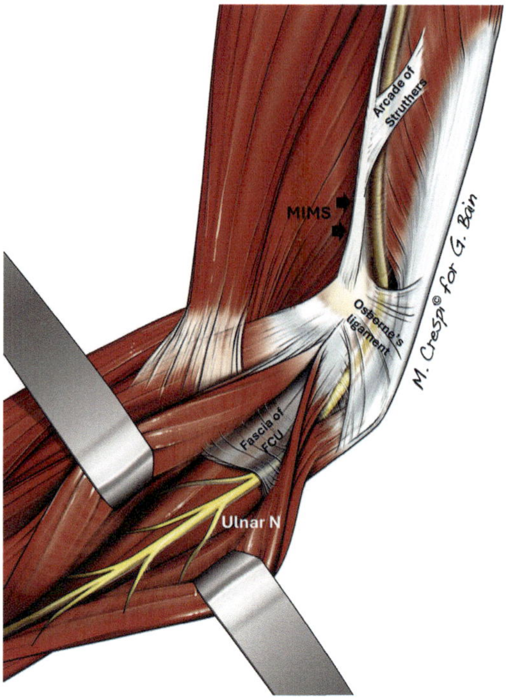

Fig. 17.1 Potential sites of ulnar nerve entrapment at the elbow. (Copyright Dr. Gregory I. Bain and Max Crespi)

lar septum, is located 8–10 cm above the medial epicondyle and can be a site of ulnar nerve compression [1]. As the ulnar nerve enters the cubital tunnel behind the medial epicondyle, compression may occur due to the thickened Osborne ligament (cubital tunnel retinaculum), osteophytes from elbow osteoarthritis, or an anomalous anconeus epitrochlearis muscle. Distally, the aponeurosis between the two heads of the flexor carpi ulnaris (FCU) is another potential site of entrapment.

Although the medial intermuscular septum (MIMS) rarely causes compression in idiopathic cases, it can become problematic after anterior transposition of the nerve, so its excision is recommended during surgery.

Branches of the medial antebrachial cutaneous nerve may occasionally cross the ulnar nerve at an average distance of 2.9 cm distal to the medial epicondyle, with a range from 1.0 to 4.5 cm [2]. Therefore, during the skin incision for ulnar nerve release at the elbow, special care must be taken to avoid iatrogenic injury to this structure, which is at high risk due to its anatomical proximity.

1.3 Anatomical Variation of Ulnar Nerve and Compression Structures

The anconeus epitrochlearis is a small accessory muscle found in some individuals, extending from the medial epicondyle to the olecranon. When present and hypertrophied, it has the potential to compress the ulnar nerve, leading to clinical symptoms.

An unusual anatomical variation may occur along the ulnar nerve's course proximal to the elbow. This variation involves a cutaneous nerve branch originating approximately 40 mm proximal to the medial epicondyle, arising from the radial aspect of the main ulnar nerve trunk. The branch follows a superficial path, extending distally and passing anterior to the medial epicondyle without penetrating the flexor muscle fascia [3].

Although rare, the ulnar nerve can be positioned anteriorly at the elbow. In cases where an empty cubital tunnel is encountered during dissection, further exploration may reveal the ulnar nerve passing posteriorly and penetrating through the intermuscular septum 3–5 cm proximal to the medial epicondyle. From there, it runs anterior to the pronator-flexor mass before entering the forearm between the ulnar and humeral heads of the flexor carpi ulnaris [4].

1.4 Treatment Options

1.4.1 Nonoperative Management

Early-stage cubital tunnel syndrome, characterized by symptoms without muscle weakness or atrophy, can often be managed with nonoperative approaches such as activity modification, night splinting, and nerve gliding exercises. In a clinical trial involving 51 participants with mild to moderate ulnar nerve entrapment, researchers found that providing guidance on avoiding prolonged movements or positions significantly reduced subjective discomfort. However, the addition of night splinting and nerve gliding exercises did not yield further improvements beyond the information alone [5].

1.4.2 Operative Management

Several surgical options exist for the treatment of cubital tunnel syndrome, including simple decompression of ulnar nerve, decompression with anterior transposition (subcutaneous, intramuscular, or submuscular), medial epicondylectomy, and endoscopic ulnar nerve release. These procedures aim to alleviate pressure on the ulnar nerve by either releasing or repositioning it, depending on the severity of compression and individual patient factors.

Simple decompression VS *ulnar nerve transposition*

Numerous meta-analyses have compared the outcomes of simple decompression versus decompression with ulnar nerve transposition [6–9]. The findings consistently demonstrate no significant difference between the two techniques in terms of clinical and neurophysiological improvements. However, transposition is associated with a higher incidence of complications compared to simple decompression. Simple decompression was also associated with shorter operative time, lower overall costs compared to subcutaneous ulnar nerve transposition, and reduced expenses related to sick leave [10]. These factors make simple decompression a more cost-effective option in the treatment of cubital tunnel syndrome.

Open VS *endoscopic ulnar nerve release*

Several clinical studies and a meta-analysis comparing open simple decompression and endoscopic ulnar nerve release found no statistically significant differences in terms of clinical recovery, pain scores, postoperative satisfaction, postoperative hematoma rates, or the need for secondary surgical procedures. However, patients who underwent endoscopic ulnar nerve release experienced less scar tenderness and elbow pain compared to those who had open simple decompression [11–15].

1.5 Evolution of Endoscopic Techniques in Ulnar Nerve Decompression

Endoscopic cubital tunnel decompression was first described by Tsai et al. in 1995 [16]. Through endoscopic visualization, the ulnar nerve can be released from the arcade of Struthers proximally to the flexor carpi ulnaris (FCU) muscle heads distally. Early outcomes demonstrated favorable results with minimal complications and a smaller incision compared to open decompression in situ. Various specialized instruments have been developed for this procedure, which can be categorized into three types:

1. Task-specific equipment, such as Storz instruments (Karl Storz, Tuttlingen, Germany) and the Agee device (3 M, Orthopedic Products, St. Paul, Minnesota, USA)
2. The use of endoscope and cannula, including those from Integra LifeSciences (Plainsboro, New Jersey, USA) and Ace Glass (Louisville, Kentucky, USA)
3. The use of endoscope combined with adaptation of basic surgical instruments such as Senn retractors and Langenbeck retractors [17]

2 Indications and Contraindications

2.1 Indications for Endoscopic Decompression

- Idiopathic cubital tunnel syndrome

2.2 Contraindications

- Lesions or masses compressing the ulnar nerve.
- Hostile nerve bed (e.g., extensive scarring from previous trauma).
- Severe elbow contracture.
- Concomitant conditions requiring ulnar nerve transposition, such as corrective surgery for humeral or elbow malalignment.
- Recurrent cubital tunnel syndrome.
- Limited external shoulder rotation.
- Ulnar nerve hypermobility (e.g., subluxation or dislocation during elbow movement) is considered a relative contraindication by some surgeons. In such cases, the surgeon may opt to either perform an endoscopic ulnar nerve transposition or convert to open surgery to ensure optimal nerve stabilization and prevent further complications.
- Lack of surgeon expertise in the endoscopic technique (relative contraindication).

3 Surgical Technique

3.1 Patient Positioning and Anesthesia

The most common patient positioning for endoscopic cubital tunnel decompression is the supine position, with the arm abducted and externally rotated on an arm table. A kidney tray is typically used to elevate the elbow from the arm table, facilitating the insertion of the endoscope and surgical instruments while ensuring optimal access and visualization. A tourniquet is applied to the most proximal part of the arm to minimize blood flow during the procedure. Care is taken to ensure that the tourniquet does not obstruct the proximal release of the ulnar nerve, allowing for adequate exposure and decompression while maintaining a clear surgical field.

The most common methods for pain control during endoscopic ulnar nerve release are general anesthesia or regional anesthesia. However, the wide-awake, local anesthesia, no tourniquet (WALANT) technique is also a viable option.

3.2 Wide-Awake, Local Anesthesia, and No Tourniquet (WALANT) for Endoscopic Ulnar Nerve Release

The WALANT technique can be effectively applied for endoscopic ulnar nerve release. This approach offers several advantages, including a more comfortable patient experience, elimination of the need for preadmission testing and fasting, improved time efficiency, and reduced costs. Moreover, it is a safer alternative for patients with comorbidities, as it eliminates the risks associated with general anesthesia, potentially expanding the eligibility for surgery in this patient population. However, WALANT may not be suitable for patients who experience significant anxiety or who are unable to communicate effectively with the surgeon due to language or cognitive barriers [18]. WALANT surgery is often less "dry" than procedures with a tourniquet, as vasoconstriction takes about 26 min, and local anesthetic can blur endoscopic visualization. An antifog solution helps reduce condensation on the lens. Clear communication with the patient is important; they may feel pressure when the cannula passes through the cubital tunnel, but pain indicates inadequate anesthesia or nerve impingement.

3.3 Surgical Technique Using Storz Equipment (Karl Storz) (Fig. 17.2)

1. A 2 cm longitudinal skin incision is made over the retrocondylar groove, located between the medial epicondyle and the olecranon.
2. The ulnar nerve is identified by incising the roof of the cubital tunnel, providing access for decompression.
3. After identifying the ulnar nerve at the retrocondylar groove, tunneling forceps are used to create a space between the subcutaneous tissue and fascia, extending from the medial epicondyle to 10–12 cm proximally and 8–10 cm distally (Fig. 17.3).
4. A "hooded" 4 mm, 30° endoscope is introduced into the incision. The hooded component is used to elevate and retract the soft tissues, improving visualization of the ulnar nerve and its surrounding structures.
5. Under endoscopic guidance, the forearm fascia and the fibrous raphe between the two muscular heads of the flexor carpi ulnaris (FCU) over the ulnar nerve are cut using blunt-tipped Metzenbaum scissors. The ulnar nerve is fully released from its overlying soft tissues until the motor branches of the FCU are exposed, approximately 8 cm distal to the medial epicondyle (Fig. 17.4).
6. The endoscope is also utilized to decompress the proximal ulnar nerve in a similar fashion. The deep fascia and the arcade of Struthers above the ulnar nerve are divided, extending up to 10 cm proximal to the medial epicondyle.
7. No excision of the medial intermuscular septum (MIMS) is required unless the nerve is going to be transposed, or there is clear evidence of impingement along the course of the ulnar nerve.
8. Hemostasis is achieved using long bipolar cautery to control any bleeding during the procedure, ensuring a clear operative field.

Postoperatively, a bulky compressive dressing is applied for 2–3 days, after which it is replaced with a simple dressing. Patients are encouraged to move their elbow within their comfort limits and are expected to achieve a full range of motion within 1 week. Strenuous exercise is restricted for the first week. Patients can typically return to sports or moderate to heavy-duty work at 6 weeks, depending on their recovery progress.

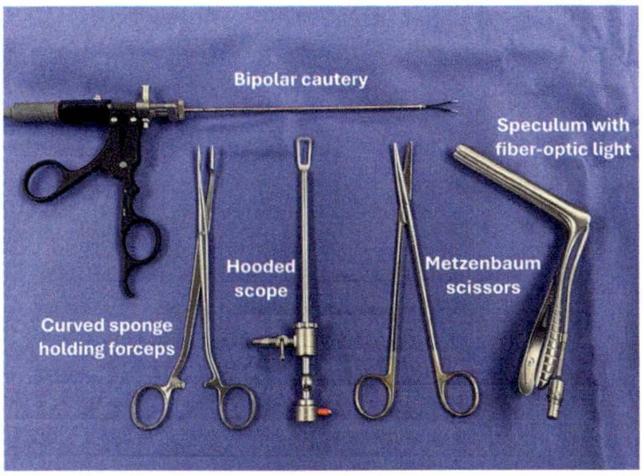

Fig. 17.2 Endoscopic ulnar nerve release equipment. (Copyright Dr. Gregory I. Bain)

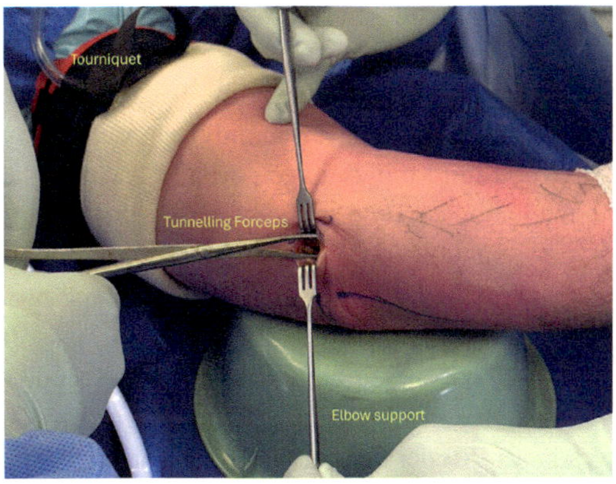

Fig. 17.3 Creating space between subcutaneous tissue and fascia using tunneling forceps. (Copyright Dr. Gregory I. Bain)

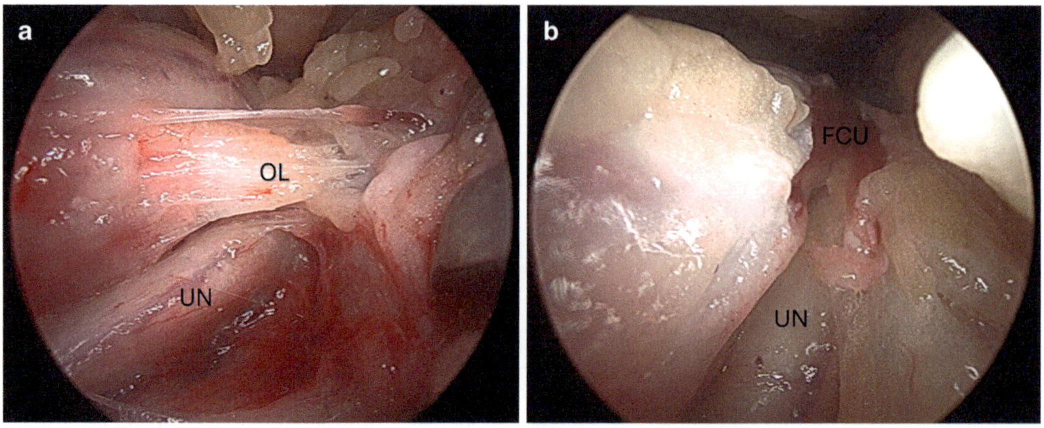

Fig. 17.4 (**a**) Endoscopic view of Osborne's ligament and (**b**) fascia of flexor carpi ulnaris, the potential ulnar nerve compression sites. (UN Ulnar nerve, OL Osborne's ligament, FCU Flexor carpi ulnaris). (Copyright Dr. Gregory I. Bain)

3.4 Evaluation of Ulnar Nerve Subluxation

After completing the endoscopic ulnar nerve release, the stability of the ulnar nerve should be carefully assessed through the full range of elbow motion. This ensures that the nerve remains properly positioned and is not subluxating over the epicondyle during elbow flexion.

An intraoperative classification system for ulnar nerve subluxation following decompression has been proposed, along with corresponding treatment guidelines [19]:

Grade 1: Minimal nerve mobility. The ulnar nerve remains within the retrocondylar groove, may exhibit mild toggling, or partially ascends the medial epicondyle without surpassing it (partial subluxation). Intraoperative findings include a deep retrocondylar groove, and preoperative findings typically show minimal soft tissue laxity (Beighton score <5/9). No additional treatment is required for this grade.

Grade 2: Moderate nerve hypermobility. The ulnar nerve ascends the medial epicondyle but does not completely overcome it (partial subluxation). Intraoperative findings often include a shallow retrocondylar groove, and preoperative assessments reveal inherent soft tissue laxity (Beighton score $\geq$ 5/9). Medial epicondylectomy may be considered in these cases, though it is optional.

Grade 3: Severe nerve hypermobility. The ulnar nerve ascends and completely surpasses the medial epicondyle (complete anterior dislocation). Treatment for this grade typically involves either a medial epicondylectomy or anterior transposition of the ulnar nerve.

Although the decision to perform ulnar nerve transposition is typically based on intraoperative assessment of ulnar nerve stability during elbow flexion, a randomized controlled trial revealed that even in cases of ulnar nerve instability during flexion, transposition and simple decompression yielded similar clinical outcomes. However, ulnar nerve transposition was associated with a higher complication rate compared to simple decompression in this patient group [20].

3.4.1 Indications for Endoscopic Ulnar Nerve Anterior Transposition [21]

- Hostile nerve bed, such as excessive scarring from previous trauma or the presence of large osteophytes in elbow osteoarthritis.
- Cubitus valgus deformity.
- Ulnar nerve hypermobility.
- Recurrent cubital tunnel syndrome, particularly in cases where incomplete nerve release or a new compressive site is suspected.

3.4.2 Endoscopic Ulnar Nerve Anterior Transposition [22]

The medial intermuscular septum (MIMS) must be excised, as MIMS can potentially serve as a new site of impingement along the transposed ulnar nerve's course (Fig. 17.5).

To mobilize the ulnar nerve before transposition, an additional subcutaneous volar portal is created just medial to the medial epicondyle (Fig. 17.6). A nylon tape is introduced through this portal to facilitate manipulation of the nerve. The ulnar nerve, along with its accompanying vessels, is dissected from the surrounding soft tissue under endoscopic guidance. Once freed, the ulnar nerve is transposed into a subcutaneous space anterior to the medial condyle, which is developed using tunnel forceps or a spatula (Fig. 17.7).

After positioning the ulnar nerve in its new location, the entire course of the nerve is inspected to ensure smooth movement without kinking or compression. To prevent the nerve from relocating behind the epicondyle, the medial condyle is rasped to promote adhesion to adjacent soft tissue. Additionally, subcutaneous tissue is sutured to the medial condyle to secure the nerve in its new position. Before closure, the stability of the nerve is checked throughout the full range of elbow motion. Hemostasis is achieved by deflating the tourniquet.

The wound is closed in layers, and postoperatively, the elbow is maintained in a flexed position for 10 days using an arm sling. Gentle active

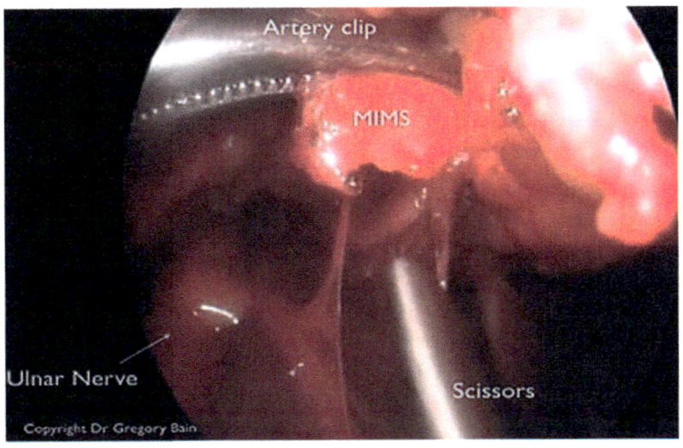

Fig. 17.5 Endoscopic resection of medial intermuscular septum (MIMS). (Copyright Dr. Gregory I. Bain)

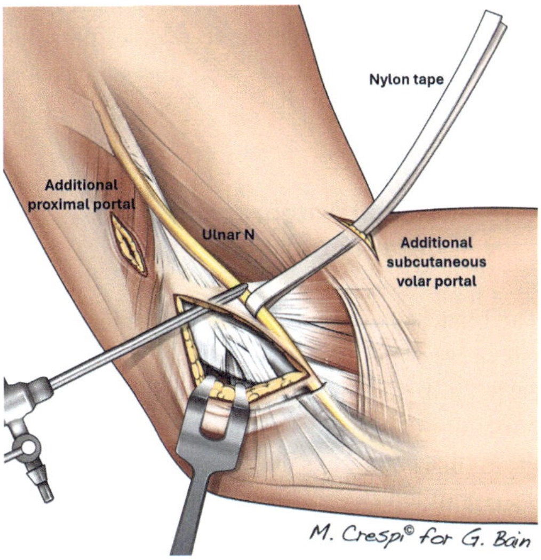

Fig. 17.6 An additional proximal portal can be created to place a retractor during medial intermuscular septum resection. An additional subcutaneous volar portal can be used to mobilise the ulnar nerve anteriorly. (Copyright Dr. Gregory I. Bain and Max Crespi)

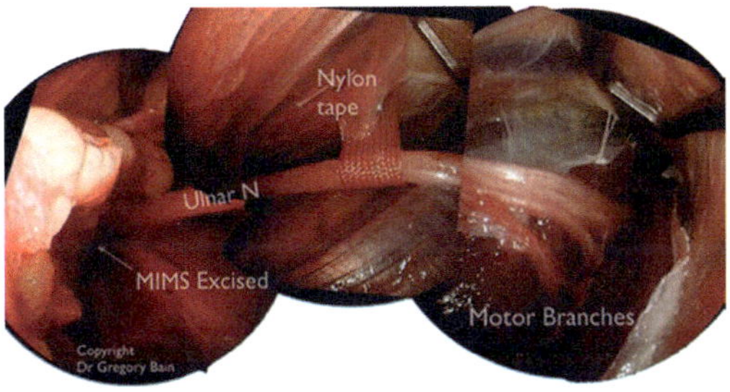

Fig. 17.7 Endoscopic view of anterior transposition of the ulnar nerve. (Copyright Dr. Gregory I. Bain)

elbow mobilization is permitted outside the sling during this period, but patients are advised to refrain from fully straightening the elbow until day 11. Light activities can be resumed after 10 days, while moderate to heavy tasks or a return to sports should be avoided for 6–12 weeks.

4 Potential Complications

A safety cadaveric study has demonstrated that the technique can be safely and completely performed [23]. Although endoscopic ulnar nerve release is associated with fewer complications compared to open ulnar nerve release, potential complications still exist with the endoscopic approach.

4.1 Medial Antebrachial Cutaneous Nerve Injury

The branches of the medial antebrachial cutaneous nerve, while at lower risk than in open surgery, still require careful attention, as the proximity of these nerves to the operating field means that endoscopy does not entirely eliminate the risk of injury.

4.2 Subcutaneous Hematoma

During the separation of subcutaneous tissue to create a soft tissue plane for endoscopic visualization, this step should be performed with care to minimize tissue trauma. Any potential bleeding vessels should be coagulated using bipolar cautery, avoiding cutting to prevent unnecessary bleeding. Prior to wound closure, the tourniquet should be deflated to allow identification and coagulation of any remaining bleeding vessels. Additionally, applying a bulky dressing for 2–3 days postoperatively helps to compress the surgical site and reduce the potential space for subcutaneous hematoma formation.

4.3 Ulnar Nerve Injury

During endoscopic decompression, ulnar nerve branches are at risk of injury. The cutting or dissection of compressed structures should always be performed under direct endoscopic visualization. If the tips of the scissors become obscured or cannot be clearly visualized, the entire instrument should be carefully withdrawn from the skin incision without closing the blades inside the wound, to avoid inadvertent injury to the ulnar nerve or its branches.

5 Conclusion

Endoscopic cubital tunnel release offers a minimally invasive alternative to traditional open surgery for treating cubital tunnel syndrome. This approach allows for effective decompression of the ulnar nerve with a smaller incision, faster recovery, and reduced scar tenderness and elbow pain. Although surgical outcomes between endoscopic and open techniques show no significant differences in clinical recovery, the endoscopic method demonstrates advantages in patient comfort and postoperative recovery. However, careful attention to nerve stability, anatomical variations, and potential complications is critical to optimizing surgical success and minimizing risks.

References

1. Polatsch DB, Melone CP Jr, Beldner S, Incorvaia A. Ulnar nerve anatomy. Hand Clin. 2007;23(3):283–9, v. https://doi.org/10.1016/j.hcl.2007.05.001.
2. Mirza A, Mirza JB, Lee BK, Adhya S, Litwa J, Lorenzana DJ. An anatomical basis for endoscopic cubital tunnel release and associated clinical outcomes. J Hand Surg Am. 2014;39(7):1363–9. https://doi.org/10.1016/j.jhsa.2014.04.030.
3. Chow JC, Papachristos AA, Ojeda A. An aberrant anatomic variation along the course of the ulnar nerve above the elbow with coexistent cubital tunnel syndrome. Clin Anat. 2006;19(7):661–4. https://doi.org/10.1002/ca.20351.

4. Satteson ES, Li Z. Anteriorly positioned ulnar nerve at the elbow: a rare anatomical event: case report. J Hand Surg Am. 2015;40(5):984–6. https://doi.org/10.1016/j.jhsa.2015.02.006.
5. Svernlov B, Larsson M, Rehn K, Adolfsson L. Conservative treatment of the cubital tunnel syndrome. J Hand Surg Eur. 2009;34(2):201–7. https://doi.org/10.1177/1753193408098480.
6. Caliandro P, La Torre G, Padua R, Giannini F, Padua L. Treatment for ulnar neuropathy at the elbow. Cochrane Database Syst Rev. 2016;11(11):CD006839. https://doi.org/10.1002/14651858.CD006839.pub4.
7. Chen HW, Ou S, Liu GD, Fei J, Zhao GS, Wu LJ, et al. Clinical efficacy of simple decompression versus anterior transposition of the ulnar nerve for the treatment of cubital tunnel syndrome: a meta-analysis. Clin Neurol Neurosurg. 2014;126:150–5. https://doi.org/10.1016/j.clineuro.2014.08.005.
8. Macadam SA, Gandhi R, Bezuhly M, Lefaivre KA. Simple decompression versus anterior subcutaneous and submuscular transposition of the ulnar nerve for cubital tunnel syndrome: a meta-analysis. J Hand Surg Am. 2008;33(8):1314. e1–12. https://doi.org/10.1016/j.jhsa.2008.03.006.
9. Zlowodzki M, Chan S, Bhandari M, Kalliainen L, Schubert W. Anterior transposition compared with simple decompression for treatment of cubital tunnel syndrome. A meta-analysis of randomized, controlled trials. J Bone Joint Surg Am. 2007;89(12):2591–8. https://doi.org/10.2106/JBJS.G.00183.
10. Bartels RHMA, Termeer EH, van der Wilt GJ, van Rossum LGM, Meulstee J, Verhagen WIM, et al. Simple decompression or anterior subcutaneous transposition for ulnar neuropathy at the elbow: a cost-minimization analysis–Part 2. Neurosurgery. 2005;56(3):531–6. https://doi.org/10.1227/01.NEU.0000154128.36178.43.
11. Byvaltsev VA, Stepanov IA, Kerimbayev TT. A systematic review and meta-analysis comparing open versus endoscopic in situ decompression for the treatment of cubital tunnel syndrome. Acta Neurol Belg. 2020;120(1):1–8. https://doi.org/10.1007/s13760-019-01149-9.
12. Ozturk T, Zengin EC, Sener U, Sener M. Endoscopic versus open in situ decompression for the management of cubital tunnel syndrome. Acta Orthop Traumatol Turc. 2022;56(2):125–30. https://doi.org/10.5152/j.aott.2022.21143.
13. Schwarm FP, Nagl J, Graf K, Reinges MHT, Uhl E, Krishnan KG, et al. A prospective randomized study comparing retractor-endoscopic vs. open release of carpal tunnel and cubital tunnel syndromes. Clin Neurol Neurosurg. 2022;222:107437. https://doi.org/10.1016/j.clineuro.2022.107437.
14. Shekouhi R, Chughtai M, Benjamin JA, Saengchote SA, Chim H. Patient-reported outcome measures after endoscopic cubital tunnel release with at least 1-year postoperative follow-up. Hand (N Y). 2025;20(2):170–8. https://doi.org/10.1177/15589447231199798.
15. Watts AC, Bain GI. Patient-rated outcome of ulnar nerve decompression: a comparison of endoscopic and open in situ decompression. J Hand Surg Am. 2009;34(8):1492–8. https://doi.org/10.1016/j.jhsa.2009.05.014.
16. Tsai TM, Bonczar M, Tsuruta T, Syed SA. A new operative technique: cubital tunnel decompression with endoscopic assistance. Hand Clin. 1995;11(1):71–80. https://doi.org/10.1016/S0749-0712(21)00010-1.
17. Jaroenporn W, Predeeprompan P, Vechasilp J, Vathana T, Limthongthang R. Cost-saving minimal incision endoscopic-assisted cubital tunnel release using simple surgical instruments: case series. Cureus. 2019;11(10):e5914. https://doi.org/10.7759/cureus.5914.
18. Tosti R, Rekant MS. Wide awake local anesthesia no tourniquet endoscopic cubital tunnel release. J Hand Surg Am. 2022;47(10):1022. e1–e5. https://doi.org/10.1016/j.jhsa.2022.04.004.
19. Mirza A, Mirza JB, Thomas TL Jr. Classification and treatment of ulnar nerve subluxation following endoscopic cubital tunnel release. J Hand Surg Glob Online. 2020;2(4):232–9. https://doi.org/10.1016/j.jhsg.2020.05.001.
20. Bartels RH, Verhagen WI, van der Wilt GJ, Meulstee J, van Rossum LG, Grotenhuis JA. Prospective randomized controlled study comparing simple decompression versus anterior subcutaneous transposition for idiopathic neuropathy of the ulnar nerve at the elbow: part 1. Neurosurgery. 2005;56(3):522–30; discussion –30. https://doi.org/10.1227/01.neu.0000154131.01167.03.
21. Fok MW, Cobb T, Bain GI. Endoscopic cubital tunnel decompression: state of the art. J ISAKOS. 2021;6(6):367–74. https://doi.org/10.1136/jisakos-2020-000506.
22. Morse LP, McGuire DT, Bain GI. Endoscopic ulnar nerve release and transposition. Tech Hand Up Extrem Surg. 2014;18(1):10–4. https://doi.org/10.1097/BTH.0000000000000030.
23. Bain GI, Bajhau A. Endoscopic release of the ulnar nerve at the elbow using the Agee device: a cadaveric study. Arthroscopy. 2005;21(6):691–5. https://doi.org/10.1016/j.arthro.2005.02.018.

Part V

Arthritis and Stiffness

Elbow Osteoarthritis: Etiology and Pathogenesis

18

Cunyi Fan

1 Background

The muscles that encase the elbow joint exert considerable stress upon it during periods of load bearing, with the potential to reach magnitudes threefold that of the body's weight in the act of lifting. Under the duress of dynamic loading, these forces might soar to more than six times the body's weight. Given the elbow joint's modest contact area, this leads to a substantial burden on the hyaline cartilage, especially pronounced during the axial extension phase. The repetitive onslaught of stress beyond the physiological threshold can precipitate the erosion and fracturing of the cartilage, culminating in the emergence of intra-articular loose bodies and the peripheral proliferation of osteophytes [1, 2]. In the elbow joint, the condition is more commonly characterized by the presence of osteophytes and capsular contracture, while joint narrowing is more frequently observed in other joints. Current studies have found that elbow osteoarthritis appears to begin primarily in the lateral part of the elbow, with erosion of the radial head cartilage occurring earlier than the ulnohumeral joint and slowly moving medially, with the ulnohumeral already involved by the time symptoms of degeneration appear [3].

2 Etiology

Osteoarthritis (OA) is a significant age-related disease, recognized as the fourth leading cause of chronic disability. Approximately 40% of individuals over the age of 60 are diagnosed with this condition. In developed countries, OA is the most common reason for joint replacement, and its socioeconomic burden is expected to grow due to increasing longevity and obesity rates [4]. Elbow osteoarthritis is relatively uncommon compared to OA in the shoulder or lower limbs. Primary elbow OA is particularly rare, affecting only around 2% of the population [5, 6]. However, it remains the second most common cause of elbow stiffness after trauma.

3 Multifactorial Contribution

Multiple factors, such as genetics, aging, joint loading, joint malalignment, and obesity, are considered to play significant roles in the progression of osteoarthritis [3]. These factors interact synergistically to disrupt the balance between anabolic and catabolic processes in cartilage tissue. When cartilage degradation exceeds the self-

Supplementary Information The online version contains supplementary material available at https://doi.org/10.1007/978-981-95-3732-7_18.

C. Fan (✉)
National Medical Center for Orthopaedic, Shanghai 6th People's Hospital, Shanghai Jiaotong University, School of Medicine, Shanghai, China

I.-H. Jeon et al. (eds.), *Elbow Arthroscopy*, https://doi.org/10.1007/978-981-95-3732-7_18

repair mechanisms, it leads to a gradual loss of both the structure and function of the entire joint. Aging leads to changes in the mechanical properties of cartilage, increasing its susceptibility to degeneration. Inflammatory mechanisms are involved in the pathophysiology of osteoarthritis (OA), with inflammatory mediators inducing chondrocytes to produce proteases, nitric oxide, and other factors that inhibit matrix synthesis and promote apoptosis [7].

4 Risk Factors for Primary Elbow OA

Individuals engaged in physically demanding work, athletes involved in throwing sports, and those dependent on crutches or wheelchairs are at increased risk of developing primary elbow OA due to increased joint stress [8]. Men are observed to have four times the likelihood of developing elbow osteoarthritis compared to women, with a preference for the dominant arm, frequently the right one [6]. The typical age for the onset of symptoms is around 50 years; however, even those as young as 20 have been noted to exhibit signs of degeneration [9, 10].

5 Pathogenesis of Elbow Arthritis

5.1 Molecular Mechanisms and Genetic Pathways

Primary osteoarthritis is an enduring affliction of the synovial joints, marked by the gradual deterioration of the hyaline cartilage and the subsequent exposure of the underlying subchondral bone. The articular cartilage gradually breaks down and softens, followed by the regeneration of new cartilage and bone at the joint margins (osteophytes), with cyst formation and sclerosis in the subchondral bone. Concurrent synovitis and capsular fibrosis contribute to elbow swelling, stiffness, and chronic pain [9]. Osteoarthritis is a multifaceted condition, yet genetic factors have been implicated as playing a pivotal role in the modulation of OA-associated pathways. These include the regulation of cartilage and bone turnover, remodeling, body weight, muscle mass, and the body's response to injury [11]. The research spotlight has been cast on genes that uphold the structural integrity of the cartilage extracellular matrix, namely COL2A1, COL9A3, and COL11A1, as well as genes that participate in chondrocyte signal transduction pathways, and genes linked to inflammatory cytokines, including IL-1 and TNF-α [12]. The utilization of candidate gene analysis and genome-wide association studies has facilitated the development of insightful case-control studies focused on osteoarthritis. Moreover, significant advancements have been achieved in recent years in understanding the role of epigenetic modifications and their interplay with genetic polymorphisms [13]. Beyond epigenetics, inflammatory mechanisms are integral to the pathophysiology of OA. Joint damage can be precipitated by a constellation of risk factors or conditions, including age, obesity, injury, and, as previously noted, genetic predisposition, culminating in a self-perpetuating cycle of local tissue degradation and chronic, low-grade inflammation that inexorably leads to OA-related functional impairment. Inflammation arises from the activation of the immune system in response to tissue damage [3]. The presence of damage-associated molecular patterns, resulting from cartilage breakdown, acts as triggers for chondrocytes, fibroblast-like synoviocytes, and synovial macrophages to secrete critical inflammatory mediators, encompassing cytokines (e.g., TNF-α, IL-1β, IL-6), growth factors, chemokines, prostaglandins, leukotrienes, adipokines, and more. Toll-like receptors (TLRs) and the receptor for advanced glycation end products (RAGE) are the principal pattern recognition receptors (PRRs) engaged in this process [14]. The detrimental alterations are mediated by matrix metalloproteinases (MMPs) and a disintegrin and metalloproteinase with thrombospondin motifs (ADAMTSs). The failure of reparative mechanisms leads to an amplified and unresolved inflammatory response, hypertrophic chondrocytes, apoptosis, a disruption of homeostasis, and, ultimately, the manifestation of clinical osteoarthritis.

5.2 Repetitive Injury in Overhead Athletes

The elbow is subject to significant mechanical stress during physical activity, and injuries are particularly common among "overhead athletes," such as volleyball, golf, tennis, and baseball players, whose performance involves repetitive, forceful throwing or swinging motions [15]. Contact sports like rugby and martial arts, as well as sports involving falls, such as gymnastics, also contribute to a high risk of elbow trauma. Athletes may unwittingly push their elbow mechanics beyond the point of tolerance, imposing additional stress that leads to injury, altered joint kinetics, and, ultimately, osteoarthritis. In both adults and adolescents, repetitive use and trauma can contribute to the development of osteoarthritis, with young athletes being particularly susceptible to osteochondritis dissecans of the capitellum [16]. Secondary changes, including the formation of osteophytes in the olecranon and coronoid processes, intra-articular loose bodies, and chondromalacia of the radius and capitellum, are frequent and may occur at a relatively young age, particularly in those involved in throwing sports, such as javelin throwers or shot-put athletes [16]. Over time, many athletes develop osteoarthritic changes that can lead to pain and a reduced range of motion throughout the joint [17]. A comprehensive patient history and thorough clinical examination are critical for an accurate diagnosis, as other injuries or dislocations may mimic the symptoms of osteoarthritis. For instance, osteochondritis dissecans should be considered in athletes whose elbows are exposed to chronic shear stress, such as basketball players who are prone to microtrauma or ischemic events [18]. Pain during elbow extension may indicate olecranon traction spurs or synovial impingements, while restricted forearm rotation may point to conditions like radio-ulnar synostosis. A past incident of elbow injury, osteochondritis dissecans, synovial osteochondromatosis, or other issues leading to joint instability or misalignment can also escalate the risk for osteoarthritis [14, 19]. Genetic factors have been found to play a role in the development of primary elbow osteoarthritis, influencing pathways related to bone metabolism, body weight, muscle mass, and injury response. However, further research is needed to fully understand these mechanisms [11].

6 Post-traumatic Osteoarthritis: A Common Variant

Post-traumatic osteoarthritis, a variant more frequently encountered than its primary counterpart, is often the plight of younger, more physically active individuals. Its etiology is multifaceted, encompassing intrinsic elements such as joint incongruity, adhesive bands, impingement, cartilage decay, or a complex interplay of factors, as well as extrinsic factors like heterotopic ossification or contractures of the soft tissues surrounding the joint [20]. This form of osteoarthritis can stem from an initial cartilage injury or be the lingering consequence of inadequately resolved trauma, perpetuating elbow instability. Such disruptions in the joint's mechanics accelerate the wear of cartilage. Athletes who engage in the repetitive motions of throwing with their upper limbs may experience medial elbow laxity, which can precipitate a pattern of repetitive hyperextension on the lateral side, culminating in the formation of the tell-tale posteromedial osteophytes and intra-articular loose bodies [21]. These anomalies within the joint can elicit a spectrum of mechanical symptoms—ranging from impingement and locking to crepitus—and are a significant source of elbow stiffness.

Post-traumatic osteoarthritis may occur as a result of traumatic injuries, which can affect men and women of all ages, although it is most prevalent in young males [22]. The risk of developing this pathology largely depends on the severity and nature of the injury, as well as the mechanisms through which the trauma is sustained. For example, intra-articular distal humerus fractures are commonly associated with degenerative joint complications over time [23]. Similarly, ligament instability, which disrupts joint kinetics, can exacerbate preexisting conditions, accelerating the degenerative process [24]. More severe injuries, particularly in young athletes, may result in capitellar osteochondritis dissecans (OCD), a condition that affects the entire articular cartilage structure [25]. Patients with post-traumatic arthritis often report pain throughout the entire range of motion, a hallmark symptom of the disease [26].

7 Radiocapitellar Joint: The Origin Site of Elbow OA

Elbow osteoarthritis is now widely recognized to initiate within the confines of the radiocapitellar joint [9]. This joint, boasting a smaller articular surface compared to its ulnohumeral counterpart, disproportionately absorbs 55% of the axial load when the forearm assumes a neutral position [27]. The intense concentration of stress at this site often catapults the radiocapitellar joint to the forefront in exhibiting the earliest radiographic indicators of degeneration. Telltale signs of wear typically manifest at the posteromedial region of the radial head and along the posterior edge of the crest that delineates the trochlea from the capitellum. As the disease progresses, the posteromedial ulnohumeral joint becomes ensnared in the degenerative cascade [28].

References

1. An KN, Himeno S, Tsumura H, Kawai T, Chao EY. Pressure distribution on articular surfaces: application to joint stability evaluation. J Biomech. 1990;23(10):1013–20. https://doi.org/10.1016/0021-9290(90)90316-u.
2. Adams JE, Wolff LH 3rd, Merten SM, Steinmann SP. Osteoarthritis of the elbow: results of arthroscopic osteophyte resection and capsulectomy. J Shoulder Elb Surg. 2008;17(1):126–31. https://doi.org/10.1016/j.jse.2007.04.005.
3. Ravalli S, Pulici C, Binetti S, Aglieco A, Vecchio M, Musumeci G. An overview of the pathogenesis and treatment of elbow osteoarthritis. J Funct Morphol Kinesiol. 2019;4(2):30. https://doi.org/10.3390/jfmk4020030.
4. Musumeci G, Loreto C, Imbesi R, Trovato FM, Di Giunta A, Lombardo C, et al. Advantages of exercise in rehabilitation, treatment and prevention of altered morphological features in knee osteoarthritis. A narrative review. Histol Histopathol. 2014;29(6):707–19. https://doi.org/10.14670/HH-29.707.
5. Kroonen LT, Piper SL, Ghatan AC. Arthroscopic management of elbow osteoarthritis. J Hand Surg Am. 2017;42(8):640–50. https://doi.org/10.1016/j.jhsa.2017.05.023.
6. Gramstad GD, Galatz LM. Management of elbow osteoarthritis. J Bone Joint Surg Am. 2006;88(2):421–30. https://doi.org/10.2106/JBJS.E.00568.
7. Kielbowski K, Herian M, Bakinowska E, Banach B, Sroczynski T, Pawlik A. The role of genetics and epigenetic regulation in the pathogenesis of osteoarthritis. Int J Mol Sci. 2023;24(14) https://doi.org/10.3390/ijms241411655.
8. Stanley D. Prevalence and etiology of symptomatic elbow osteoarthritis. J Shoulder Elb Surg. 1994;3(6):386–9. https://doi.org/10.1016/S1058-2746(09)80024-4.
9. Kwak JM, Jeon IH. Surgical management for primary osteoarthritis of the elbow. J Orthop Surg (Hong Kong). 2021;29(1):2309499020988174. https://doi.org/10.1177/2309499020988174.
10. Morrey BF. Primary degenerative arthritis of the elbow. Treatment by ulnohumeral arthroplasty. J Bone Joint Surg Br. 1992;74(3):409–13. https://doi.org/10.1302/0301-620X.74B3.1587890.
11. Spector TD, MacGregor AJ. Risk factors for osteoarthritis: genetics. Osteoarthr Cartil. 2004;12(Suppl A):S39–44. https://doi.org/10.1016/j.joca.2003.09.005.
12. Yucesoy B, Charles LE, Baker B, Burchfiel CM. Occupational and genetic risk factors for osteoarthritis: a review. Work. 2015;50(2):261–73. https://doi.org/10.3233/WOR-131739.
13. Loughlin J. Genetic contribution to osteoarthritis development: current state of evidence. Curr Opin Rheumatol. 2015;27(3):284–8. https://doi.org/10.1097/BOR.0000000000000171.
14. Felson DT. Risk factors for osteoarthritis. Clin Orthop Relat Res. 2004;427(Suppl):S16–21. https://doi.org/10.1097/01.blo.0000144903.51849.f0.
15. Fleisig GS, Andrews JR, Dillman CJ, Escamilla RF. Kinetics of baseball pitching with implications about injury mechanisms. Am J Sports Med. 1995;23(2):233–9. https://doi.org/10.1177/036354659502300218.
16. Koh J, Dietz J. Osteoarthritis in other joints (hip, elbow, foot, ankle, toes, wrist) after sports injuries. Clin Sports Med. 2005;24(1):57–70. https://doi.org/10.1016/j.csm.2004.08.011.

17. Schmitt H, Hansmann HJ, Brocai DR, Loew M. Long term changes of the throwing arm of former elite javelin throwers. Int J Sports Med. 2001;22(4):275–9. https://doi.org/10.1055/s-2001-13814.
18. Kajiyama S, Muroi S, Sugaya H, Takahashi N, Matsuki K, Kawai N, et al. Osteochondritis Dissecans of the Humeral Capitellum in young athletes: comparison between baseball players and gymnasts. Orthop J Sports Med. 2017;5(3):2325967117692513. https://doi.org/10.1177/2325967117692513.
19. Felson DT, Goggins J, Niu J, Zhang Y, Hunter DJ. The effect of body weight on progression of knee osteoarthritis is dependent on alignment. Arthritis Rheum. 2004;50(12):3904–9. https://doi.org/10.1002/art.20726.
20. Brewley EE, Gorman RA 2nd, Christmas KN, Simon P, Chapel RJ, Mighell MA. Use of a modified Outerbridge-Kashiwagi procedure for the treatment of posttraumatic elbow sequelae. J Shoulder Elb Surg. 2019;28(7):1387–94. https://doi.org/10.1016/j.jse.2019.02.002.
21. Wilson FD, Andrews JR, Blackburn TA, McCluskey G. Valgus extension overload in the pitching elbow. Am J Sports Med. 1983;11(2):83–8. https://doi.org/10.1177/036354658301100206.
22. McAuliffe JA. Surgical alternatives for elbow arthritis in the young adult. Hand Clin. 2002;18(1):99–111. https://doi.org/10.1016/s0749-0712(02)00008-2.
23. O'Driscoll SW. Elbow arthritis: treatment options. J Am Acad Orthop Surg. 1993;1(2):106–16.
24. Wysocki RW, Cohen MS. Primary osteoarthritis and posttraumatic arthritis of the elbow. Hand Clin. 2011;27(2):131–7, v. https://doi.org/10.1016/j.hcl.2011.02.001.
25. Heijink A, Vanhees M, van den Ende K, van den Bekerom MP, van Riet RP, Van Dijk CN, et al. Biomechanical considerations in the pathogenesis of osteoarthritis of the elbow. Knee Surg Sports Traumatol Arthrosc. 2016;24(7):2313–8. https://doi.org/10.1007/s00167-015-3518-7.
26. Soojian MG, Kwon YW. Elbow arthritis. Bull NYU Hosp Jt Dis. 2007;65(1):61–71.
27. Hwang JT, Kim Y, Shields MN, Bachman DR, Berglund LJ, Fitzsimmons AT, et al. Effects of axial forearm instability on force transmission across the elbow. J Shoulder Elb Surg. 2019;28(1):170–7. https://doi.org/10.1016/j.jse.2018.07.016.
28. Murata H, Ikuta Y, Murakami T. An anatomic investigation of the elbow joint, with special reference to aging of the articular cartilage. J Shoulder Elb Surg. 1993;2(4):175–81. https://doi.org/10.1016/1058-2746(93)90060-T.

Arthroscopic Osteocapsular Arthroplasty for Elbow Osteoarthritis

19

K. C. Roth, A. E. van der Windt, J. W. Colaris, and D. Eygendaal

1 Background

The elbow joint is particularly prone to stiffness due to its highly congruent bony anatomy, the presence of three distinct articulations within the same synovial cavity, and the close relationship between the joint capsule, ligaments, and surrounding musculature [1, 2]. The principal biological mechanism underlying the elbow's propensity for contracture is the capsule's tendency to undergo an inflammatory process, as observed in osteoarthritis [3]. Various anatomical factors can limit extension and flexion, as described in Fig. 19.1. Anteriorly, elbow extension can be restricted by contracture of the skin, flexor muscles, or the anterior capsule. Posteriorly, it can be limited by bony impingement. Elbow flexion can be restricted posteriorly by contracture of the triceps, posterior capsule, or the posterior band of the medial collateral ligament, and anteriorly by osseous impingement. Additionally, ulnar nerve neuropathy can indirectly contribute

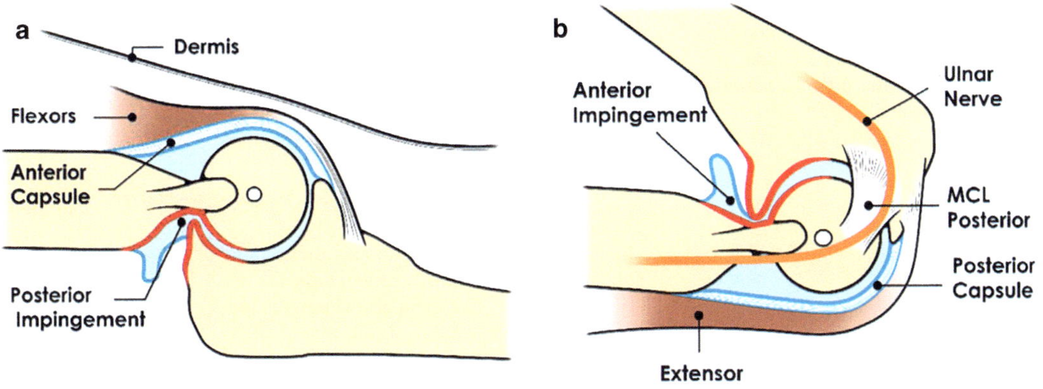

Fig. 19.1 Anatomical factors causing restricted extension (**a**) and flexion (**b**). (From: Marinelli et al. [4])

K. C. Roth · A. E. van der Windt · J. W. Colaris
D. Eygendaal (✉)
Department of Orthopaedics and Sports Medicine, Erasmus MC, University Medical Center Rotterdam, CA, Rotterdam, The Netherlands
e-mail: denise@eygendaal.nl

I.-H. Jeon et al. (eds.), *Elbow Arthroscopy*, https://doi.org/10.1007/978-981-95-3732-7_19

to contracture, as the resulting pain will restrict the patient's ability to mobilize the elbow [4].

2 Classifications of Elbow Stiffness

Numerous researchers have proposed various frameworks for categorizing elbow stiffness [4–8]. Two taxonomies are highlighted, which are most relevant in clinical practice.

In a 2003 publication, Jupiter et al. divided post-traumatic elbow stiffness into two groups: *simple and complex*. Simple stiffness is defined by mild to moderate contracture, no prior surgery, minimal heterotopic ossification, and a well-preserved bony anatomy. In contrast, complex stiffness is associated with nerve dysfunction, prior nerve transposition, retained hardware, substantial heterotopic ossification, articular incongruity, and an arc of motion less than 80°. This classification system aids in assessing the risks and benefits of surgical intervention, as the complex form is linked to higher surgical complication rates and necessitates greater technical expertise [7].

Inspired by the widely utilized ISAKOS shoulder stiffness taxonomy [9], the ISAKOS Pathoanatomical Classification of Elbow Stiffness was published in 2019 [5] and is presented in Table 19.1. According to this framework, elbow stiffness can be categorized into four subtypes: *intra-articular, capsular, extra-articular, and neurological.* For all patients with elbow stiffness being considered for surgery, a preoperative CT scan is recommended. If there is post-traumatic deformity, post-traumatic osteoarthritis, or a malunion, a 3D CT scan might be valuable, which involves scanning both elbows and superimposing a virtual model of the unaffected side onto the affected side to better identify pathology. For patients with a clinical suspicion of a neurological disorder, the clinical neurophysiology department can provide electromyography, nerve conduction studies, and nerve ultrasounds preoperatively.

Table 19.1 ISAKOS Pathoanatomical Classification of Elbow Stiffness

1. Intra-articular	2. Capsular	3. Extra-articular	4. Neurologic
Osteoarthritis, osteochondral defects, avascular necrosis, intra-articular malunion, synovitis, articular adhesions/fibrosis, loose bodies	*Ligaments:* Contracture, calcifications	*Muscles:* Muscle contracture	*Central:* Behavioral dystonia, spasticity
	Capsule: Contracture, calcifications	*Tendons and bursa:* Tear, calcifications, bursitis	*Peripheral:* Ulnar, radial, median nerve; cutaneous nerves
	Congruity: Instability, subluxation, dislocation	*Other:* Heterotopic ossifications, skin contracture, extra-articular malunion	*Sensory and autonomic:* Charcot joint, CRPS

3 Indications for Surgery

The functional range of motion (ROM) required for activities of daily living (ADL) has been a subject of ongoing discussion. Morrey et al. (1981) initially proposed that most ADL could be accomplished with 100° of elbow flexion (30°–130°) and 100° of forearm rotation (50° pronation and 50° supination) [10]. However, more recent studies indicate that contemporary tasks may demand a wider ROM. For instance, Sardelli et al. (2011) observed that operating a cellular phone requires 130° of elbow flexion (17°–147°), typing on a keyboard necessitates 65° of pronation, and turning a doorknob involves 77° of supination [11]. Functionally, limitations in elbow flexion often pose greater challenges than restrictions in extension, especially in the elderly [12]. Furthermore, many occupations and athletic activities demand a broader ROM than the values proposed by Morrey. For these individuals, even slight reductions in ROM can present significant difficulties [2]. Consequently, the decision to pursue surgical intervention is highly individualized, depending on the specific ROM required for occupational, athletic, or recreational activities [13]. Table 19.2 outlines the indications and (relative) contraindications for arthroscopic treatment.

For stiffness caused by soft tissue contractures, initial treatment with physiotherapy (PT) and splinting is recommended. If significant improvement in range of motion is not achieved within 3–6 months, surgical intervention may be considered. In contrast, when range of motion is limited by osseous deformities, such as osteophytosis, early surgical treatment is recommended. A treatment algorithm for the symptomatic stiff elbow is provided in Fig. 19.2 [1].

Table 19.2 Indications and contraindications for arthroscopic arthrolysis

Indications	Relative contraindications
1. Persistent pain and inability to perform functional tasks despite 3–6 months of conservative management 2. Joint locking or catching caused by loose bodies. Preoperative CT imaging, including 3D reconstruction, is critical for evaluation 3. Symptomatic restrictions in ROM, lesser than the traditionally proposed thresholds of 30°–130° of elbow flexion and 50°–50° of forearm rotation, may warrant surgical intervention if they interfere with daily activities, occupational tasks, sports, or hobbies 4. Patients should demonstrate a commitment to preserving the achieved range of motion through adherence to home exercise programs and physical therapy	1. Ulnar nerve-related issues, including entrapment, instability, or difficulty localizing the nerve 2. Severe flexion contracture (<90°), often associated with extensive extra-articular soft-tissue adhesions, which necessitates ulnar nerve release 3. History of multiple previous surgical incisions, which may complicate the procedure 4. Rotational impairments or proximal radioulnar (PRU) pathology, as these conditions cannot be adequately addressed arthroscopically 5. Extensive heterotopic ossifications 6. Pathology located outside the joint capsule (extra-articular)

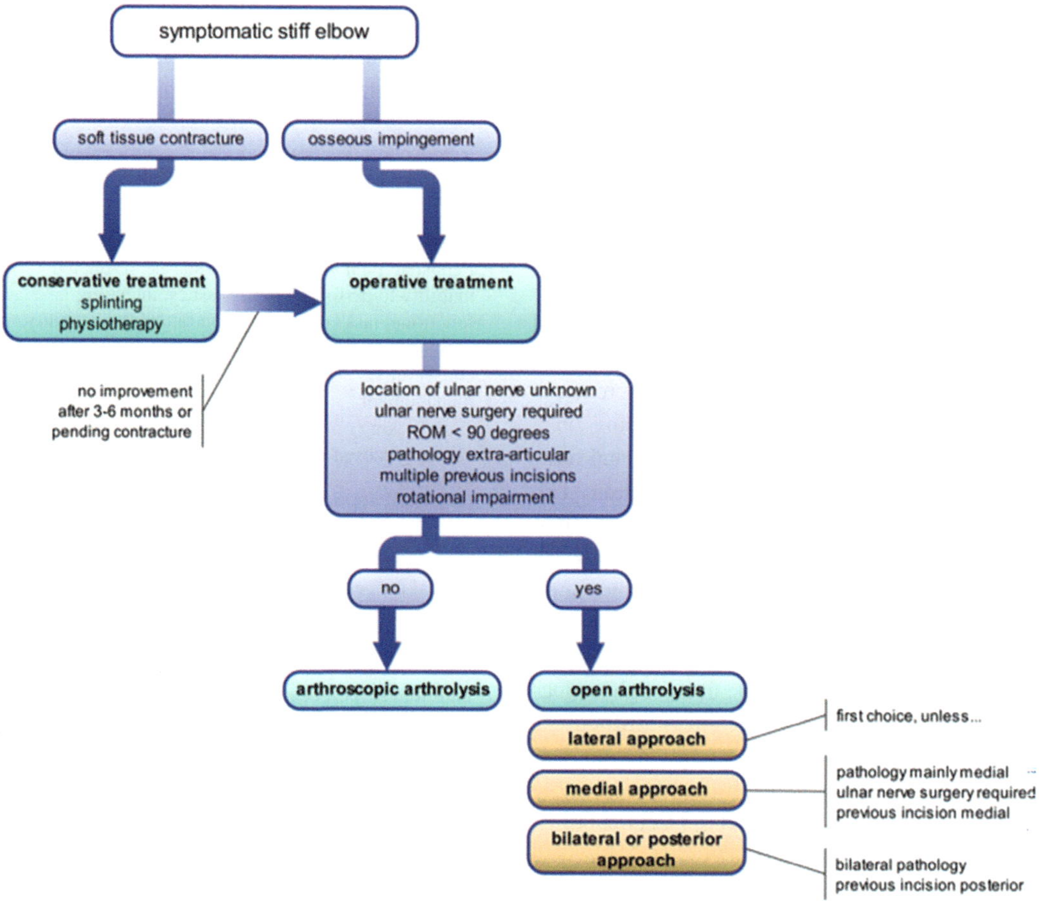

Fig. 19.2 Treatment algorithm for the symptomatic stiff elbow. (From: Siemensma et al. [1])

4 Outcomes and Complications

Arthroscopic arthrolysis offers several potential advantages over open surgery, including improved visualization, reduced postoperative pain and swelling, faster recovery with less scarring, and a lower risk of infection [14]. A recent review comparing the outcomes of open and arthroscopic treatments for elbow stiffness found similar success rates (91.8% for arthroscopic and 88.8% for open procedures) [1]. Both treatments showed comparable improvements in the Mayo Elbow Performance Score (MEPS): 29 points for open surgery and 26 points for arthroscopic surgery. In terms of range of motion, open surgery resulted in a greater improvement of 70° (from 43° to 113°), compared to 39° (from 68° to 108°) with arthroscopic treatment. This difference is attributed to the fact that severe contractures were primarily addressed through open surgery. Nevertheless, arthroscopic treatment was associated with significantly lower complication rates (9.1% vs. 18.1%) and revision rates (1.6% vs. 6.3%).

A recent study further demonstrated that arthroscopic treatment yielded slightly greater functional gains in patients with post-traumatic stiffness compared to those with osteoarthritis [15]. In the post-traumatic group, the mean preoperative flexion-extension was 120°–40° (80° total), which improved to 140°–10° (130° total) at a 27-month follow-up. In the osteoarthritis group, the preoperative flexion-extension was

117°–34° (82° total), improving to 133°–19° (114° total). This resulted in a functional gain of 62.5% in the post-traumatic group and 39% in the osteoarthritis group, with the latter still representing a clinically meaningful improvement. Additionally, the MEPS improved from 67 to 95 points (a gain of 28) in the post-traumatic group, while the osteoarthritis group showed an improvement from 59 to 85 points (a gain of 26). In line with these findings, another study found that arthroscopic arthrolysis is especially effective for early stages of osteoarthritis [14].

Furthermore, postoperative range of motion can be sustained over time. In a study by Kim and Shin, a 43° improvement was maintained over a 42.5-month follow-up, with most of the improvement occurring within the first year and no significant loss thereafter [16].

5 Arthroscopic Capsular Release and Debridement of Osteoarthritis: Step-by-Step Surgical Procedure

Arthroscopic osteocapsular arthroplasty of the elbow involves the three-dimensional reshaping of bones, removal of loose bodies, and capsular release to restore motion, improve function, and alleviate pain [17]. Due to the risk of nerve injury, O'Driscoll recommends arthroscopic contracture releases only when they pose equal or lower risk than open surgery. He proposed a "safety-driven" technique designed to minimize nerve damage without compromising the effectiveness of the procedure [17]. Several elements of this technique have been incorporated into our surgical approach.

5.1 Step-by-Step Surgical Procedure

Step 0. Preoperative Considerations

- Determine whether the elbow stiffness is simple or complex, according to Jupiter's classification.
- Identify which of the four potential causes of elbow stiffness are present: intra-articular, capsular, extra-articular, and/or neurological disorders. Arthroscopy can only address intra-articular and capsular causes.
- Evaluate the patient's motivation and readiness for an intensive postoperative rehabilitation program to maintain range of motion.

Step 1. Patient Preparation

- Perform a "Time-Out Procedure" and administer antibiotic prophylaxis.
- *Patient positioning:* Position the patient in lateral decubitus on a beanbag mattress, with the arm placed on a U-shaped support, allowing free elbow mobilization during surgery. Ensure the elbow is free from external pressure, particularly on the anterior capsule, to protect neurovascular structures (see Fig. 19.3). Position the contralateral arm cranially in a "sleeping position," resting along the patient's pillow, secured with a sheet and clamp. Thus, no arm support is needed for the unaffected arm to enhance your working space needed for arthroscopy.
- *Surgical site marking:* Mark the ulnar nerve and portal entry points for guidance (Fig. 19.4).

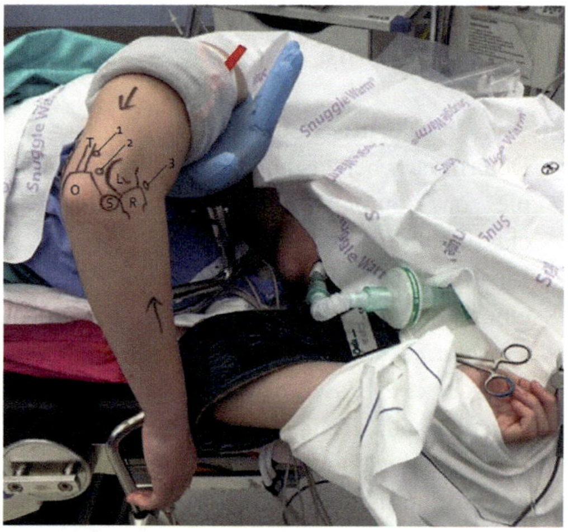

Fig. 19.3 Patient positioning

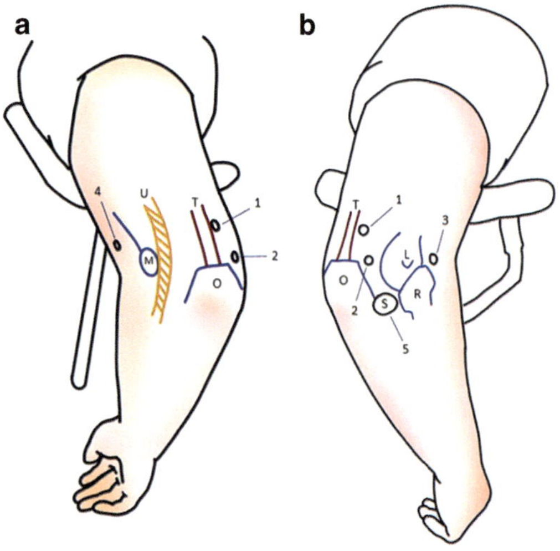

Fig. 19.4 Portals for arthroscopic arthrolysis (**a**) Medial view (**b**) Lateral view. (From: Siemensma et al. [1])

Step 2. Assessment Under Anesthesia

- Prior to surgery, assess elbow range of motion and stability through a physical examination under anesthesia [18].
- Assess flexion/extension and pronation/supination ranges.
- Evaluate for MCL (medial collateral ligament) instability.
- Check for posterolateral rotatory ligamentous instability (PLRI) of the lateral ulnar collateral ligament (LUCL).

Step 3. Nerve Management

- Exsanguinate the limb before inflating the tourniquet using an elasticated bandage.
- For patients with ulnar nerve issues (such as entrapment, instability, or difficulty localizing the nerve) or potential scarring from prior surgery or post-traumatic arthritis, we recommend performing an open ulnar nerve release before starting arthroscopy [19]. A limited open ulnar nerve decompression through a 2 cm incision can help prevent neuritis [17].
- Ensure proper protection of the posterior interosseous nerve (PIN) using inside-out techniques and careful portal placement.

Step 4. Portal Creation and Joint Distension

- Distend the joint by injecting saline into the posterior fossa through the triceps muscle to displace the capsule and neurovascular structures away from the bony structures. Successful injection causes bulging of the posterolateral corner.
- Create five standard portals: three posterior (posterolateral, proximal posterolateral, olecranon fossa) and two anterior (proximal anteromedial and anterior superior lateral).
- Always maintain awareness of the nerve locations. While joint distension moves the anterior capsule and neurovascular structures away from the joint surface, it does not alter the relative position of the capsule to the nerves. See Table 19.3 for portal placement considerations in different compartments.

Step 5. Posterior Compartment Exploration and Debridement

- Access the posterior compartment via the straight posterior portal for camera insertion, using the posterolateral portal as the working portal.
- Perform posterior capsulectomy and release, along with debridement of adhesive tissue in the posterior fossa to enhance visualization and improve flexion.

Table 19.3 Considerations during portal placement

	Compartment		
	Posterior	Radiocapitellar	Anterior
Portal placement			
Arthroscope	Straight posterior	Posterolateral	Anteromedial
Working portal	Posterolateral	Elbow soft spot	Anterolateral
Access locations			
1	3 cm proximal to the olecranon tip	Radial side of the olecranon tip	Anterior and proximal to the medial epicondyle
2	Radial side of the olecranon tip	Elbow soft spot	Anterior and proximal to the lateral epicondyle
Considerations			
1	Avoiding triceps central band	Slightly extend elbow during insertion to prevent subcutaneous placement	Palpate medial intermuscular septum confirming proper placement
2	Blade insertion at 45° angle to posterior olecranon plane; penetrate capsule using curved clamp, confirmed by popping sensation and fluid outflow	Skin-only incision to prevent MABCN damage; insert trocar toward joint, while slightly lifting the forearm, while maintaining contact with the anterior humerus surface	Insert needle from the lateral side under arthroscopic view
3			Caution at anterior capsule near the radial head to avoid PIN damage
Visualization			
1	Fossa olecrani	Posterolateral compartment	Coronoid fossa
2	Posterolateral space	Radial head	Capitellum
3	Olecranon tip	Proximal radioulnar joint	Radial head
4	Ulnohumeral joint		Anterior capsule
5	Ulnar joint side		Coronoid process
Goals			
1	Fibrous tissue debridement for improving view and elbow extension	Loose body removal	Synovectomy from lateral portal
2	Osteophytectomy reducing posterior impingement and improving extension	Removal of fibrous tissue	Removal of osteophytes from coronoid process
3	Loose body removal		Blunt release of anterior capsule

From: Siemensma et al. [1]

- Remove any loose bodies and hypertrophic osteophytes from the tip of the olecranon and the roof of the olecranon fossa, ensuring no impingement remains.
- Special care is required during debridement of the ulnar aspect of the olecranon due to its proximity to the ulnar nerve. Debridement should be performed only under direct visualization of the shaver, with suction deactivated to minimize nerve injury risk.
- Perform dynamic assessment of motion intraoperatively after posterior debridement to determine if additional resection is required [20].

Step 6. Radiocapitellar Compartment

- Excise fibrous tissue and adhesions.
- Resect osteophytes from the posterior aspect of the capitellum.
- *Reshape* the radial head to restore its anatomical contour.
- Extract any loose bodies present in the joint.
- If necessary, create an additional portal.

Step 7. Anterior Compartment Debridement and Release

- *Portal entry:* Access the anterior compartment via the proximal anteromedial portal. Palpate the ulnar nerve and the medial intermuscular septum. Create a portal anterior to the septum at a safe distance from the ulnar nerve. Make a skin incision followed by blunt dissection to reach the capsule. Introduce the trocar and arthroscope, ensuring avoidance of the ulnar and median nerves.
- *Creation of anterolateral portal:* Use the outside-in technique, guided by a needle, ensuring awareness of the radial nerve during portal creation.
- Perform osteophyte reduction of the coronoid process. Release the capsular recess using a shaver.
- Remove fibrous tissue, intra-articular foreign bodies, and osteophytes using forceps or an arthroscopic reamer.
- *Capsular release:* Perform a sharp release of the proximal capsular attachment on the radial side. The remaining capsule is bluntly detached using a shearing maneuver with a switching stick or a detached shaver.
- Create sufficient intracapsular space by stripping the capsule off the humerus, stopping when the brachialis muscle fibers are visible to avoid neurovascular injury [21].
- Take care to minimize the risk of nerve injury, particularly to the posterior interosseous and median nerves.

5.2 Postoperative Care

- Apply a compression bandage for 48 h.
- *Weight-bearing:* Allow weight-bearing as tolerated, based on the patient's pain levels.
- *Range of motion:* Allow full range of motion direct postoperatively.
- *Exercise instructions:* Begin passive exercises on day 1 post-surgery, performing 10 repetitions of flexion-extension movements 6 times daily. These exercises should be done while lying down and assisted by the opposite hand.
- *Pain management:* Adequate pain medication is necessary for early movement.
- *Physiotherapist guidance:* Initial physiotherapy should be conducted during the hospital stay, followed by home physiotherapy within 2–3 days post-discharge.

5.3 Tips and Tricks

- For those less experienced in elbow arthroscopy, it is recommended to begin with a posterior arthroscopic approach and perform the anterior release via an open technique.
- Thorough preoperative planning is essential to identify which of the four potential causes of elbow stiffness are present: intra-articular, capsular, extra-articular, and/or neurological disorders.
- Perform repeated dynamic assessments of motion intraoperatively after debridement to determine if additional resection is required.
- A useful trick to minimize the risk of ulnar nerve complications during posteromedial debridement, is to ensure the shaver is always under direct visualization and to deactivate the suction during this phase of the procedure.
- Perform blunt release of anterior capsule (with a disconnected shaver).

- It is a key point to maintain a low threshold for converting to an open procedure if anterior visualization is significantly obstructed by synovitis or fibrous tissue, as clear visualization is critical for safe and effective surgery.

References

1. Siemensma MF, van der Windt AE, van Es EM, Colaris JW, Eygendaal D. Management of the stiff elbow: a literature review. EFORT Open Rev. 2023;8(5):351–60. https://doi.org/10.1530/EOR-23-0039.
2. Attum B, Obremskey W. Posttraumatic elbow stiffness: a critical analysis review. JBJS Rev. 2016;4(9):e4. https://doi.org/10.2106/JBJS.RVW.15.00084.
3. Keschner MT, Paksima N. The stiff elbow. Bull NYU Hosp Jt Dis. 2007;65(1):24–8.
4. Marinelli A, Guerra E, Bain G. Classification of elbow stiffness. J ISAKOS. 2024;9(2):234–9. https://doi.org/10.1016/j.jisako.2023.10.011.
5. Guerra E, Kelberine FM, Marinelli A, Rotini R, Bain G. The stiff elbow: classification and treatment algorithm. In: Bain G, Eygendaal D, van Riet RP, editors. Surgical techniques for trauma and sports related injuries of the elbow. Berlin/Heidelberg: Springer Berlin Heidelberg; 2020. p. 173–80.
6. Morrey BF. The posttraumatic stiff elbow. Clin Orthop Relat Res. 2005;431:26–35. https://doi.org/10.1097/01.blo.0000152897.68636.19.
7. Jupiter JB, O'Driscoll SW, Cohen MS. The assessment and management of the stiff elbow. Instr Course Lect. 2003;52:93–111.
8. Kamineni S. Arthrolysis of the post-traumatic stiff elbow. In: Stanley D, Kay NRM, editors. Surgery of the elbow. London: Arnold; 1998. p. 228–34.
9. Bain GI, Clitherow HDS. The pathogenesis and classification of shoulder stiffness. In: Itoi E, Arce G, Bain GI, Diercks RL, Guttmann D, Imhoff AB, et al., editors. Shoulder stiffness: current concepts and concerns. Berlin/Heidelberg: Springer Berlin Heidelberg; 2015. p. 3–19.
10. Morrey BF, Askew LJ, Chao EY. A biomechanical study of normal functional elbow motion. J Bone Joint Surg Am. 1981;63(6):872–7. https://doi.org/10.2106/00004623-198163060-00003.
11. Sardelli M, Tashjian RZ, MacWilliams BA. Functional elbow range of motion for contemporary tasks. J Bone Joint Surg Am. 2011;93(5):471–7. https://doi.org/10.2106/JBJS.I.01633.
12. Ruch DS, Shen J, Chloros GD, Krings E, Papadonikolakis A. Release of the medial collateral ligament to improve flexion in post-traumatic elbow stiffness. J Bone Joint Surg Br. 2008;90(5):614–8. https://doi.org/10.1302/0301-620X.90B5.19999.
13. Keener JD, Galatz LM. Arthroscopic management of the stiff elbow. J Am Acad Orthop Surg. 2011;19(5):265–74. https://doi.org/10.5435/00124635-201105000-00004.
14. Hy C, D E, B T. Elbow arthroscopy – indications and technique. J Clin Orthop Trauma. 2021;19:147–53. https://doi.org/10.1016/j.jcot.2021.05.022.
15. Sos C, Petit A, Brunet J, Rabarin F, Saint Cast Y, Raimbeau G, et al. Comparison of results of arthroscopic arthrolysis between traumatic and degenerative elbow stiffness. Orthop Traumatol Surg Res. 2023;109(2):103436. https://doi.org/10.1016/j.otsr.2022.103436.
16. Kim SJ, Shin SJ. Arthroscopic treatment for limitation of motion of the elbow. Clin Orthop Relat Res. 2000;375:140–8. https://doi.org/10.1097/00003086-200006000-00017.
17. O'Driscoll SW, Blonna D. Osteocapsular arthroplasty of the elbow: surgical technique. JBJS Essent Surg Tech. 2014;3(3):e15. https://doi.org/10.2106/JBJS.ST.M.00002.
18. Park MJ, Chang MJ, Lee YB, Kang HJ. Surgical release for posttraumatic loss of elbow flexion. JBJS Essent Surg Tech. 2011;1(3):e16. https://doi.org/10.2106/JBJS.ST.K.00008.
19. Pederzini LA, Di Palma F. Arthroscopic capsular release and debridement of osteoarthritis: how I do it! In: Bain G, Eygendaal D, van Riet RP, editors. Surgical techniques for trauma and sports related injuries of the elbow. Berlin/Heidelberg: Springer Berlin Heidelberg; 2020. p. 181–4.
20. Schreiner AJ, Schweikardt N, Guhring D, Ahrend MD, Dobele S, Ahmad SS, et al. Arthroscopic arthrolysis leads to improved range of motion and health-related quality of life in post-traumatic elbow stiffness. J Shoulder Elb Surg. 2020;29(8):1538–47. https://doi.org/10.1016/j.jse.2020.01.099.
21. San Pastor PC. Arthroscopic Arthrolysis of stiff elbow. Arthrosc Tech. 2020;9(6):e817–e21. https://doi.org/10.1016/j.eats.2020.02.015.

20 Clinical Outcomes of Arthroscopic Osteocapsular Arthroplasty in Elbow Osteoarthritis

Jia Guo and In-Ho Jeon

1 Background

Primary elbow osteoarthritis (OA) typically originates at the posteromedial radial head (beveled rim), where it articulates with the zona conoidea of the lateral trochlear ridge of the humerus, and subsequently progresses to involve the ulnohumeral joint (Fig. 20.1) [1]. The key pathological changes include osteophyte formation, capsular contracture, and medial collateral ligament (MCL) involvement, which are the main surgical targets. In the early stages, patients typically experience impingement

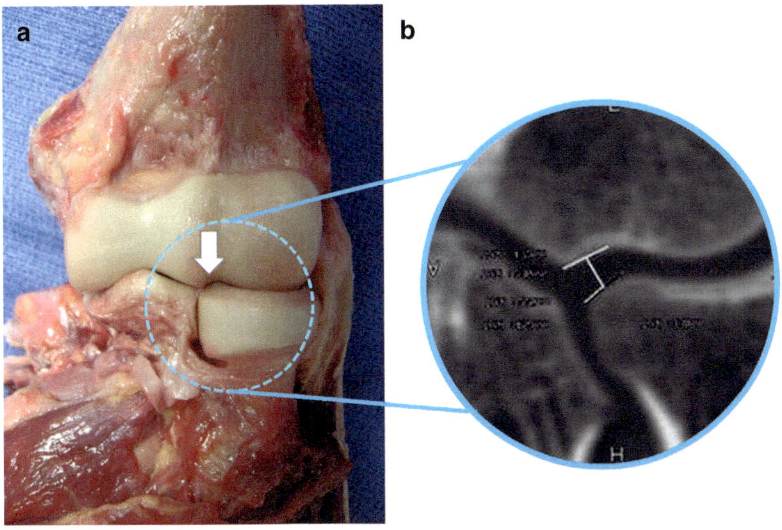

Fig. 20.1 Zona conoidea of the elbow: articulation between the radial head and lateral trochlea of the elbow. (**a**) Zona conoidea (white arrow) marked cadaveric photo. (**b**) Measurement of distance between the lateral trochlear rim and radial head bevel in CT scan [1]

Supplementary Information The online version contains supplementary material available at https://doi.org/10.1007/978-981-95-3732-7_20.

J. Guo (✉) · I.-H. Jeon
Department of Orthopaedic Surgery, Asan Medical Center, University of Ulsan, College of Medicine, Seoul, Republic of Korea

I.-H. Jeon et al. (eds.), *Elbow Arthroscopy*, https://doi.org/10.1007/978-981-95-3732-7_20

pain at terminal extension and flexion. As OA progresses to more advanced stages, pain may occur at rest or in the mid-arc of motion, often accompanied by further restriction of joint movement.

While open surgery has been a traditional method of choice, the arthroscopic approach has more recently gained attention as a minimally invasive alternative, with the potential to reduce soft tissue disruption and facilitate faster postoperative recovery.

2 Indications and Contraindications

Arthroscopic osteocapsular arthroplasty (OCA) is indicated for patients with elbow OA who present with functional limitations and impingement pain caused by osteophyte formation and capsular contracture. The decision to perform arthroscopic OCA should be individualized, considering both radiologic findings and clinical presentation. Patients with mild, early-stage radiographic changes, often characterized by the presence of osteophytes or loose bodies contributing to mechanical impingement and without evident joint space narrowing, may still be appropriate candidates for arthroscopic OCA [2].

In contrast, advanced-stage osteoarthritis, particularly with marked joint space narrowing, is generally associated with poorer clinical outcomes, and is therefore considered a relative contraindication to arthroscopic intervention [3]. Similarly, significant anatomical distortion, whether due to congenital deformity or post-traumatic changes, as well as a history of submuscular ulnar nerve transposition, may be relative contraindications, depending on surgeon's experience and expertise.

According to the Kwak classification system [3], optimal candidates for arthroscopic OCA include patients with grade I (uni-fossa involvement) and grade II (bi-fossa involvement) elbow OA. While grade III, characterized by joint space narrowing, is generally less suitable for arthroscopic management, patient selection should still be individualized based on symptom severity and functional limitations (Fig. 20.2).

	Grade 0	Grade I (uni-fossa)		Grade II (bi-fossa)	Grade III
		IA	IP		
Fossa Involvement	None	Anterior	Posterior	Both	Any
Joint Involvement	Intact				Narrowing
CT Image					

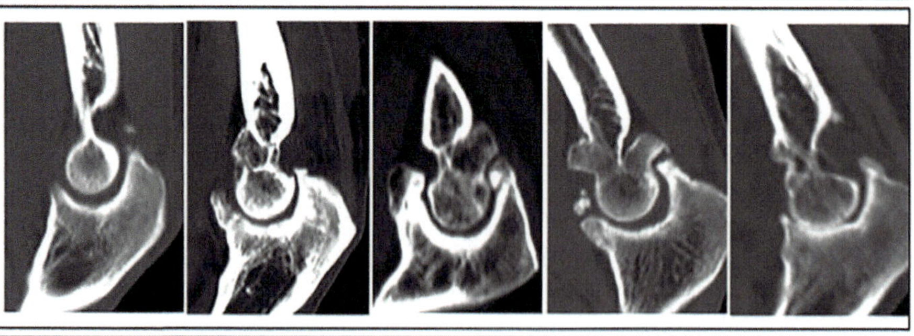

Definition	
Involved Fossa	More than 50% osteophyte in the fossa
Joint Narrowing	Less than 1mm in the more than 50% of articular space

Fig. 20.2 Computed tomography (CT)-based classification for elbow osteoarthritis. (Adapted from: Kwak JM, Osteoarthritis Cartilage. 2019 Jul.) [3]

3 Surgical Techniques

3.1 Patient Setup

The author prefers the lateral decubitus position under general anesthesia, as it allows the elbow to be positioned to full intraoperative evaluation of flexion and extension. Precise anatomical marking of landmarks, including the lateral epicondyle, radial head, medial epicondyle, and ulnar nerve, is crucial before surgery.

In cases of elbow stiffness with severe flexion loss (flexion <90°), prophylactic ulnar nerve decompression through a minimal incision should be considered prior to arthroscopic OCA. Decompression spanning 3 cm is recommended, extending proximally and distally from the cubital tunnel [4].

The author prefers to address the posterior compartment first, as it provides better access to the medial and lateral gutters before joint swelling develops.

3.2 Establishing a View and Working Space

Standard portals (including the direct posterior, posterolateral, and soft spot portals) are typically used, while accessory portals can be established to facilitate the use of an intra-articular retractor.

The first and most challenging step is to visualize articular structures and establish anatomic orientation. Access the joint by penetrating thick scar tissue with a switching stick through the direct posterior viewing portal, and then advance the arthroscope. A 4 mm shaver is introduced through the posterolateral portal to debride proliferative synovium and expose key anatomic landmarks in the posterior compartment. Once articular structures, such as olecranon tip and orientation, are clearly identified, spur resection can be performed.

3.3 Osteophyte Removal and Subsequent Soft-Tissue Release

3.3.1 Posterior Compartment

In the posterior compartment, osteophytes are typically found at the olecranon tip and along the medial and lateral borders of the ulna. An intra-articular retractor, introduced through an accessory portal, can be used to improve working space and reduce the risk of ulnar nerve injury. It is crucial to remove osteophytes from the olecranon fossa, its margins, the olecranon tip, and its sides to improve the elbow extension. Passive extension should be assessed under direct arthroscopic visualization to ensure that no bony impingement remains in the ulnohumeral joint (Figs. 20.3 and 20.4).

For flexion limitations, posteromedial capsular release is most important. During release of the posteromedial gutter, the anatomy of ulnar nerve must be thoroughly understood and carefully protected (Table 20.1).

In cases of rotational stiffness, resection of radial head osteophytes and excision of fibrotic scar tissue at the posterior radiocapitellar and proximal radioulnar joints may be considered to improve forearm rotation. A posterolateral portal is typically utilized as the viewing portal, while the soft-spot portal serves as the working portal during these procedures. If additional release is required, a proximal radioulnar joint portal can be established to enhance surgical access and tissue excision.

3.3.2 Anterior Compartment

The arthroscope is introduced through the proximal anteromedial portal, while the proximal anterolateral portal is established under direct visualization and serves as the working portal. An anterolateral portal may be established as an accessory portal using the inside-out technique, advancing from the proximal anteromedial portal toward

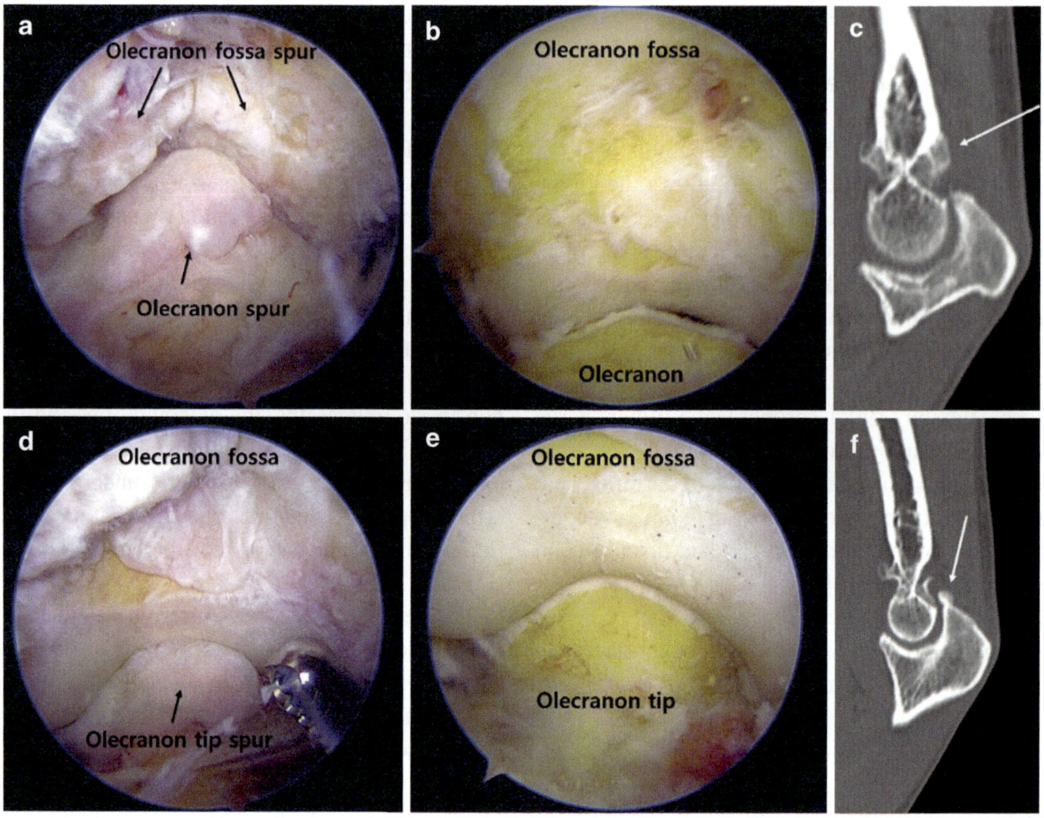

Fig. 20.3 (**a**, **d**) Osteophyte of olecranon fossa and olecranon tip. (**b**, **e**) Exposed olecranon fossa and olecranon after removal of osteophytes. (**c**, **f**) Corresponding CT sagittal images

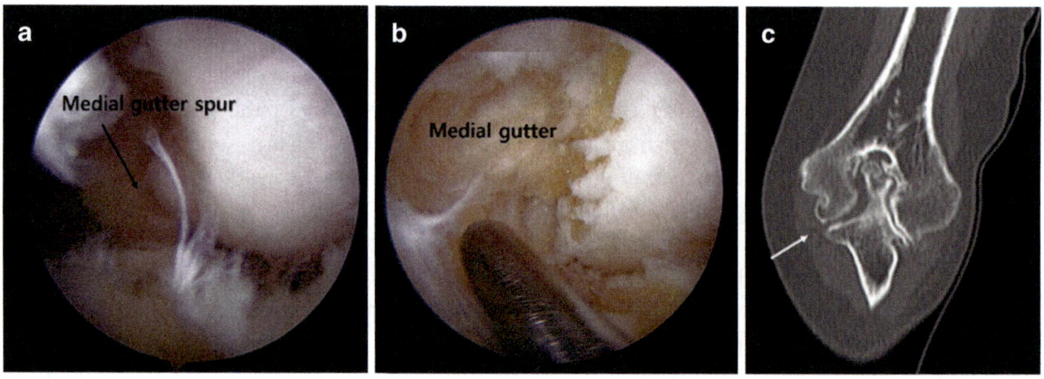

Fig. 20.4 (**a**) Osteophyte at posteromedial gutter. (**b**) Exposed posteromedial gutter after osteophyte removal. (**c**) Corresponding CT coronal image

a direct lateral orientation. This technique can reduce the risk of injury to neurovascular structures (video 20.1). To optimize visualization and create additional working space, retractors may be employed. Excision of loose bodies, hypertrophic synovial tissue, and fibrous adhesions is performed using a shaver. However, preservation of the joint capsule until the final stage of the procedure is recommended to limit fluid extravasation and reduce subsequent soft-tissue swelling.

Osteophytes in the radial fossa, coronoid fossa, and at the coronoid process should be carefully identified and removed using a 4.0 mm burr (Figs. 20.5, 20.6, and 20.7). To minimize the risk of neurovascular injury, suction devices should be avoided when operating with burrs or shavers.

Following osteophyte removal, capsular or adhesion release is performed. A persistent extension deficit following posterior compartment procedures is usually due to anterior capsular contracture. Releasing the anterior capsule from its humeral attachment can improve extension while minimizing the risk of nerve injury.

Anterior capsular release must be performed with caution to avoid injury to the median and radial nerves, which lie just anterior to the brachialis muscle and radial head, respectively. The radial nerve runs through the interval between the brachialis and brachioradialis muscles approximately 2–3 cm proximal to the radial head. A small fat pad located anterior to the radial neck serves as a useful warning anatomic landmark during arthroscopy (Fig. 20.8). In cases of severe capsular fibrosis, the distortion of initial anatomic structures increases the risk of radial nerve injury, so special care is needed.

Table 20.1 Key points for ulnar nerve protection during posteromedial capsular release

Tip	Key point
Mini-open ulnar nerve exposure and protection	Prophylactic ulnar nerve decompression and tagging can be performed prior to posteromedial capsular release
Minimal suction use	Limit the use of suction near the medial olecranon to minimize the risk of iatrogenic traction or injury to the ulnar nerve
Careful release of posteromedial gutter	When using a burr, ensure it faces away from the ulnar nerve Prioritize nerve protection over aggressive bone resection in the posteromedial gutter

Although the capsule may be thickened due to fibrosis, it can be effectively removed using a shaver until the brachialis muscle becomes visible. During this process, the shaver should be oriented toward the joint and directed from distal to proximal. It is particularly important to clearly identify the space between the capsule and the brachialis muscle (Fig. 20.9). An intraarticular retractor can be used to protect neurovascular structures and provide better working space. Once the brachialis muscle is visualized, capsular release should proceed until the middle of the radial head is reached (Fig. 20.10). At this point, a fatty layer surrounding the radial nerve serves as a consistent anatomical marker, and it is safe to switch to a reverse basket retractor to minimize nerve injury (Fig. 20.8). The capsule can be removed thoroughly (capsulectomy) or incised (capsulotomy), depending on the severity of stiffness.

After completing the procedure, the range of motion is reassessed.

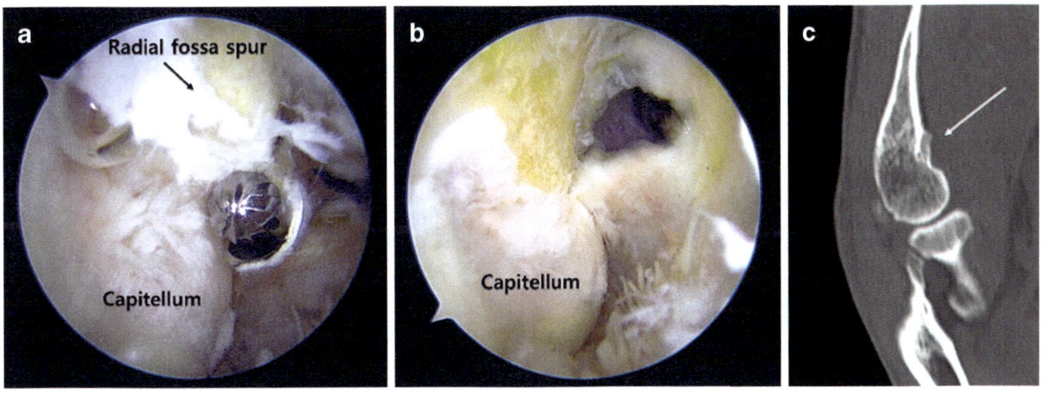

Fig. 20.5 (**a**) Osteophyte at the radial head fossa. (**b**) Exposed radial head fossa after osteophyte removal. (**c**) Corresponding CT sagittal image

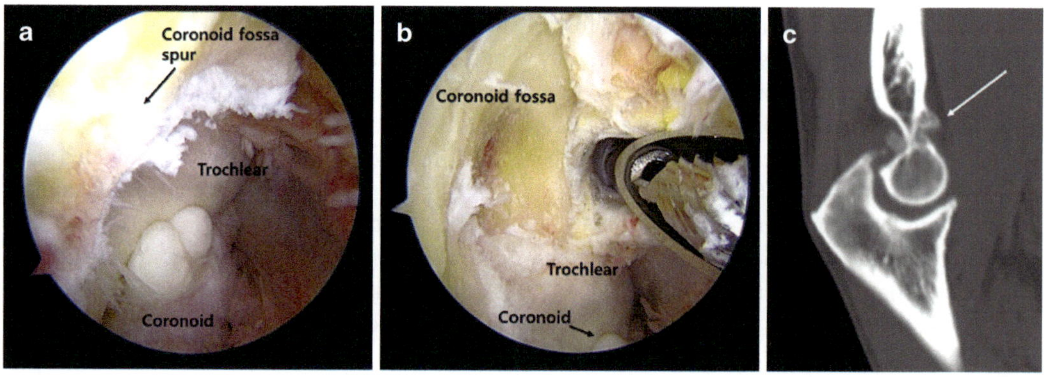

Fig. 20.6 (**a**) Osteophyte at the coronoid fossa. (**b**) Exposed coronoid fossa after osteophyte removal. (**c**) Corresponding CT sagittal image

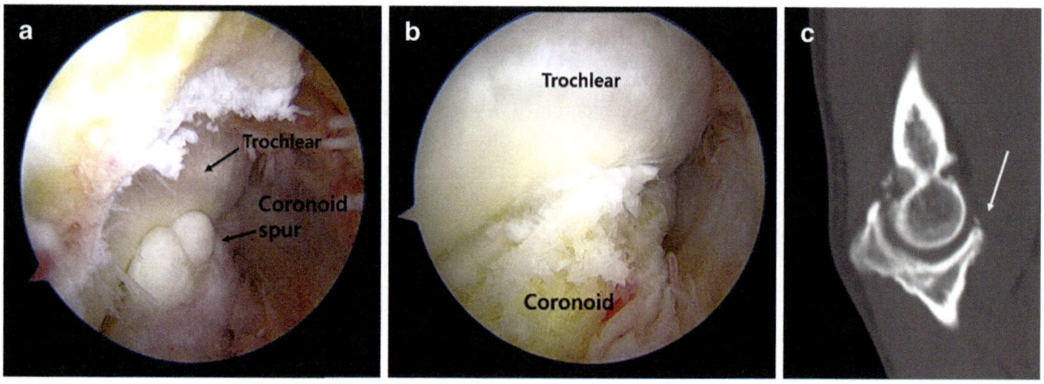

Fig. 20.7 (**a**) Coronoid osteophyte at the anterior aspect of ulnohumeral joint. (**b**) After excision of the coronoid tip osteophyte. (**c**) Corresponding CT sagittal image

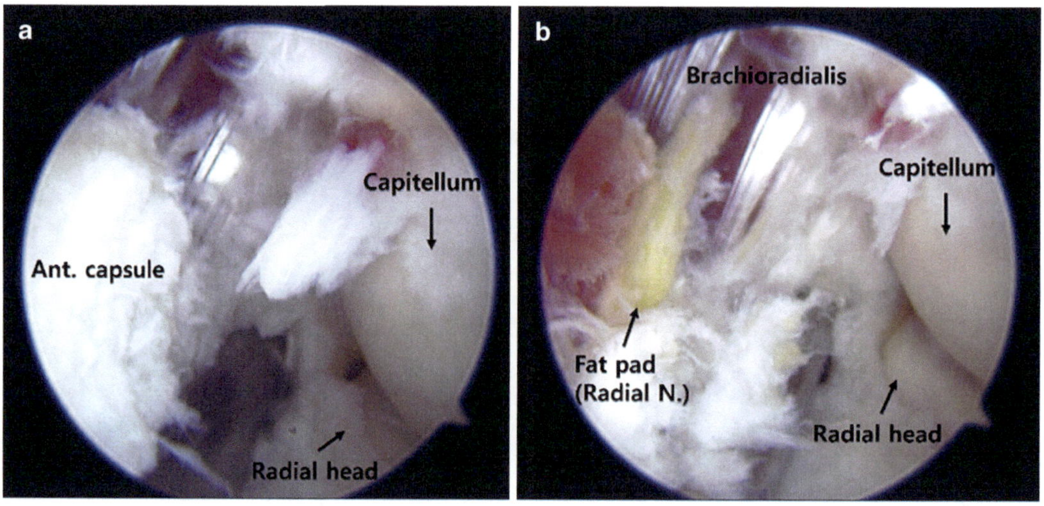

Fig. 20.8 (**a**) Before debridement of the anterior capsule. (**b**) A small fat pad located just in front of the radial neck, serving as a useful marker for the radial nerve during arthroscopy

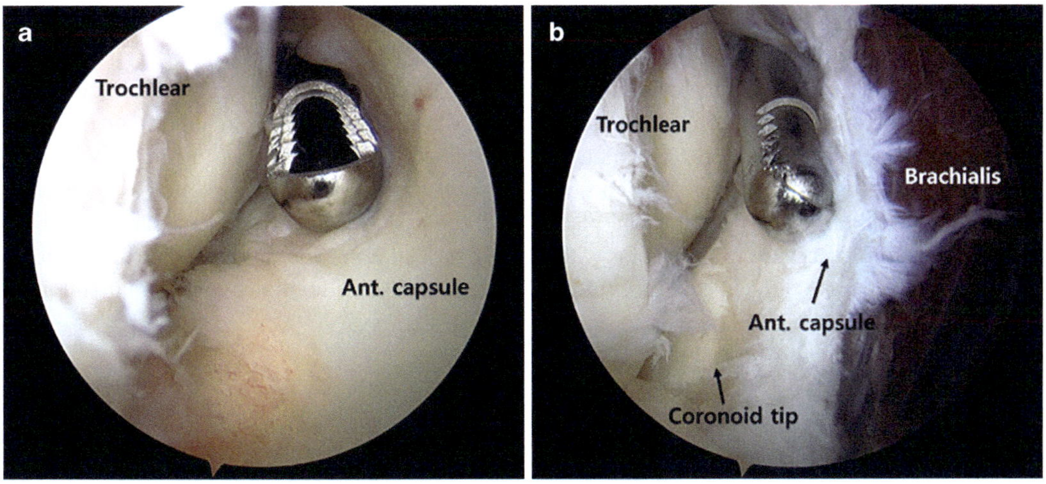

Fig. 20.9 (**a**) Before debridement of the anterior capsule. (**b**) It is important to clearly identify the space between the capsule and the brachialis muscle during an anterior capsulectomy

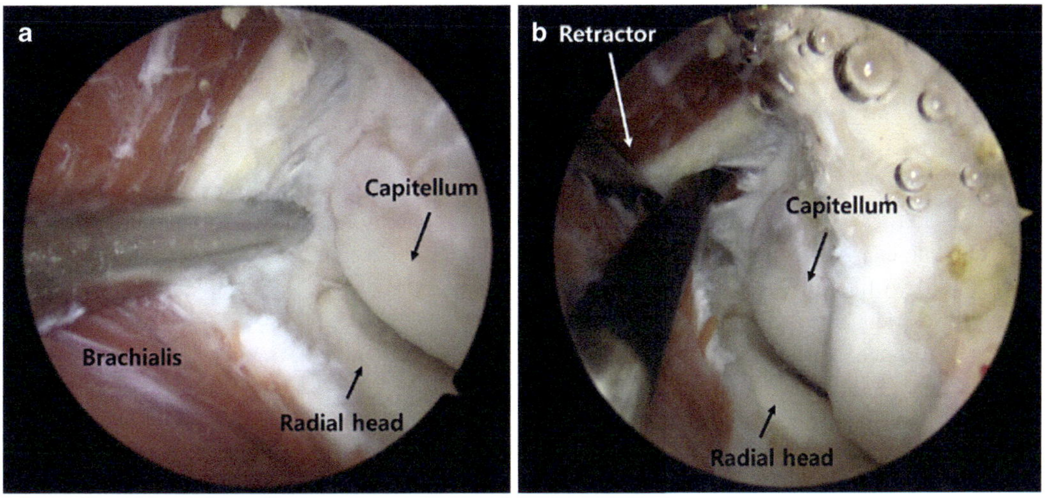

Fig. 20.10 (**a**) The capsule should be excised thoroughly rather than merely incised, continuing until the release is complete on both the medial and lateral sides. (**b**) A retractor can be used to confirm the capsule's location and apply gentle traction to facilitate safe removal

4 Postoperative Care

Constant elevation of arm and immobilization for first 24 h are recommended to reduce postoperative swelling. Following this period, active-assisted passive range-of-motion exercises can be initiated. To prevent inadvertent postoperative elbow instability, a hinged elbow brace should be applied during these exercises.

During postoperative rehabilitation, it is crucial to regularly monitor for neurological symptoms, especially regarding the ulnar nerve. Oral medications, such as NSAIDs, should be used to manage pain and facilitate effective rehabilitation exercise.

5 Complications

As with any surgery procedure, complications may occur during or after arthroscopic procedures. Neurological injuries are more common in arthroscopic procedures of elbow than in those of knee or shoulder because of its superficial placement with less soft tissue coverage. Patients with a history of elbow surgery, rheumatoid arthritis, or joint contractures are at higher risk iatrogenic neurologic injury. Although complications involving the median and radial nerves have been reported alongside those of the ulnar nerve, proper use of retractors can help prevent these nerve injuries.

6 Outcomes

Many studies have reported favorable outcomes for arthroscopic treatment of elbow osteoarthritis (Table 20.2). A comparative study by Kwak et al. demonstrated that arthroscopic osteocapsular arthroplasty yields outcomes comparable to those of the open procedure in cases of primary elbow osteoarthritis without severe ulnohumeral joint narrowing [5].

Table 20.2 Reported clinical outcomes after arthroscopic osteocapsular arthroplasty for elbow osteoarthritis

	No. of elbows	Mean follow up period (months)	Arc of F–E, Pre (°)	Arc of F–E, Post (°)	Clinical score, Pre	Clinical score, Post	Complications	Revision surgery
Adams et al. (2008) [6]	42	44.1	96.97 ± 24.8	123.20 ± 17.16	MEPS: 67.5 ± 12.9	MEPS: 84.4 ± 16.1	2	1
MacLean et al. (2013) [7]	21	66	125	127	N	N	0	0
Lim et al. (2014) [8]	43	38.4	84	104	VAS: 4.5, MEPS: 57.4	VAS: 2.2, MEPS: 88	2	5
Galle et al. (2016) [9]	31	41.0	102 ± 21	124 ± 18	VAS: 6 ± 3 0.5, MEPS: 57 ± 18	VAS: 2 ± 2.1, MEPS: 88 ± 14	0	1
Kwak et al.(2019) [5]	52	35.4	66.5 ± 22.6	108.0 ± 24.0	VAS: 6.4 ± 1.3, MEPS: 44.3 ± 12.2	VAS: 4.1 ± 2.0, MEPS: 73.8 ± 16.7	0	2
So et al. (2023) [10]	56	62.2	89.4 ± 20.2	105.4 ± 20.4	VAS: 4.9 ± 2.3, MEPS: 62.3 ± 10.6	VAS: 1.4 ± 1.8, MEPS: 87.8 ± 12.1	3	2

References

1. Jeon IH, Chun JM, Lee CS, Yoon JO, Kim PT, An KN, et al. Zona conoidea of the elbow: another articulation between the radial head and lateral trochlear of the elbow. J Bone Joint Surg Br. 2012;94(4):517–22. https://doi.org/10.1302/0301-620x.94b4.27842.
2. Blonna D, Lee GC, O'Driscoll SW. Arthroscopic restoration of terminal elbow extension in high-level athletes. Am J Sports Med. 2010;38(12):2509–15. https://doi.org/10.1177/0363546510376727.
3. Kwak JM, Kim H, Sun Y, Kholinne E, Koh KH, Jeon IH. Arthroscopic osteocapsular arthroplasty for advanced-stage primary osteoarthritis of the elbow using a computed tomography-based classification. J Shoulder Elb Surg. 2020;29(5):989–95. https://doi.org/10.1016/j.jse.2019.09.036.
4. Kelly EW, Morrey BF, O'Driscoll SW. Complications of elbow arthroscopy. J Bone Joint Surg Am. 2001;83(1):25–34. https://doi.org/10.2106/00004623-200101000-00004.
5. Kwak JM, Kholinne E, Sun Y, Lim S, Koh KH, Jeon IH. Clinical outcome of Osteocapsular arthroplasty for primary osteoarthritis of the elbow: comparison of arthroscopic and open procedure. Arthroscopy. 2019;35(4):1083–9. https://doi.org/10.1016/j.arthro.2018.11.057.
6. Adams JE, Wolff LH 3rd, Merten SM, Steinmann SP. Osteoarthritis of the elbow: results of arthroscopic osteophyte resection and capsulectomy. J Shoulder Elb Surg. 2008;17(1):126–31. https://doi.org/10.1016/j.jse.2007.04.005.
7. MacLean SB, Oni T, Crawford LA, Deshmukh SC. Medium-term results of arthroscopic debridement and capsulectomy for the treatment of elbow osteoarthritis. J Shoulder Elb Surg. 2013;22(5):653–7. https://doi.org/10.1016/j.jse.2013.01.030.
8. Lim TK, Koh KH, Lee HI, Shim JW, Park MJ. Arthroscopic débridement for primary osteoarthritis of the elbow: analysis of preoperative factors affecting outcome. J Shoulder Elb Surg. 2014;23(9):1381–7. https://doi.org/10.1016/j.jse.2014.01.009.
9. Galle SE, Beck JD, Burchette RJ, Harness NG. Outcomes of elbow arthroscopic Osteocapsular arthroplasty. J Hand Surg Am. 2016;41(2):184–91. https://doi.org/10.1016/j.jhsa.2015.11.018.
10. So SP, Kwak JM, Lee JB, Ben H, Kim KH, Koh KH, et al. Serial changes in clinical outcomes after arthroscopic Osteocapsular arthroplasty for primary elbow osteoarthritis: a medium-term follow-up study. Orthop J Sports Med. 2023;11(5):23259671231162398. https://doi.org/10.1177/23259671231162398.

21 Arthroscopic Transfossa Approach for Osteocapsular Arthroplasty in Elbow Osteoarthritis

Jae-Man Kwak, Erica Kholinne, and In-Ho Jeon

1 Background

Loss of elbow motion due to trauma or arthritis is common and significantly compromises functional capacity of the upper extremity [1–3]. Arthroscopic osteocapsular arthroplasty (OCA) of the elbow is a procedure involving three-dimensional reshaping of the bones, removal of any loose bodies, and capsulectomy to restore motion and function as well as to reduce or eliminate pain [4]. This technique has become a more common procedure in recent years since it is generally believed to provide results that are at least comparable to those of traditional open procedures, but it allows better visualization of intra-articular lesions, a quicker recovery, and better cosmetic results. Although there is little doubt regarding the efficacy of arthroscopic contracture release, the procedure is technically challenging and there are serious concerns about the risk of nerve injury. However, arthroscopic OCA is technically dependent especially in advanced anterior capsular contracture into anterior compartment with risk of neurovascular structures [5–8]. Ulnar nerve subluxation and prior transposition increase the risk of ulnar nerve injury during the creation of anteromedial portal as the main viewing portal in arthroscopic OCA. In addition, less intuitive visualization compared with traditional open procedures contributes to a prolonged learning curve.

The concept of "transfossa" has originally been used for "OK procedure" by eliminating fossa with bony spurs in olecranon and coronoid fossa. However, it is not recommendable to routinely excessive eliminating fossa in arthroscopic transfossa approach but only limited resection mainly for visualization purpose with saving bony column of distal humerus as much and then, resurfacing around connecting fossa which is the principle of OCA. Since the direction of visualization through the fossa gives more intuitive understanding of anterior pathology.

Supplementary Information The online version contains supplementary material available at https://doi.org/10.1007/978-981-95-3732-7_21.

J.-M. Kwak (✉)
Department of Orthopedic Surgery, Uijeongbu Eulji Medical Center, College of Medicine, Eulji University, Uijeongbu, Republic of Korea

E. Kholinne
Faculty of Medicine, Universitas Trisakti, Jakarta, Indonesia

I.-H. Jeon
Department of Orthopedic Surgery, Asan Medical Center, University of Ulsan College of Medicine, Seoul, Republic of Korea

2 Indications

The typical indication for the arthroscopic transfossa approach includes that of conventional arthroscopic osteocapsular arthroplasty, which is

I.-H. Jeon et al. (eds.), *Elbow Arthroscopy*, https://doi.org/10.1007/978-981-95-3732-7_21

J.-M. Kwak et al. / Osteoarthritis and Cartilage xxx (xxxx) xxx

	Grade 0	Grade I (uni-fossa)		Grade II (bi-fossa)	Grade III
		IA	IP		
Fossa Involvement	None	Anterior	Posterior	Both	Any
Joint Involvement	Intact				Narrowing

CT Image

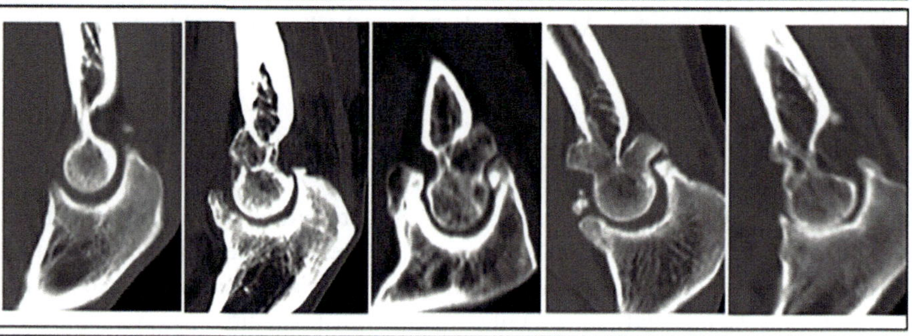

Definition	
Involved Fossa	More than 50% osteophyte in the fossa
Joint Narrowing	Less than 1mm in the more than 50% of articular space

Fig. 21.1 Kwak and Jeon classification for Elbow OA

functional loss of elbow motion caused by trauma, heterotopic ossification (HO), malunion, arthritis, osteochondritis dissecans, neurologic imbalance, or prior surgery [6, 8–12]. However, transfossa approach allows successful management of severe capsular contracture by accessing directly the anterior compartment through the olecranon fossa, and ulnar nerve problem such as ulnar nerve subluxation and prior transposition surgery, since the procedure saves anteromedial portal of the joint. Especially, it would be perfect indication for the posterior dominant spur of elbow OA (Grade IP, Kwak and Jeon classification, Fig. 21.1) [13]. For patients with a functional arc of motion, defined as flexion from 30° to 130° preoperatively, the indication for surgery is painful impingement and/or functional impairment due to the need for terminal elbow extension. The arthroscopic transfossa approach can be more useful in advanced stiff elbows that have severe capsular contracture and/or a large amount of bony spurs or loose bodies in the anterior compartment that make it difficult to access the anterior compartment. It is also effectively applicable for the management of extension-dominant stiff elbows that have pathology mostly in the posterior compartment and mainly require anterior capsular resection in the anterior compartment.

3 Contraindications

Contraindications of the arthroscopic transfossa approach also follow the indications of arthroscopic osteocapsular arthroplasty and include (I) heterotopic ossification that is inseparable from a nerve and (II) the need for implant removal. A relative contraindication is substantial distortion of anatomy or anatomic landmarks for the anterolateral portal. Severe capsular contracture, prior subcutaneous transposition of the ulnar nerve, failed prior contracture release, and/or extensive scarring from skin grafts or flaps are not contraindications.

4 Step-by-Step Surgical Procedure

4.1 Patient Positioning

General anesthetic is administered, and the patient is placed in the lateral decubitus position with the arm resting on a custom-made arm holder specifically designed for elbow arthroscopy. Wrap a tourniquet around the arm [6, 14, 15]. The shoulder is flexed to between 90° and 100°, and the elbow rests at 90° of flexion (Fig. 21.2). For conventional arthroscopic OCA, the patient positioning is critical so that adequate access to the coronoid and coronoid fossa is possible without the working instruments hitting the chest of the patient that usually happens with anteromedial portal. The arthroscopic transfossa approach reduces the problem since it allows saving the anteromedial portal.

4.2 Surgical Steps

The surgical step basically follows "safety-driven strategy," as Dr. O'Driscoll first described [16–18], and is used in a standardized sequence of four steps: (I) Get in and establish a view, (II) create a space in which to work, (III) bone removal, and (IV) capsulectomy in each compartment. However, in the arthroscopic transfossa approach, the bony procedure should be completed in both compartments, and capsule release should be done next in both compartments, since these two compartments are going to be connected after making the transfossa portal.

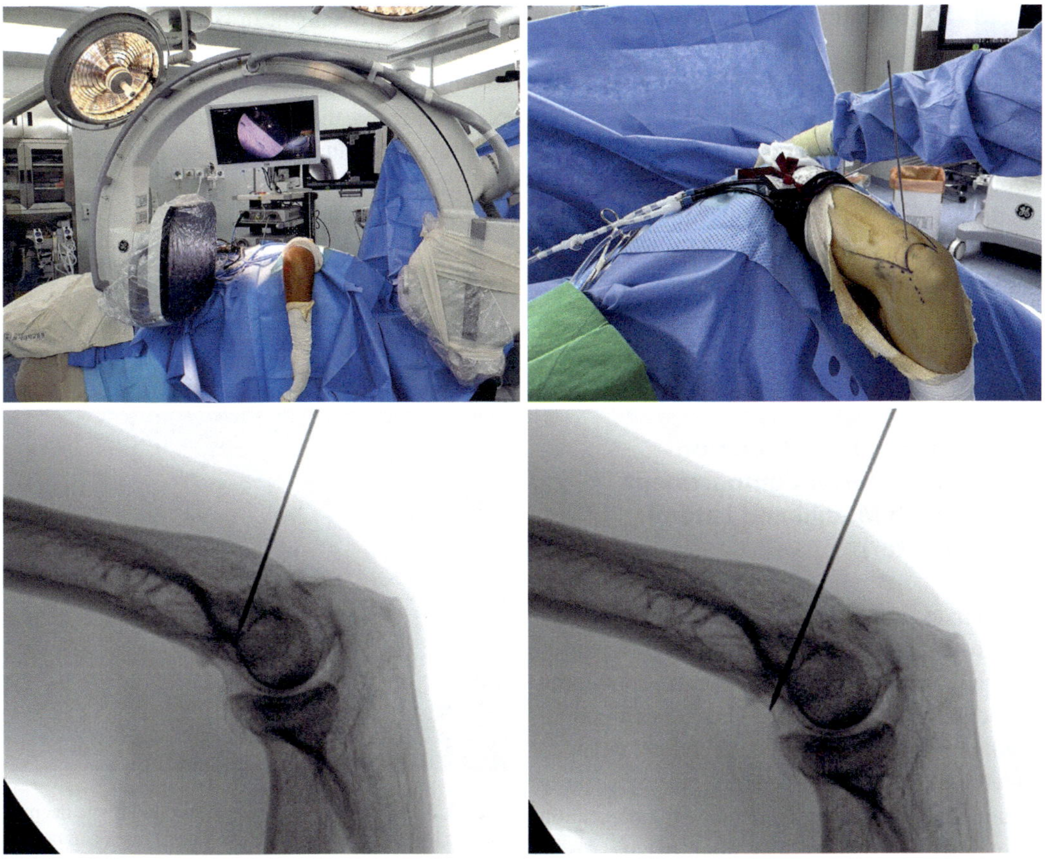

Fig. 21.2 For marking, a 2.0 mm or thicker K-wire or a cannulated drill guide pin can be used. Following this, initial enlargement is performed using a cannulated drill, which serves as the basic enlargement point

4.3 Creation of Posterior and Posterolateral Portal

Begin work in the posterior compartment with the arthroscope in the posterolateral portal and the working instrument in the posterior portal. Starting posteriorly allows you to address those parts of the elbow that are most challenging if swelling occurs, including the medial and lateral gutters.

4.4 Surgical Marking of the Deep Portion of Olecranon Fossa

After clearance of bursa tissue and some part of the fat pad, the surgeon can access the olecranon fossa. Watching the olecranon fossa from posterolateral portal, the assistant manipulates the patient's arm to make full extension several time. In the meantime, surgeons recognize the point where the olecranon tip is heading to (Video 21.1). If it is not obvious what the olecranon tip is, measure the olecranon diameter using the probe and temporarily mark the center of olecranon with electrocautery device. If you get the heading point of the olecranon tip where the deep portion of olecranon fossa is, bony marking is possible by making small hole using 2.0 mm K-wire. C-arm-guided confirmation can be followed (Fig. 21.2).

4.5 Osteophyte Resection in Posterior Compartment (with Medial and Lateral Gutter)

Osteophytes are universally present in hypertrophic osteoarthritis and are common in posttraumatic arthritis. A retractor is commonly placed through the proximal posterolateral portal to minimize the risk of tissues becoming wrapped up around the burr especially when working around the ulnar nerve. To recreate the olecranon fossa, identify the original floor of the fossa, which is already marked, and remove osteophytes from it and from the surrounding margins. The olecranon is restored to its normal shape by removing osteophytes from the tip and the sides (Video 21.2).

4.6 Connecting and Widening of the Fossa

After the bony clearance around fossa, deepening the fossa centering the marked deep fossa can be performed using arthroscopic burr (Fig. 21.3, Video 21.3). Once you are approaching the anterior compartment, periosteum like white tissue will be discovered. Debridement of transfossa using the electrocautery device is recommended if the diameter of the hole is about 5–6 mm, which allows the 4.5 mm scope to pass through (Video 21.4). Preoperative CT scan can give information about the depth of fossa and number of bony spurs in coronoid fossa. If the bony spur is dominant in coronoid fossa, a few more millimeters widening would be acceptable to eliminate the bony spurs in coronoid fossa. In older patients, the fossa is usually paper-thin, and this procedure can be completed within a few minutes.

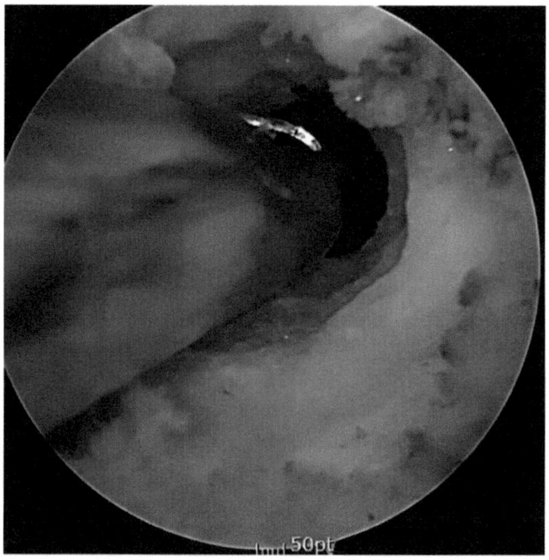

Fig. 21.3 After the bony clearance around fossa, deepening the fossa centering the marked deep fossa can be performed using arthroscopic burr. It is recommended to use the direct posterior portal as the working portal and the posterolateral portal as the viewing portal

4.7 Creation of Anterolateral Portal as Working Portal

Only anterolateral portal is usually enough in arthroscopic transfossa approach. The anterolateral portal is at the level of the radiocapitellar joint articulation. At that level in the arm, the radial nerve lies anterior to the center of radial head. Radial and posterior interosseous nerve injuries caused by placement of the anterolateral portal have been reported. "Needle-and-knife technique," as reported by O'Driscoll et al., is the recommended method for safe anterolateral portal placement [17, 18].

While viewing the lateral capsule and radiocapitellar joint with the arthroscope through the transfossa portal, a spinal needle is inserted through the skin incision for the anterolateral portal and into the joint (Video 21.5). A 70° scope would be essential to visualize lateral capsule and radiocapitellar joint. The orientation of the needle is adjusted until it lies directly anterior to the radiocapitellar articulation. The assistant holds the needle to maintain that position and orientation.

4.8 Osteophyte Resection in Anterior Compartment

Osteophyte of coronoid can usually be easily removed by transverse osteotomy using the osteotome from the anterolateral portal. The line for osteotomy should be located 1–2 mm above the anterior capsular insertion. Be cautious not to involve the anterior capsule, which is an important indicator of the original coronoid height (Fig. 21.4, Video 21.6). Loose bodies also can be removed through the working portal.

If the coronoid spur is not very dominant, further resection is usually not necessary. If further coronoid spur resection is required, the widening of anterior rim of the hole can be applied. At this point, the tip of arthroscope should be slightly out for showing the anterior rim of coronoid fossa (Fig. 21.5).

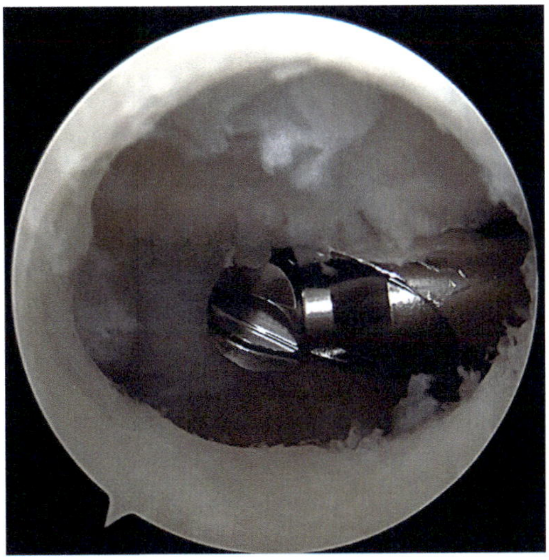

Fig. 21.4 Through the anterolateral portal, the anterior compartment of the elbow can be easily accessed, and the anterior margin of the transfossa portal can be debrided using arthroscopic burr

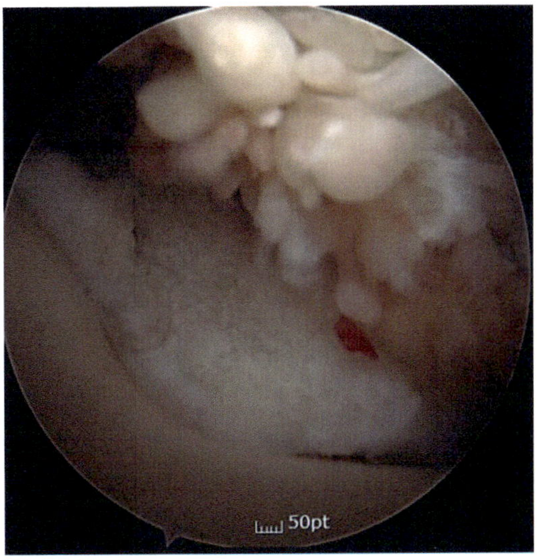

Fig. 21.5 The resected coronoid osteophyte viewing from transfossa portal. The safe line for osteophyte resection of coronoid should be located 1–2 mm above the anterior capsular insertion. Be caution not to involve the anterior capsule that is an important indicator original coronoid height

4.9 Capsular Release in Anterior Compartment

Capsular release should be started from the bone at the capsule insertion (Fig. 21.6, Video 21.7). When detaching the capsule from the bone using electrocautery, the head of the device should be facing the bone but only contact the capsule at the bone-to-capsule junction, and point-by-point shooting can prevent potential neurovascular damage. If the anterior capsule is not the main pathology, capsular detachment from the bone with forced full extension is usually enough.

4.10 Capsular Release in Posterior Compartment

Release the capsule according to the severity of the flexion loss. If the patient lacks flexion, as is usually the case, the posterior capsulectomy includes not only release along the supracondylar ridges but also posteromedial and posterolateral capsular releases. The extent of the capsular release in each gutter depends on the severity of the loss of flexion. With severe loss of flexion, continue the release through the posterior bundle of the medial collateral ligament on the medial side and to the radial head on the lateral side. If a decompression of the ulnar nerve is performed, the posteromedial capsule release can be performed through that incision.

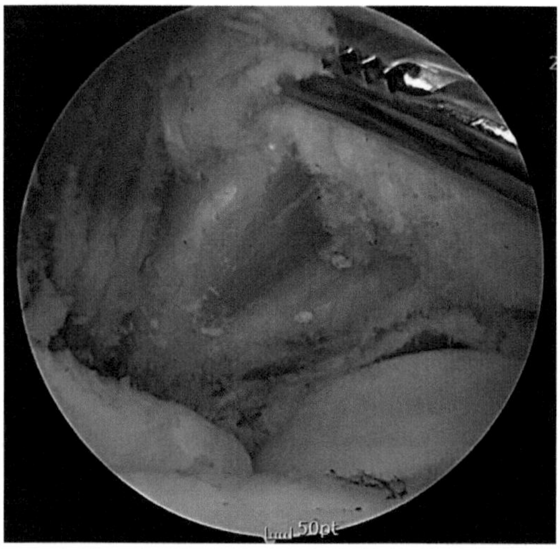

Fig. 21.6 The released anterior capsule. The capsule was released from the bony attachment using electrocautery device or arthroscopic shaver. The instrument should be kept facing the bony side throughout the entire capsular release procedure

4.11 Wound Closure

Postoperatively, check the nerve function before performing a regional block and commencing continuous passive motion. Early range of motion exercise is started through a range of motion equal to that achieved during surgery. Instruct the patient to perform exercises every hour for 5 min to minimize soft-tissue or nerve problems due to continuous pressure or stretching.

Caution Points

- *Neurovascular safety*: Maintain a safe distance from the ulnar nerve during portal placement and capsular release [19–23].
- *Fluid management*: Avoid excessive intra-articular fluid pressure to prevent extravasation and compartment syndrome.
- *Stepwise approach*: Address osteophyte resection before capsular contractures to minimize bleeding and maintain visualization.
- *Anatomical variations*: Be aware of anatomical distortions due to prior surgeries or trauma, which may alter standard portal placement.

5 Key Procedure Highlight

When creating the transfossa portal, gradual enlargement is necessary. For marking, a 2.0 mm or thicker K-wire or a cannulated drill guide pin can be used. Following this, initial enlargement is performed using a cannulated drill, which serves as the basic enlargement point. Subsequently, an arthroscopic burr is used to gradually enlarge the portal in a circular motion. It is recommended to use the direct posterior portal as the working portal and the posterolateral portal as the viewing portal.

References

1. Blonna D, Bellato E, Marini E, Scelsi M, Castoldi F. Arthroscopic treatment of stiff elbow. ISRN Surg. 2011;2011:378135. https://doi.org/10.5402/2011/378135.
2. Jupiter JB, O'Driscoll SW, Cohen MS. The assessment and management of the stiff elbow. Instr Course Lect. 2003;52:93–111.
3. Koh KH, Lim TK, Lee HI, Park MJ. Surgical treatment of elbow stiffness caused by post-traumatic heterotopic ossification. J Shoulder Elb Surg. 2013;22:1128–34. https://doi.org/10.1016/j.jse.2013.04.019.
4. Kwak JM, Kholinne E, Sun Y, Lim S, Koh KH, Jeon IH. Clinical outcome of Osteocapsular arthroplasty for primary osteoarthritis of the elbow: comparison of arthroscopic and open procedure. Arthroscopy. 2019;35:1083–9. https://doi.org/10.1016/j.arthro.2018.11.057.
5. Bachman DR, Fitzsimmons JS, O'Driscoll SW. Safety of arthroscopic vs. Open/combined heterotopic ossification removal around the elbow. Arthroscopy. In Press. 2019; https://doi.org/10.1016/j.arthro.2019.09.010.
6. Dodson CC, Nho SJ, Williams RJ 3rd, Altchek DW. Elbow arthroscopy. J Am Acad Orthop Surg. 2008;16:574–85. https://doi.org/10.5435/00124635-200810000-00003.
7. Field LD, Altchek DW, Warren RF, O'Brien SJ, Skyhar MJ, Wickiewicz TL. Arthroscopic anatomy of the lateral elbow: a comparison of three portals. Arthroscopy. 1994;10:602–7. https://doi.org/10.1016/s0749-8063(05)80055-6.
8. Gramstad GD, Galatz LM. Management of elbow osteoarthritis. J Bone Joint Surg Am. 2006;88:421–30. https://doi.org/10.2106/jbjs.E.00568.
9. Blonna D, Lee GC, O'Driscoll SW. Arthroscopic restoration of terminal elbow extension in high-level athletes. Am J Sports Med. 2010;38:2509–15. https://doi.org/10.1177/0363546510376727.
10. Gay DM, Raphael BS, Weiland AJ. Revision arthroscopic contracture release in the elbow resulting in an ulnar nerve transection: a case report. J Bone Joint Surg Am. 2010;92:1246–9. https://doi.org/10.2106/jbjs.I.00555.
11. Ilahi OA, Strausser DW, Gabel GT. Post-traumatic heterotopic ossification about the elbow. Orthopedics. 1998;21:265–8.
12. Jupiter JB, Ring D. Operative treatment of post-traumatic proximal radioulnar synostosis. J Bone Joint Surg Am. 1998;80:248–57. https://doi.org/10.2106/00004623-199802000-00012.
13. Kwak JM, Kholinne E, Sun Y, Alhazmi AM, Koh KH, Jeon IH. Intraobserver and interobserver reliability of the computed tomography-based radiographic classification of primary elbow osteoarthritis: comparison with plain radiograph-based classification and clinical assessment. Osteoarthr Cartil. 2019;27:1057–63. https://doi.org/10.1016/j.joca.2019.03.004.
14. Hackl M, Lappen S, Burkhart KJ, Leschinger T, Scaal M, Muller LP, Wegmann K. Elbow positioning and joint insufflation substantially influence median and radial nerve locations. Clin Orthop Relat Res. 2015;473:3627–34. https://doi.org/10.1007/s11999-015-4442-3.
15. Hodax JD, Blood TD, Kleinhenz DT, Gorman M, Biercevicz A, DaSilva M. An anatomic evaluation of arthroscopic access to the radial head. Arthroscopy. 2017;33:953–8. https://doi.org/10.1016/j.arthro.2017.01.031.
16. O'Driscoll SW, Blonna D. Osteocapsular arthroplasty of the elbow: surgical technique. Essent Surg Tech. 2013;3:e15 11. https://doi.org/10.2106/JBJS.ST.M.00002.
17. Park SE, Bachman DR, O'Driscoll SW. The safety of using proximal anteromedial portals in elbow arthroscopy with prior ulnar nerve transposition. Arthroscopy. 2016;32:1003–9. https://doi.org/10.1016/j.arthro.2015.12.043.
18. Thaveepunsan S, Shields MN, O'Driscoll SW. The needle-and-knife technique: a safe technique for anterolateral portal placement in elbow arthroscopy. Orthop J Sports Med. 2019;7:2325967118817232. https://doi.org/10.1177/2325967118817232.
19. Blonna D, Wolf JM, Fitzsimmons JS, O'Driscoll SW. Prevention of nerve injury during arthroscopic capsulectomy of the elbow utilizing a safety-driven strategy. J Bone Joint Surg Am. 2013;95:1373–81. https://doi.org/10.2106/jbjs.K.00972.
20. Kelly EW, Morrey BF, O'Driscoll SW. Complications of elbow arthroscopy. J Bone Joint Surg Am. 2001;83:25–34. https://doi.org/10.2106/00004623-200101000-00004.
21. Lee EK, Namdari S, Hosalkar HS, Keenan MA, Baldwin KD. Clinical results of the excision of heterotopic bone around the elbow: a systematic review. J Shoulder Elb Surg. 2013;22:716–22. https://doi.org/10.1016/j.jse.2012.11.020.
22. Marshall PD, Fairclough JA, Johnson SR, Evans EJ. Avoiding nerve damage during elbow arthroscopy. J Bone Joint Surg Br. 1993;75:129–31.
23. Steinmann SP. Elbow arthroscopy: where are we now? Arthroscopy. 2007;23:1231–6. https://doi.org/10.1016/j.arthro.2007.08.008.

Arthroscopic Partial Radial Head Resection for Elbow Osteoarthritis

22

Michael Hackl and Sebastian Lappen

1 Background

Radial head resection is a surgical procedure performed for a range of conditions, including osteoarthritis, inflammatory arthritis, or, in rare instances, radial head fractures. In the context of osteoarthritis, this procedure is more commonly performed for post-traumatic arthritis, particularly following fractures, rather than for primary osteoarthritis. The decision to proceed with radial head resection is influenced by various factors, including the extent of joint degeneration, deformity of the radial head, associated wear of the capitellum, and the patient's functional requirements. While radial head resection is a valid option for treating certain cases, it is not typically the first choice. Preservation of the radial head is often preferred to maintain joint function and delay more extensive interventions. However, it may be considered when conservative treatment or radial head preserving techniques such as arthroscopic debridement or proximal radial shortening osteotomy fail to provide sufficient symptom relief.

Radial head resection can be performed using traditional open techniques or minimally invasive arthroscopic methods, tailored to the clinical context. The use of arthroscopic techniques is becoming increasingly common, reflecting a broader trend toward minimally invasive procedures. Arthroscopy provides significant advantages, including reduced blood loss, lower risk of infection, faster recovery times, and easier evaluation of concomitant pathologies, making it an appealing option for both surgeons and patients. Despite these benefits, arthroscopy is technically demanding and requires substantial expertise, which may limit its adoption on a wider scale.

2 Anatomy and Biomechanics of the Radial Head

The radial head plays a critical role in elbow joint mechanics and upper limb function. Articulating with the capitellum of the humerus and contacting the radial notch of the ulna, it is integral to the proximal radioulnar joint, enabling forearm pronation and supination. The radial neck connects the head to the radius and serves as a transitional zone that aids in mobility while ensuring structural support. Ligamentous attachments, particularly the annular ligament, secure the radial head against the radial notch and stabilize the joint during forearm rotation.

Radial head resection demands a thorough understanding of the anatomy due to the radial head's critical role in elbow stability and load

M. Hackl (✉) · S. Lappen
Department of Orthopaedic and Trauma Surgery, University Medical Centre Mannheim, Medical Faculty Mannheim, University of Heidelberg, Mannheim, Germany
e-mail: michael.hackl@medma.uni-heidelberg.de

I.-H. Jeon et al. (eds.), *Elbow Arthroscopy*, https://doi.org/10.1007/978-981-95-3732-7_22

distribution. The radial head is essential for maintaining elbow stability, particularly as a secondary stabilizer against valgus stress and lateral force transmission when the forearm is extended or loaded. Additionally, it contributes to elbow stability by tensioning the lateral collateral ligament (LCL) complex.

The radial head also plays a significant role in axial load transmission, bearing substantial force during activities such as lifting or pushing. The radial head is responsible for transmitting up to 60% of the axial force applied through the elbow, with this percentage varying based on the degree of flexion [1–3]. When the radial head is removed, the load shifts primarily to the ulnohumeral joint.

3 Indications and Contraindications

Arthroscopic partial radial head resection is indicated for various conditions affecting the elbow joint, particularly when conservative treatments fail to alleviate symptoms. The goal is to relieve pain, improve joint function, while minimizing invasiveness. Stability and congruity of the ulnohumeral joint is an absolute prerequisite when considering radial head resection. This procedure is primarily used to address issues such as:

- *Radiocapitellar osteoarthritis*: Arthroscopic partial resection of the radial head may be indicated for the management of painful radiocapitellar osteoarthritis. This procedure is often combined with arthroscopic debridement and capsular release to improve joint function and relieve pain.
- *Rheumatoid arthritis*: In advanced cases of rheumatoid arthritis affecting the elbow, arthroscopic partial excision of the radial head can be performed to relieve motion-related pain and crepitus, as well as to address joint narrowing and sclerosis.
- *Radial head fractures*: In rare cases of isolated radial head fractures without concomitant fractures or collateral ligament injuries, small (<25% of the circumference) and non-reconstructable fracture fragments can be removed arthroscopically to improve joint function if the defect does not engage with the capitulum [4].
- *Malunited radial head fragments*: When malunion occurs following ORIF of radiocapitellar fractures, resection of the malunited radial head fragments may be required to restore joint function, especially forearm rotation, and alleviate associated symptoms.

While arthroscopic partial radial head resection is effective for specific conditions, it is important to consider the patient's overall health, the extent of joint damage, and potential alternatives such as debridement/reshaping of the radial head, radial shortening osteotomy or radial head replacement. Whenever radial head fracture fragments are displaced into the soft tissues surrounding the neck/metaphysis, meticulous open dissection may be preferred for proper excision without putting the posterior interosseous nerve at risk of injury.

Radial head resection should be carefully indicated in young and high-demand patients, as excision might lead to elongation of the interosseous membrane over time and thus lead to painful ulna impaction and/or stump impingement of the proximal radius.

4 Surgical Technique

4.1 Preoperative Planning

A thorough clinical assessment is mandatory. Patients with painful (post-traumatic) osteoarthritis of the radiocapitellar joint typically experience pain upon palpation of the radiocapitellar joint space and exhibit a positive grind test. Forearm rotation may or may not be (painfully) restricted. Conventional radiographs and MRI or CT imaging is required to evaluate the severity of joint degeneration as well as concomitant pathologies (Fig. 22.1).

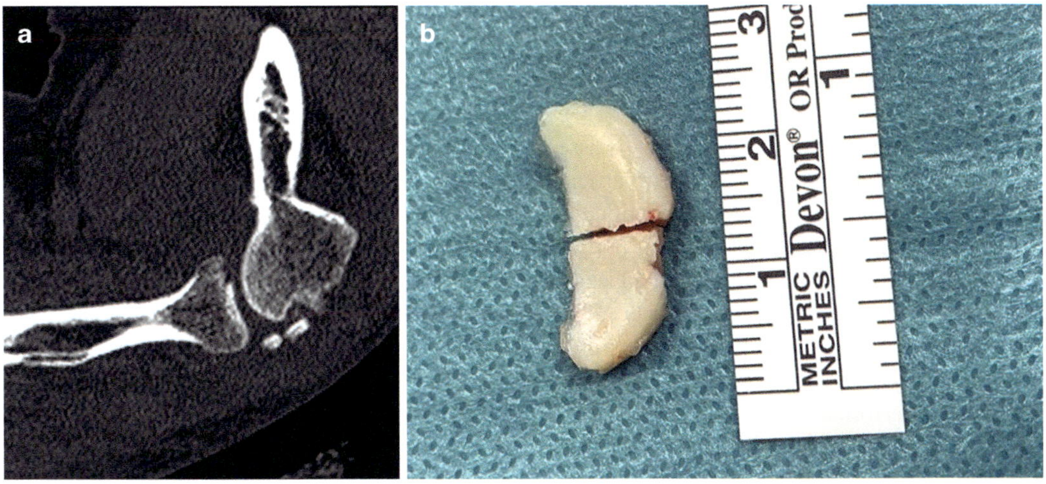

Fig. 22.1 (**a**) CT scan of a 62-year-old patient with an osteochondral fracture of the radial head. The patient presented 2 weeks following trauma. Arthroscopic partial radial head resection was indicated and performed. (**b**) Intraoperative image of the arthroscopically resected fragments

4.2 Patient Positioning and Anesthesia

The patient is typically positioned in the lateral decubitus or prone position with the arm suspended to allow unobstructed movement of the elbow joint. General anesthesia or regional blocks are used to provide adequate pain control.

4.3 Arthroscopic Portal Placement

Standard arthroscopic portals are established, including:

- The *anterolateral portal* is placed 1–2 cm proximal and anterior to the lateral epicondyle. This portal provides access to the anterior compartment of the elbow and is established first in the hands of the authors. It allows for visualization of the anterior structures, including the radial head. Proper placement of this portal is crucial to avoid damage to nearby neurovascular structures, especially the radial nerve.
- The *anteromedial portal* is placed approximately 1–2 cm proximal and anterior to the medial epicondyle and is located anterior to the lateral intermuscular septum. It is established in an inside-out fashion in the hands of the authors. This portal provides access to the anterior compartment of the elbow and is particularly useful for instrumentation and addressing structures such as loose bodies or osteophytes of the coronoid or the radial and coronoid fossa. Careful placement of this portal is essential to minimize the risk of injury to the ulnar and median nerves as well as the brachial vessels.
- A *high posterolateral portal* is established midway between the olecranon tip and the lateral epicondyle to first get an overview of the posterior aspect of the ulnohumeral joint. Loose bodies and osteophytes are here typically removed through a trans-tricipital working portal. After completion of this task, the arthroscope is moved along the lateral border of the olecranon into the posterolateral aspect of the elbow. This allows an excellent overview of the radiocapitellar joint and of the posterolateral aspect of the ulnohumeral joint.
- A *soft-spot portal* is used as a working portal to resect the typically present, hypertrophic plica and to debride and remove the radial head.

4.4 Procedure

Step 1: Diagnostic arthroscopy and adhesiolysis

The anterolateral portal is utilized to assess the ulno-trochlear and radiocapitellar articulations (Fig. 22.2). Loose bodies are identified and removed via the anteromedial working portal as needed (Fig. 22.3). Synovectomy and adhesiolysis—especially around anterior aspect of the radial head—and removal of osteophytes of the coronoid and in the coronoid and radial fossa is additionally performed.

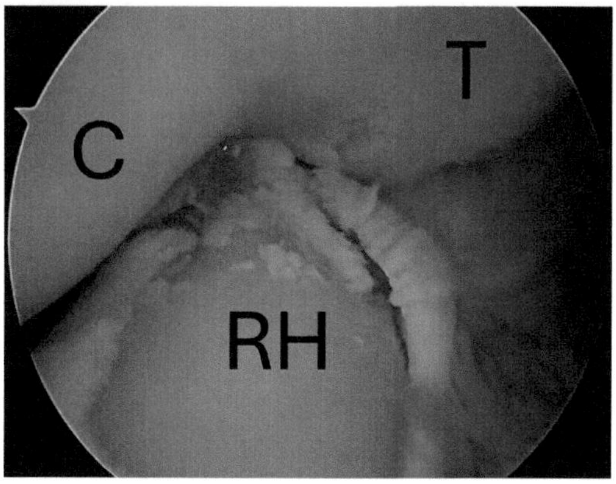

Fig. 22.2 Arthroscopic visualization of advanced radial head arthritis (RH radial head, C capitellum, T trochlea)

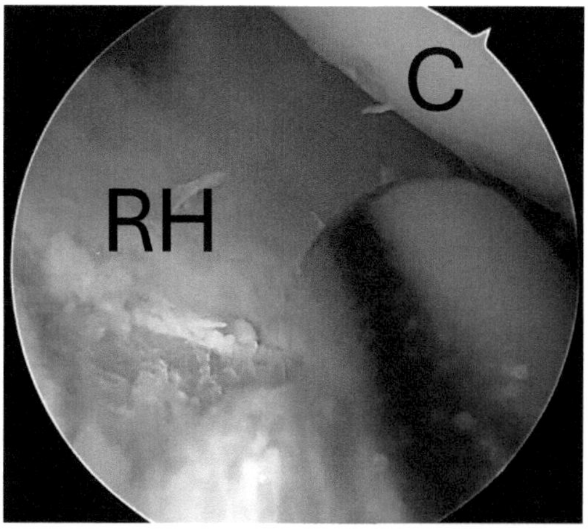

Fig. 22.3 Resection of chondral remnants with a 4 mm shaver blade through a soft-spot working portal (RH radial head, C capitellum)

After establishing the high posterolateral portal, loose bodies and osteophytes of the olecranon and the olecranon fossa are removed through a trans-tricipital working portal. After completion of this task, the arthroscope is moved into the posterolateral joint aspect.

Step 2: Surface resection

To widen the narrow radiocapitellar joint space, the chondral remnants on the articular surface of the radial head are resected with a 4 mm shaver blade through a soft-spot working portal. Forearm rotation helps to achieve full access to all aspects of the radial head (Fig. 22.3). The resection is deemed complete when at least 5 mm of space is achieved between the radial head and the capitellum.

Step 3: Radial head resection/co-plaining

A 4–5 mm arthroscopic burr is used to progressively remove the bony portion of the radial head through the soft-spot portal (Fig. 22.4). Once again, rotational maneuvers provide access to the entire radial head.

Step 4: Peripheral rim resection

The remaining peripheral rim of cartilage is excised using a combination of punches and graspers to complete the resection. Any remaining loose fragments are carefully removed, and the area is thoroughly irrigated to ensure a clean surgical field.

Step 5: Confirmation of resection adequacy

The completion of the radial head resection can be confirmed by visualizing the cortical bone of the radial shaft arthroscopically (Fig. 22.6). Additionally, an adequate radiocapitellar space can be assessed arthroscopically, using the width of a 4–5 mm burr as a reference. Radiographic or fluoroscopic imaging can then be used to verify that an 8–10 mm radiocapitellar space has been achieved, confirming that the resection is complete (Fig. 22.6).

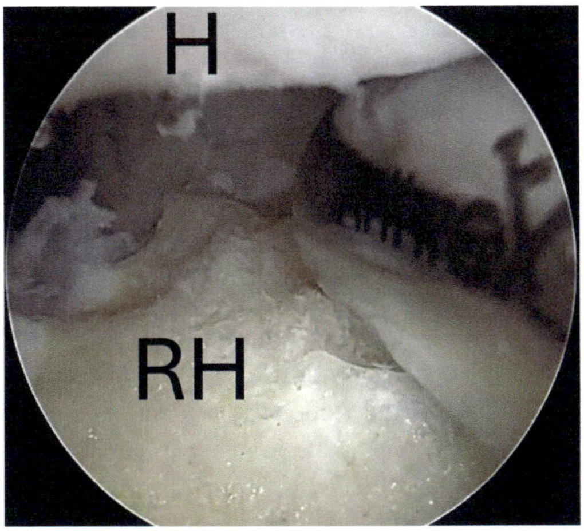

Fig. 22.4 Resection of the bony portion of the radial head with a 4–5 mm arthroscopic burr (RH radial head, H humerus)

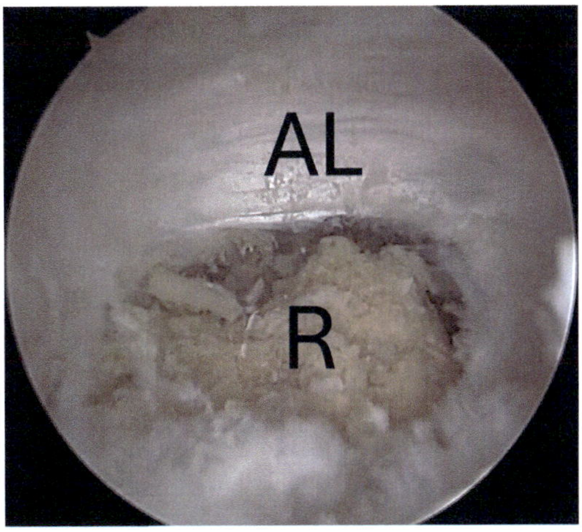

Fig. 22.5 Completed resection of the radial head (R radius, AL annular ligament)

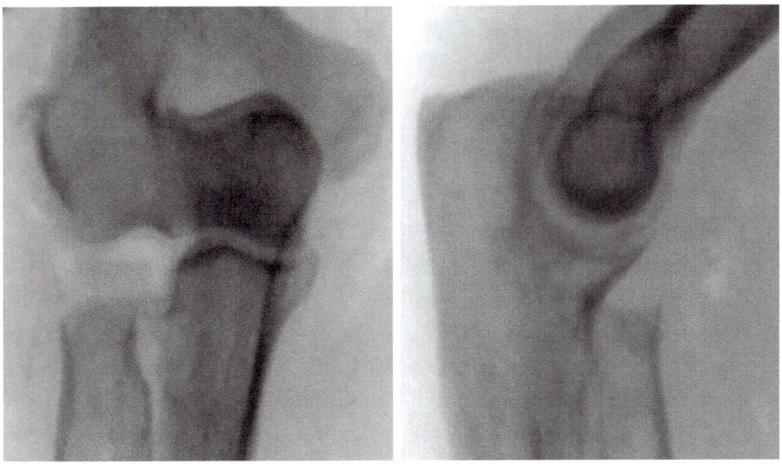

Fig. 22.6 The postoperative X-ray demonstrates the resection of the radial head with an adequately wide radiocapitellar space

4.5 Postoperative Management

Postoperatively, the elbow is immobilized briefly in a sling to allow initial healing, which is switched to a portal dressing on the fourth day. The rehabilitation plan focuses on early passive and active range-of-motion exercises from week 1 to week 6, combined with gradual strengthening. Elbow motion and forearm rotation are unrestricted. Light activities can usually resume after 6 weeks, with heavy work typically permitted after 3 months.

5 Complications and Pitfalls

Potential complications include:

- *Iatrogenic instability*: Elbow joint instability can result if the resection compromises the stabilizing structures—especially the lateral collateral ligament. Great care has to be taken to avoid inadvertent injury to the lateral capsulo-ligamentous complex when resecting the radial head with the burr.

- *Nerve injury*: Careful attention is necessary to prevent nerve damage especially when working in the anterior and posteromedial joint compartment. During radial head resection itself, the arthroscope and the shaver are in a posterolateral position and therefore the risk of nerve injury is minimized. It is crucial, however, to ensure that resection is limited to the radial neck to avoid injury to the posterior interosseous nerve.
- *Excessive or insufficient resection*: Both excessive and insufficient resection of the radial head can lead to complications. Excessive resection risks causing impingement of the remaining radius with the proximal ulna, which may lead to persistent pain during forearm rotation. Conversely, insufficient resection can result in continued contact between the radial head and capitellum, leading to joint wear and associated discomfort.

6 Tips and Tricks

- *Preventing fluid extravasation*: Take care to avoid iatrogenic tears in the capsule to prevent fluid leakage and associated swelling.
- *Enhancing visualization*: If visualization is hindered by clots, synovitis, or fluid leakage, use a blunt Wissinger rod through any portal for retraction to improve the surgical field.
- *Removing large fragments*: Use a broad-jawed grasper for the en masse removal of large fragments through the soft-spot portal.
- *Creating space in chronic cases*: Utilize small joint instruments, such as 3 mm shavers and burrs, to create adequate working space for larger surgical tools.
- *Efficient excision*: Gradually increase the size of shavers and burrs to facilitate faster and more effective excision.

7 Outcomes and Prognosis

Studies indicate that arthroscopic partial radial head resection can provide significant relief from pain, improve range of motion, and maintain joint stability. However, outcomes are closely tied to the degree of initial damage and patient adherence to rehabilitation.

McLaughlin et al. found that arthroscopic radial head resection for early, isolated radiocapitellar arthritis leads to significant improvements in motion and outcomes [5]. Patients who had radial head excision alone showed greater gains in flexion (29°) and extension (38°), with a total arc improvement of 62°, compared to 46° in those who also had ulnohumeral arthroplasty. The average Andrews-Carson score improved nearly 100 points after radial head excision. Similarly, Temporin et al. reported that in 14 patients (15 elbows) with over 2 years' follow-up, arthroscopic partial excision of the radial head reduced motion pain and increased range of motion from 115° flexion and −39° extension preoperatively to 127° flexion and −27° extension [6]. Pain resolved in all cases, and joint congruity was maintained, with only two cases showing slight narrowing after 4 years. The study concluded this method effectively alleviates symptoms and may serve as a valuable alternative to more invasive procedures. Savoie et al. performed an arthroscopic modification of the Outerbridge-Kashiwagi procedure, including radial head resection in 7 of 24 patients with significant radiocapitellar degeneration [7]. This approach achieved notable pain relief and enhanced range of motion. Radial head resection was deemed especially beneficial for cases with substantial radiocapitellar involvement, yielding favorable outcomes and functional improvements in most patients. Rotman et al. recently introduced arthroscopic matched osteoplasty of the radial head (AMOR) as a novel technique that stands out from established methods by reshaping the radial head to match the natural curvature of the capitellum, thereby maintaining joint biomechanics and stability [8]. This approach specifically targets decompression of the radiocapitellar joint while preserving the ulnohumeral joint and minimizing the risk of instability and altered kinematics. Reported outcomes showed a decrease in the mean pain score on a numeric rating scale from 8/10 to 3/10, with 75% of patients (six out of eight) expressing satisfaction and demonstrating clinical improvement. However, two patients experienced only short-term benefits, with one eventually undergoing total elbow arthroplasty due to persistent pain.

While Avisar et al. reported generally positive long-term outcomes and high patient satisfaction following radial head resection, they noted some functional limitations [9]. Patients experienced reduced elbow range of motion and grip strength in the operated hand compared to the non-operated hand, alongside minor proximal radial migration. Similarly, Singh et al. reported several complications following radial head resection, including moderate to severe postoperative pain and instances of decreased joint stability [10]. Nonetheless, the authors concluded that radial head excision offered superior functional outcomes compared to arthroplasty.

In summary, arthroscopic radial head resection has shown substantial benefits in pain reduction, improved range of motion, and preserved joint stability, making it a promising option for cases with severe radiocapitellar arthritis. However, patient outcomes are influenced by initial joint damage and adherence to rehabilitation, with some cases experiencing complications like pain, stability issues, and reduced strength.

References

1. Morrey BF, An KN, Stormont TJ. Force transmission through the radial head. J Bone Joint Surg Am. 1988;70(2):250–6.
2. Halls AA, Travill A. Transmission of pressures across the elbow joint. Anat Rec. 1964;150:243–7. https://doi.org/10.1002/ar.1091500305.
3. Hackl M, Wegmann K, Kahmann SL, Heinze N, Staat M, Neiss WF, et al. Radial shortening osteotomy reduces radiocapitellar contact pressures while preserving valgus stability of the elbow. Knee Surg Sports Traumatol Arthrosc. 2017;25(7):2280–8. https://doi.org/10.1007/s00167-017-4468-z.
4. Bhatia DN. Arthroscopic resection of the radial head. In: Bain G, Eygendaal D, van Riet RP, editors. Surgical techniques for trauma and sports related injuries of the elbow. Berlin/Heidelberg: Springer Berlin Heidelberg; 2020. p. 581–8.
5. McLaughlin RE 2nd, Savoie FH 3rd, Field LD, Ramsey JR. Arthroscopic treatment of the arthritic elbow due to primary radiocapitellar arthritis. Arthroscopy. 2006;22(1):63–9. https://doi.org/10.1016/j.arthro.2005.10.013.
6. Temporin K, Shimada K, Oura K, Owaki H. Arthroscopic partial excision of the radial head for advanced rheumatoid elbow. Orthopedics. 2022;45(4):209–14. https://doi.org/10.3928/01477447-20220225-08.
7. Savoie FH 3rd, Nunley PD, Field LD. Arthroscopic management of the arthritic elbow: indications, technique, and results. J Shoulder Elb Surg. 1999;8(3):214–9. https://doi.org/10.1016/s1058-2746(99)90131-3.
8. Rotman D, Watts AC. Arthroscopic matched osteoplasty of the radial head for painful radiocapitellar osteoarthritis: surgical technique and case series. Clin Shoulder Elb. 2024;27(3):309–15. https://doi.org/10.5397/cise.2024.00073.
9. Avisar E, Persitz J, Shohat N, Tamir E, Assaraf E, Keren T. Does radial head resection impair hand and wrist function? A long-term follow-up. J Orthop Trauma. 2021;35(12):e486–e90. https://doi.org/10.1097/bot.0000000000002126.
10. Singh AK, Jidge A, Ramteke U, Venkateswaran N, Rokade H, Mulje SM, et al. Functional outcome of elbow kinematics in radial head excision versus radial head replacement: a comparative study. Open Access Maced J Med Sci. 2019;7(9):1505–8. https://doi.org/10.3889/oamjms.2019.305.

Arthroscopic Release of the Proximal Radioulnar Joint in Elbow Osteoarthritis

23

Jun-Bum Lee, Hyun-Ki Lee, and In-Ho Jeon

1 Background

The elbow joint consists of the ulnotrochlear joint, radiocapitellar joint, and proximal radioulnar joint [1]. The proximal radioulnar joint is formed by the articulation between the ulnar notch and the radial head, with the annular ligament surrounding the radial head contributing to stability [2, 3]. The proximal radioulnar joint facilitates the pronation and supination motions of the forearm in coordination with the distal radioulnar joint [4]. Additionally, OA deformities can also affect the proximal radioulnar joint (PRUJ), with changes such as the formation of osteophytes, subchondral cysts, loose bodies in the joint space, and narrowing of the joint space observed on CT scans [5]. Clinically, patients also present with impairment in pronation and supination [6]. Limitations in rotation can cause discomfort in daily activities; for instance, restricted pronation may hinder typing on a keyboard, while restricted supination can lead to difficulties when holding a smartphone with one hand [7]. In this chapter, we aim to describe the arthroscopic release technique of the proximal radioulnar joint (PRUJ).

2 Indications for Arthroscopic PRUJ Release

The indications for arthroscopic PRUJ release are as follows:

(a) Elbow OA combined with PRUJ OA (Fig. 23.1).
(b) Patient with limitation of motion for pronation/supination (Fig. 23.2).

Middle axial CT image of PRUJ was used to assess for PRUJ OA. On the axial CT images, radiologic findings of OA such as spur formation of the radial notch, joint space narrowing, subchondral cysts, and loose bodies can be identified (Fig. 23.1).

Patients may exhibit limitations in pronation and supination. In some cases, tenderness due to bony impingement may be observed at the soft spot during extension. This can occur when osteophytes in the radial notch impinge with posterolateral trochlear osteophytes during extension (Fig. 23.2).

Supplementary Information The online version contains supplementary material available at https://doi.org/10.1007/978-981-95-3732-7_23.

J.-B. Lee (✉) · H.-K. Lee · I.-H. Jeon
Department of Orthopaedic Surgery, Asan Medical Center, University of Ulsan, College of Medicine, Seoul, Republic of Korea

I.-H. Jeon et al. (eds.), *Elbow Arthroscopy*, https://doi.org/10.1007/978-981-95-3732-7_23

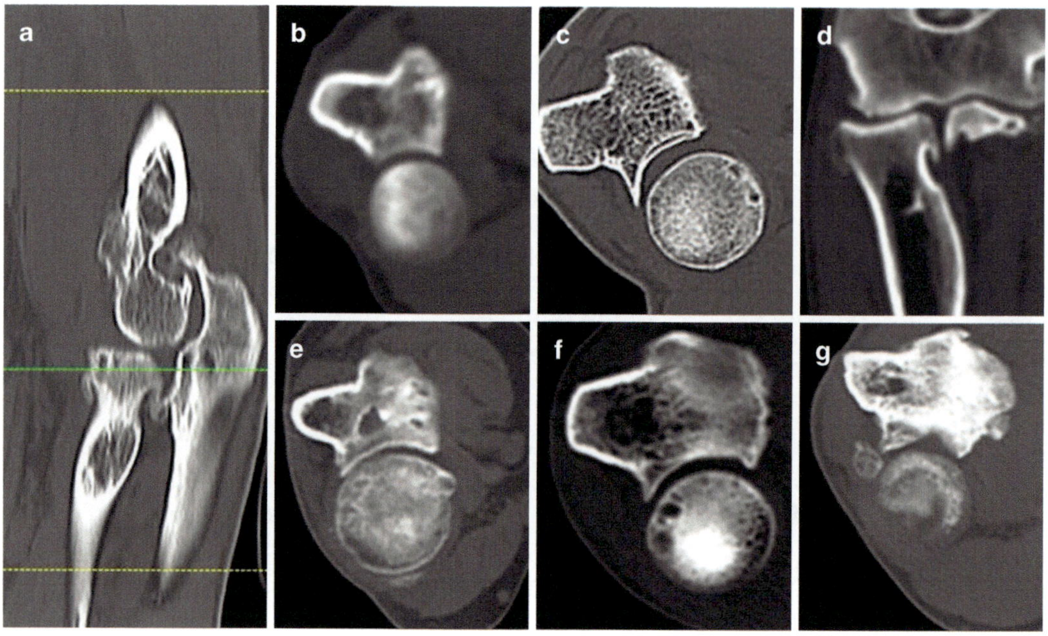

Fig. 23.1 Computed tomographic (CT) images of proximal radioulnar joint (PRUJ) osteoarthritis. (**a**) Level of the cut used to obtain a middle axial view of the PRUJ. (**b**) PRUJ without OA change. (**c**) Spur formation of radial notch of ulna. (**d**) Radial head osteophytes in the coronal view. (**e**) Joint space narrowing. (**f**) Subchondral cyst of the radial head. (**g**) Presence of a loose body

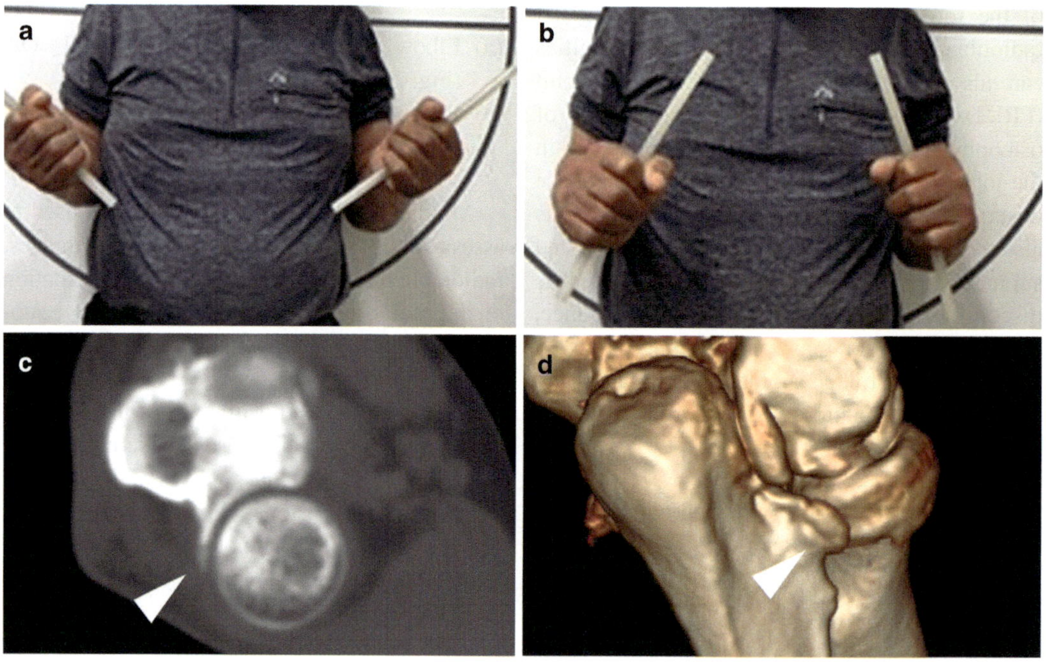

Fig. 23.2 (**a**, **b**) Clinical photos illustrating decreased pronation/supination arc. (**c**, **d**) Axial CT image and 3D reconstruction image illustrating posterior radial notch spur (the white arrowhead indicates the posterior notch spur)

3 Surgical Technique

3.1 Portal Establishment and Assessment

A total of three portals are utilized for PRUJ release: the posterolateral portal, the soft-spot portal, and the PRUJ portal. The PRUJ portal is placed at a point 1 cm below the posterior joint line of the proximal radioulnar joint (Fig. 23.3).

Before accessing the portal placement, inject 20 mL of normal saline solution into the elbow joint through an 18-gauge needle at the soft spot to distend the joint.

First, the proximal lateral portal is used as the viewing portal to access the posterior radiocapitellar joint and PRUJ joint. The soft-spot portal serves as the working portal. Due to limited space, a shaver is used for adequate soft tissue debridement to ensure a clear view. Findings of PRUJ OA are assessed at the PRUJ (Fig. 23.3).

3.2 Soft-Tissue Release

Next, an annular ligament release is performed (Fig. 23.4). The upper part of the annular ligament is released through the soft-spot portal. An intra-articular retractor can provide improved access and visualization during the procedure. Some of the lower part of the annular ligament and other distal soft tissues are resected using instruments inserted through the PRUJ portal. Adequate soft tissue release is necessary to properly expose the bony spur. The forearm is rotated in pronation/supination to assess changes in the rotation arc after the soft-tissue release.

3.3 Resection of Osteophyte

The osteophyte resection is performed using an osteotome or a high-speed burr (Fig. 23.5). It is believed that adequately removing a sufficient amount of the spur is related to a favorable surgical outcome in the presence of notch spur (Fig. 23.6). After resection of the spur, all bony fragments are also removed. Once sufficient release is achieved, pronation and supination are reassessed; if limitation of motion (LOM) persists, proximal interosseous ligament could be additionally released (Table 23.1).

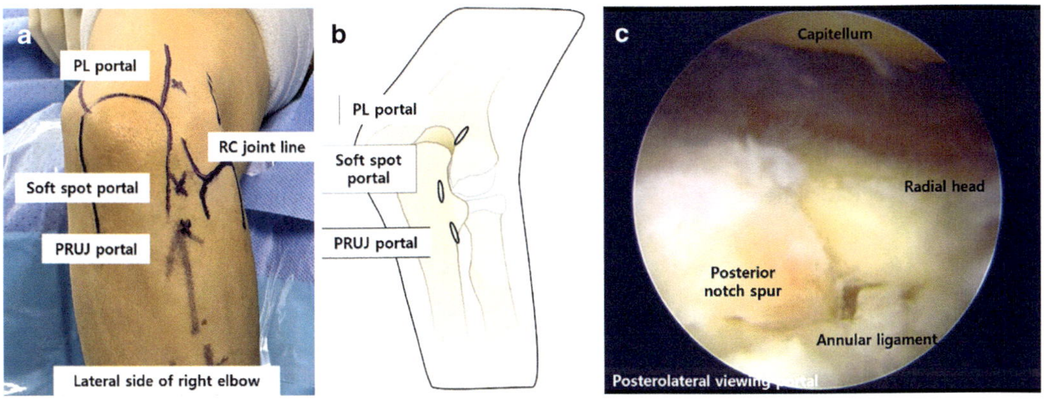

Fig. 23.3 (**a**) The patient is positioned in the lateral decubitus position with the right elbow, and the posterolateral portal is used for viewing. The soft spot portal and PRUJ portal are used as the working portal. (**b**) Illustration showed the elbow arthroscope portals for PRUJ release (**c**). The arthroscopic view from the posterolateral viewing portal,showing PRUJ OA, cartilage erosion of the radial head, and a posterior notch spur

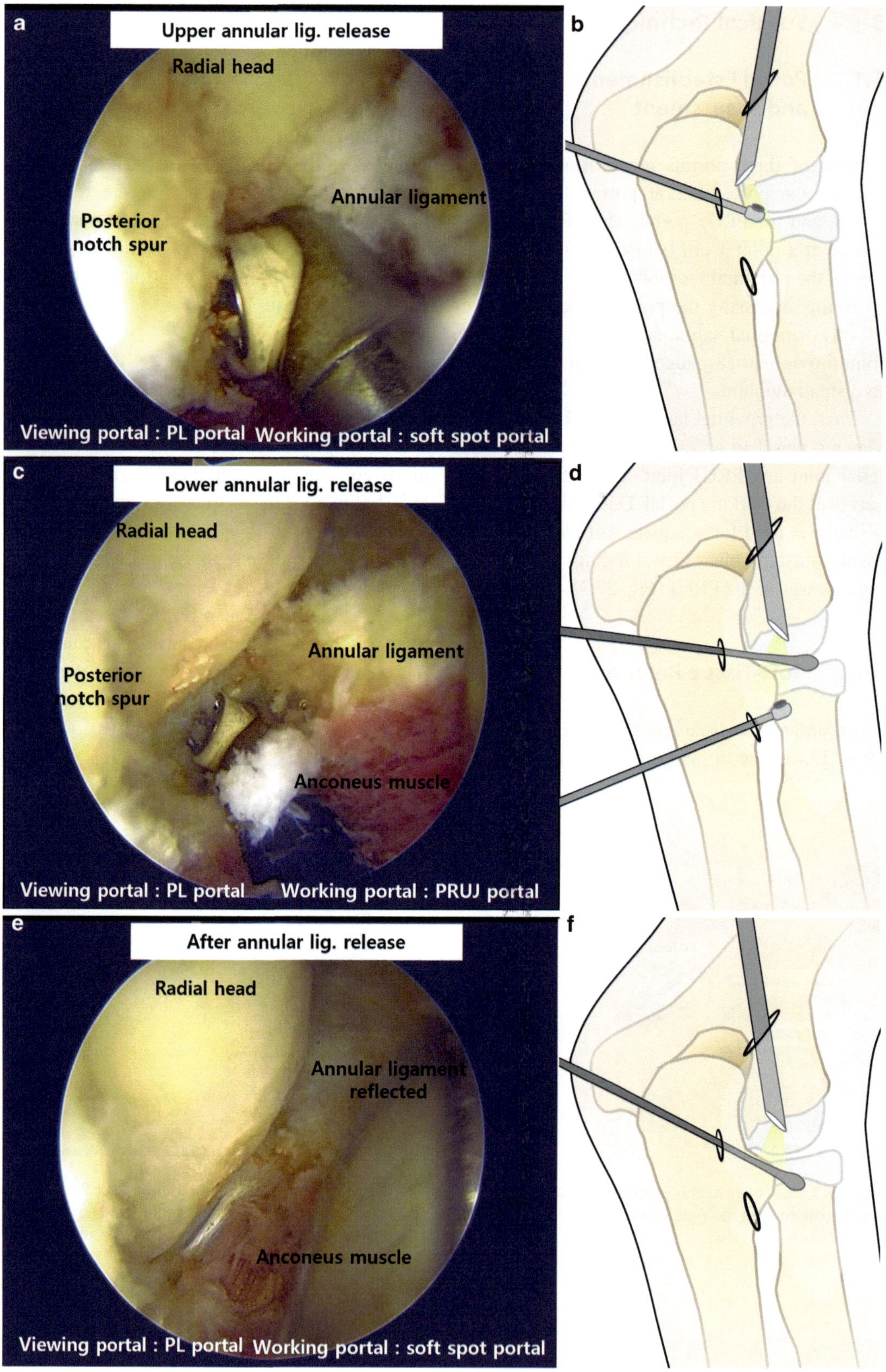
a
Upper annular lig. release
Radial head
Annular ligament
Posterior notch spur
Viewing portal : PL portal
Working portal : soft spot portal
b
c
Lower annular lig. release
Radial head
Annular ligament
Posterior notch spur
Anconeus muscle
Viewing portal : PL portal
Working portal : PRUJ portal
d
e
After annular lig. release
Radial head
Annular ligament reflected
Anconeus muscle
Viewing portal : PL portal
Working portal : soft spot portal
f

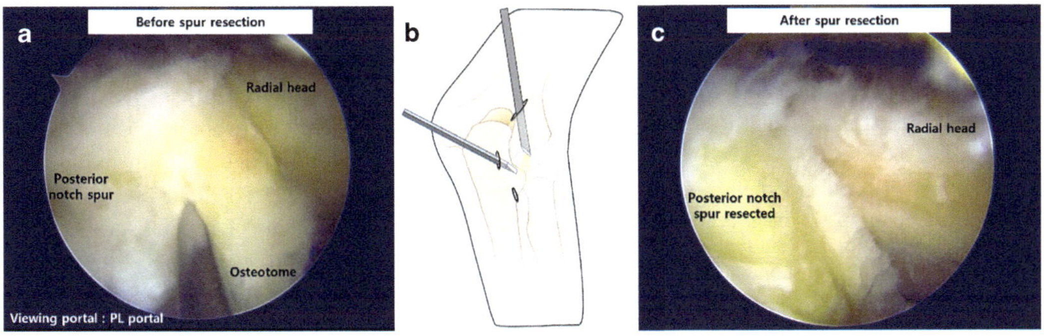

Fig. 23.5 An arthroscopic view of the right elbow in the lateral decubitus position reveals posterior notch spur. (**a**) The posterior notch spur before reduction. (**b**) Illustration showed osteotome was inserted through the soft-spot portal. (**c**) After spur resection

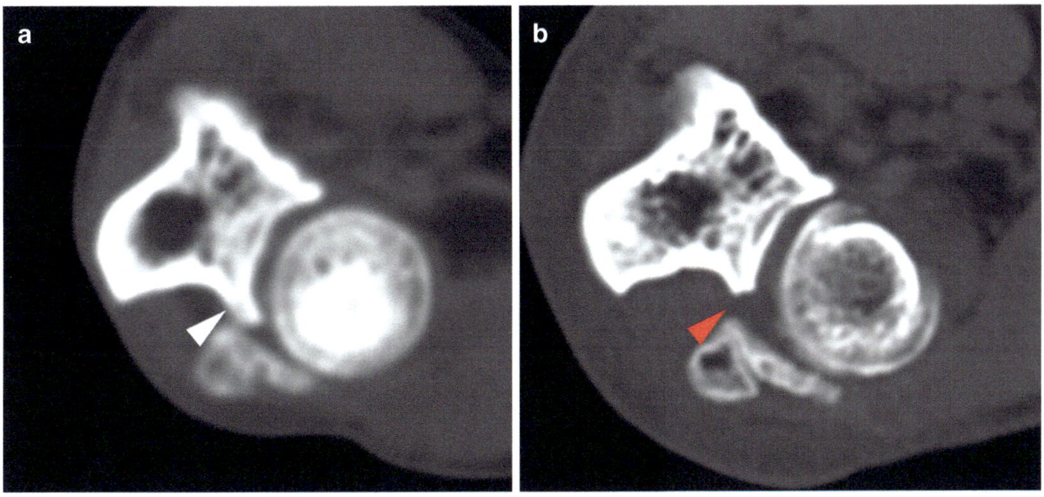

Fig. 23.6 CT axial image of PRUJ osteoarthritis. (**a**) The posterior notch spur before reduction (the white arrowhead indicates the posterior notch spur) and (**b**) after spur resection (the red arrowhead indicates the resected posterior notch spur)

Table 23.1 Advantages and limitations of arthroscopic PRUJ release

Advantages	Limitations
Minimally invasive procedure Mechanical block can be treated effectively and safely as the area lacks significant neurovascular structures that could be injured	Requires advanced knowledge of elbow anatomy, arthroscopy skills Due to the limited space in the posterolateral elbow joint, the arthroscopic instruments could be crowded inside

Fig. 23.4 An arthroscopic view of the right elbow from posterolateral portal reveals posterior notch spur of PURJ and thickened annular ligament. An electrocauterize device was inserted for annular ligament release. (**a**, **b**) Upper part annular ligament release through soft spot portal. (**c**, **d**) Lower part annular ligament release through PRUJ portal. Intra-articular retractor was inserted through the soft-spot portal and the electrocautery device was inserted through the PRUJ portal. (**e**, **f**) After annular ligament release

4 Pearls and Pitfalls (Table 23.2)

Table 23.2 Pearls and pitfalls of arthroscopic PRUJ release

Pearls	Pitfalls
Carefully selecting patients is essential for achieving successful outcome Portal placement is critical ① Due to the limited space, achieving a clear view through adequate soft-tissue debridement is a crucial first step ② Complete release of annular ligament is important for PRUJ motion improvement ③ PRUJ release and spur resection, loose body removal should be performed based on preoperative CT evaluation	Incorrect portal placement can limit visualization and complicate instrumentation in the narrow working area Aggressive extensive posterolateral release may cause PRUJ instability Anterior PRUJ release should be performed carefully, because of radial nerve injury during procedure

5 Discussion

OA changes in the PRUJ can be identified on CT axial cut images. Clinically, this presents as limitations in pronation and supination, along with tenderness in the soft-spot area. PRUJ OA is associated with the progression of elbow OA. As OA in the ulnohumeral and radiocapitellar joints progresses, PRUJ OA is often present as well. Therefore, it is important to assess for impairment in pronation and supination, as well as the presence of PRUJ OA on CT, when approaching elbow OA. This chapter describes the portal placement for accessing the PRUJ and the PRUJ release method to improve LOM associated with PRUJ OA. The portals primarily used are the posterolateral portal and the soft-spot portal, along with the addition of the PRUJ portal to access the distal PRUJ when the first two are insufficient. Due to the narrow posterolateral joint space and the close proximity of the portals, instruments can easily collide, and visibility is often restricted by soft tissue. Therefore, properly positioning the initial portals to minimize instrument interference and performing adequate intra-articular soft-tissue debridement is a crucial starting point for the procedure. Preoperative CT evaluation guides the planning of the procedure, including radial notch spur resection and loose body removal. In cases of joint space narrowing, subchondral cysts, or radial head spurs where there is LOM but no bony impingement during pronation/supination, only soft-tissue release will be performed.

To date, there have been limited studies on the clinical outcomes of PRUJ release. Future research is needed to evaluate the clinical and radiological outcomes, and to validate the significance of this technique.

References

1. Cheung EV, Adams R, Morrey BF. Primary osteoarthritis of the elbow: current treatment options. J Am Acad Orthop Surg. 2008;16(2):77–87.
2. Ehman EC, Felmlee JP, Frick MA. Imaging of the proximal and distal radioulnar joints. Magn Reson Imaging Clin N Am. 2015;23(3):417–25.
3. Weiss AP, Hastings H 2nd. The anatomy of the proximal radioulnar joint. J Shoulder Elbow Surg. 1992;1(4):193–9.
4. Malone PS, Shaw OG, Lees VC. Anatomic relationships of the distal and proximal radioulnar joints articulating surface areas and of the radius and ulna bone volumes - implications for biomechanical studies of the distal and proximal radioulnar joints and forearm bones. Front Bioeng Biotechnol. 2016;4:61.
5. Lee JB, Ben H, So SP, Alsaqri H, Lee HJ, Koh KH, et al. Osteoarthritis of proximal radioulnar joint: computed tomography-based assessment and associations with clinical findings. Orthop J Sports Med. 2024;12(9):23259671241255354.
6. Biswas D, Wysocki RW, Cohen MS. Primary and posttraumatic arthritis of the elbow. Arthritis. 2013;2013:473259.
7. Sardelli M, Tashjian RZ, MacWilliams BA. Functional elbow range of motion for contemporary tasks. J Bone Joint Surg Am. 2011;93(5):471–7.

Posttraumatic Elbow Stiffness: Arthroscopic Stiff Elbow Release

24

Hyun-Ki Lee and In-Ho Jeon

1 Background

Post-traumatic elbow stiffness occurs as a sequela of fractures, dislocations, and other traumatic bone and soft-tissue injuries around the elbow joint, leading to a restricted range of motion. Intra-articular causes may include loose bodies and complications from septic arthritis (Table 24.1) [1].

Considering persistent pain and functional impairment resulting from multifactorial causes, a comprehensive treatment strategy that accounts for joint pathology, patient-specific factors, and the unique biomechanics of the elbow is essential.

Within the first 6 months after trauma, conservative treatment is primarily used as an initial approach that includes physical therapy and continuous active stretching exercises.

Table 24.1 Intra-articular and extra-articular causes of post-traumatic stiffness of elbow

Intra-articular causes	Extra-articular causes
Loose bodies Intra-articular fracture Joint incongruity	Soft-tissue contracture Heterotopic ossification Extra-articular fracture malunion/nonunion Nonunion fractures
Complex causes (intra-articular + extra-articular)	

Modified from Morrey et al. [1]

H.-K. Lee · I.-H. Jeon (✉)
Department of Orthopaedic Surgery, Asan Medical Center, University of Ulsan, College of Medicine, Seoul, Republic of Korea

2 Indications and Contraindications

2.1 Indications

Surgical treatment is indicated when pain and functional impairments (particularly restricted range of motion) persist despite conservative management. The patient's motivation to improve elbow mobility and restore joint function plays a significant role in treatment success. The indications for arthroscopic surgery are generally similar to those of open release procedures; however, the choice of technique largely depends on the surgeon's experience and expertise.

2.2 Relative Contraindication

Ensuring appropriate portal placement for elbow arthroscopy while preserving neurovascular structures throughout the procedure is critical. If the patient has undergone anterior transposition of the ulnar nerve, open surgery is generally a more suitable approach. Additionally, in cases of severe post-traumatic elbow stiffness, anatomical distortion may make it difficult to establish proper arthroscopic portal access, which may necessitate conversion to open surgery.

I.-H. Jeon et al. (eds.), *Elbow Arthroscopy*, https://doi.org/10.1007/978-981-95-3732-7_24

2.3 Indication for Ulnar Nerve Decompression

Routine ulnar nerve decompression is not required for all patients with post-traumatic stiffness. Indications for decompression include (1) preoperative signs of ulnar neuropathy (e.g., sensory deficits, muscle atrophy, positive Tinel's sign); (2) severe flexion contracture (<90°), increasing the risk of ulnar nerve entrapment; (3) severe elbow stiffness with a flexion-extension arc of less than 60°; and (4) the presence of heterotopic ossification near the medial epicondyle or cubital tunnel.

2.4 Decompression Versus Anterior Transposition

Simple decompression is appropriate for mild ulnar neuropathy without significant anatomical changes. Anterior transposition is recommended for (1) recurrent ulnar neuropathy despite previous decompression; (2) anatomical changes involving the cubital tunnel, such as scar tissue or heterotopic ossification; and (3) severe stiffness requiring extensive capsular or medial gutter release.

3 Preoperative Evaluation

3.1 Nerve Conduction Study and Electromyography

A nerve conduction study and electromyography are generally considered if subclinical symptoms of ulnar nerve dysfunction are suspected. This may manifest as Tinel's sign present at the cubital tunnel, or objective abnormalities such as sensory disturbances, muscle atrophy, or claw hand deformities on physical examination.

3.2 Ultrasound Examination

Ultrasound is a useful tool for detecting and tracking the ulnar nerve and is occasionally used to identify masses surrounding the nerve. Preoperative nerve tracking (Fig. 24.1) and marking are particularly beneficial for patients with a history of ulnar nerve transposition, as they aid in minimizing the risk of nerve injury during surgery.

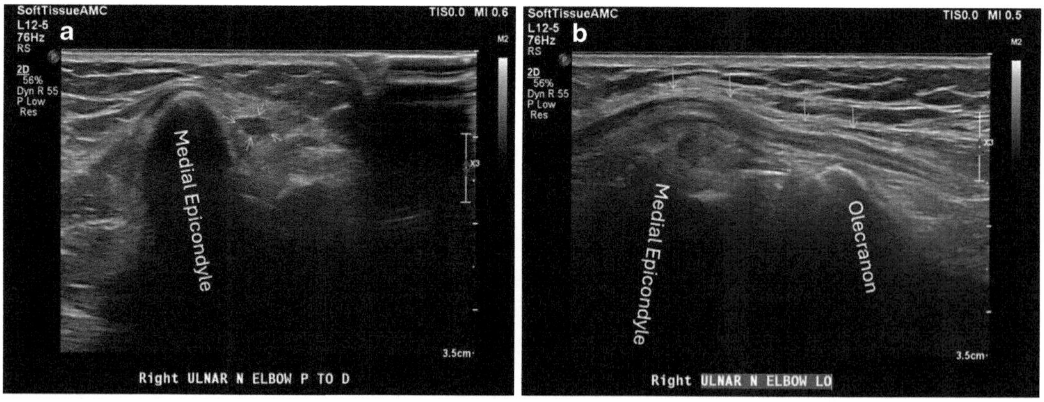

Fig. 24.1 Ultrasound imaging of the ulnar nerve (arrow) at the medial epicondyle of a patient with ulnar nerve neuropathy (37/F), short axis (**a**) with loss of fascicular pattern with hypoechoic change and longitudinal axis (**b**)

4 Stepwise Surgical Method

The lateral decubitus position is the preferred surgical position, although prone or supine positioning is also possible depending on the patient's condition. The surgery is typically performed under general anesthesia. It is essential to reassess the elbow's range of motion before and after anesthesia. Additionally, evaluating for ulnar nerve subluxation or dislocation is also important to evaluate ulnar nerve instability.

Arthroscopic procedures for the elbow are categorized into anterior and posterior compartments, with the sequence of intervention determined by the surgeon's preference and clinical considerations. The author generally prefers to start with the posterior compartment. While doing surgery, manipulation of elbow position should be done with care in cases of post-traumatic stiff elbow since iatrogenic injury to capsule, ligament, and muscle would increase the risk of heterotopic ossification. The procedure of the elbow arthroscopy usually starts from portal creation ➔ observation ➔ creation of working space ➔ soft-tissue contracture release ➔ osteotomy ➔ capsular release. Commonly, the capsular release is performed at the last step in capsule near the neurovascular structures to prevent extravasation of fluid to soft tissue and prevention of iatrogenic neurovascular injury.

4.1 Prophylactic Ulnar Nerve Decompression

Prior to addressing the anterior and posterior compartments during surgery, prophylactic ulnar nerve decompression is performed. A 2–3 cm skin incision is made between the medial epicondyle and olecranon. Using an endoscopic approach, the nerve is decompressed 3–4 cm proximal to the medial epicondyle and 3–4 cm distal to the medial epicondyle, extending toward the fibrotic arcade of the flexor carpi ulnaris. (Fig. 24.2).

In cases of performing anterior transposition, the ulnar nerve can be repositioned subcutaneously or submuscularly to prevent tethering or compression. Utilization of intraoperative nerve monitoring may help mitigate the risk of iatrogenic injury during decompression or transposition.

4.2 Posterior Compartment

Under arthroscopic guidance, anatomical landmarks including the medial/lateral epicondyles, and radial head are identified. Additional markings are made along the medial/lateral supracondylar ridges, triceps muscle boundaries, and olecranon borders.

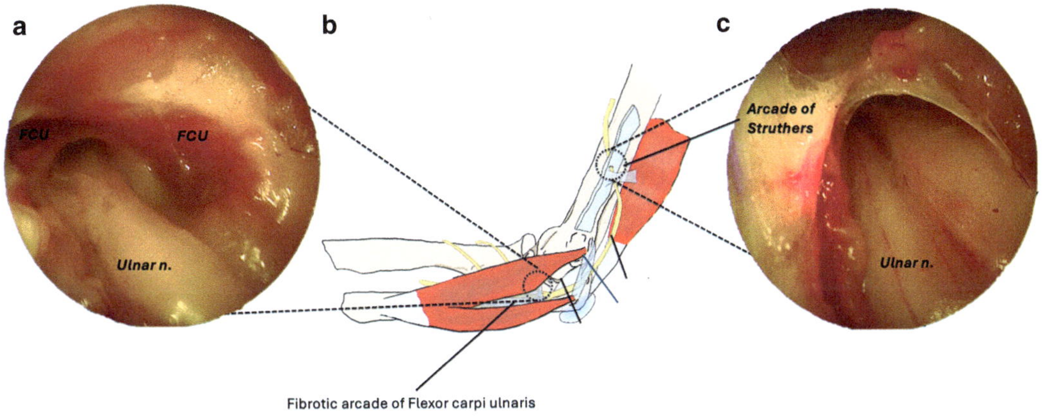

Fig. 24.2 Prophylactic ulnar nerve release. (**a**) Distal ulnar nerve release: Release of fibrotic arcade of flexor capri ulnaris. (**b**) Schematic image of ulnar nerve course near the elbow joint. (**c**) Proximal ulnar nerve release

Surgical access to the posterior compartment is achieved through three portals:

- Central posterior portal (viewing portal)
- Posterolateral portal (working portal)
- Superolateral posterior portal (accessory portal)

The central posterior portal functions as the primary viewing portal, offering visualization of the olecranon fossa (Fig. 24.3). The posterolateral portal used for debridement of fibrofatty tissue around the olecranon fossa using a shaver. Following debridement of the olecranon fossa, the thickened posterior capsule is excised in a stepwise manner, progressing from the medial gutter to the lateral gutter.

In cases of severe flexion contracture, accessing the medial gutter may be difficult. However, posteromedial capsular release (Fig. 24.4) is a critical step for achieving adequate elbow flexion. Since posteromedial contracture often results from the posteromedial fibers of the medial collateral ligament, careful consideration of the ulnar nerve's trajectory is essential to avoid iatrogenic injury. If necessary, a mini-open release of

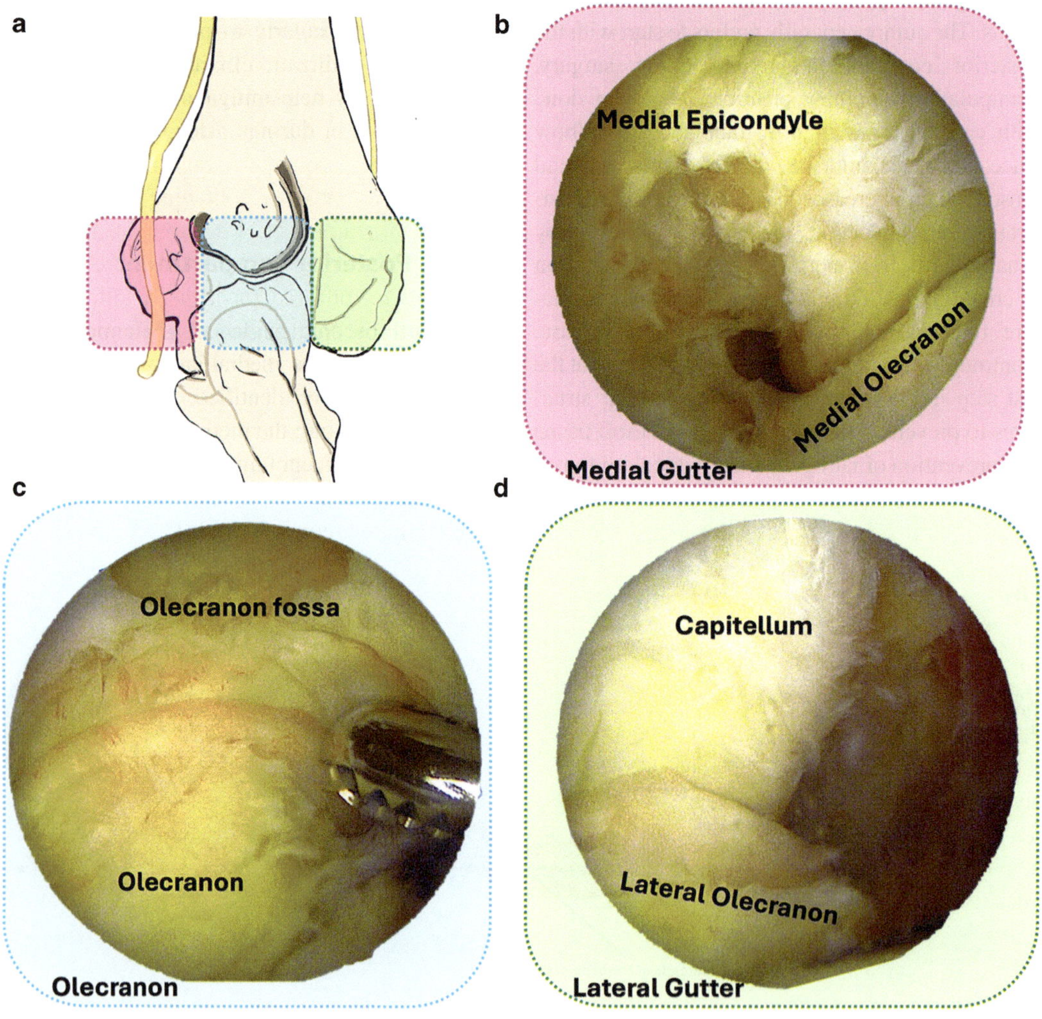

Fig. 24.3 Arthroscopic images of posterior compartment in post-traumatic stiff elbow. (**a**) Schematic image of posterior elbow compartment. (**b**) Posteromedial side (pink). (**c**) Olecranon (blue). (**d**) Posterolateral side (green): Fibrotic change and capsular adhesion is observed (b, c, d)

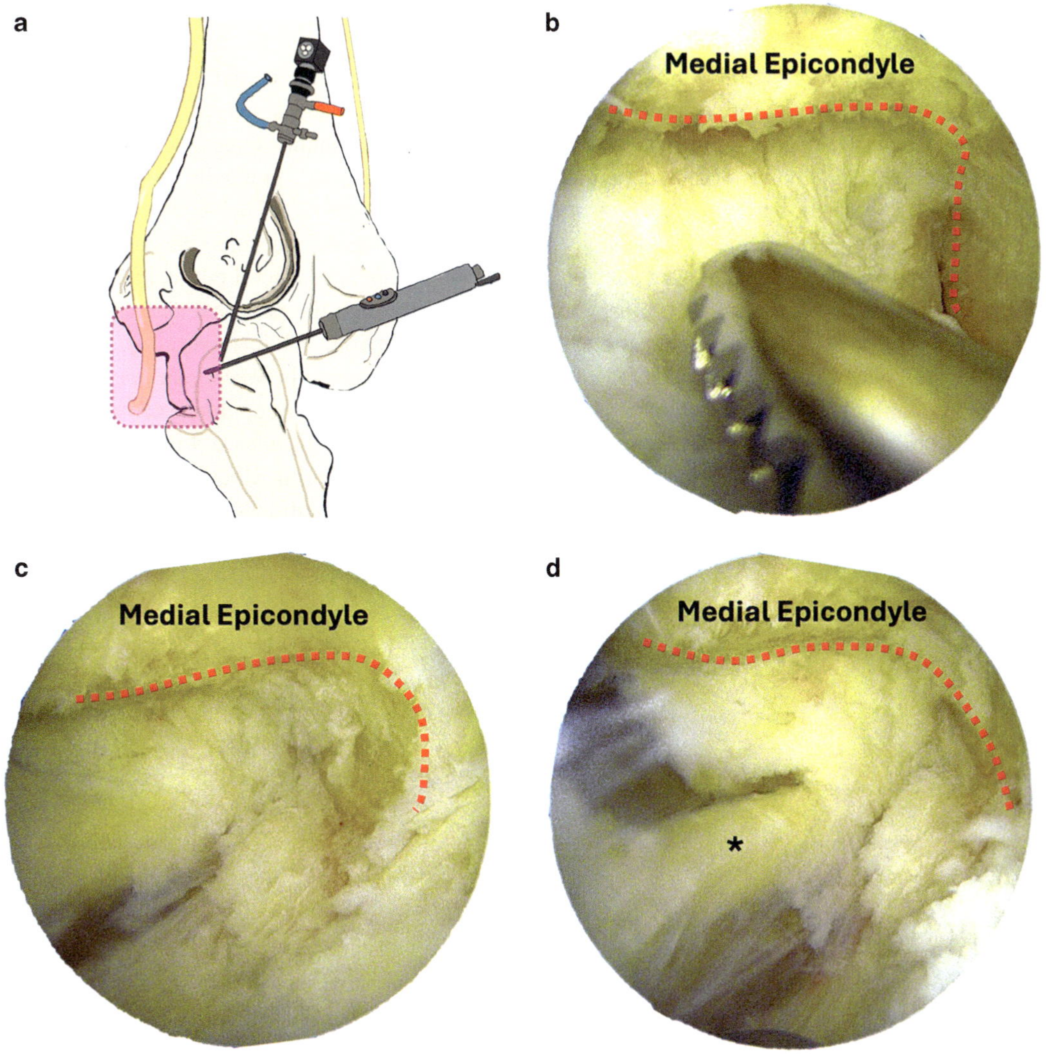

Fig. 24.4 Release of posteromedial capsule and posterior band of the medial gutter. (**a**) Schematic image of protection of ulnar nerve using nerve sling near the medial gutter. (**b**) Before release of the medial gutter. (**c**) After release of the medial gutter. (**d**) Further release of the medial gutter to fully expose the ulnar nerve (*)

the ulnar nerve can be performed before capsular release. When using a radiofrequency ablation device (Arthrocare®) for hemostasis or capsule removal, it is crucial to keep the instrument close to the bone to minimize damage to nerves and muscles.

If distal humeral fractures or postoperative adhesions between the posterior humerus and triceps are present, the triceps muscle can be elevated and released from the humeral attachment. Further lateral elevation of triceps muscle to the level of intermuscular septum help may aid in preventing postoperative flexion limitations associated with triceps adhesion. While the lateral gutter is generally considered less critical than the medial gutter, comprehensive release of both compartments to a comparable extent is recommended to achieve full elbow flexion. To optimize soft-tissue balance and facilitate adequate joint mobilization during capsular release, the use of accessory retractors and intra-articular retractors may be beneficial.

4.3 Anterior Compartment

A proximal anteromedial portal is used to insert a switching stick toward the radial head, followed by arthroscope insertion and confirmation of trocar positioning. Using the inside-out technique, a lateral portal is created, and a shaver is inserted through this portal. The inside-out technique is particularly useful when the joint is swollen, as it minimizes the risk of nerve injury during portal creation. Once the shaver is safely positioned, a proximal anterolateral portal is created for inserting an intra-articular retractor, which improves visualization by preventing the synovium from obstructing the arthroscopic view and protects the neurovascular structures.

When operating on the lateral aspect of the radial head (Fig. 24.5), full pronation of the elbow facilitates the medial displacement of the posterior interosseous nerve, thereby reducing the risk of iatrogenic injury. Also, the capsule should be excised gradually from lateral to medial to prevent radial nerve injury.

For the medial capsule, the arthroscope is moved to the anterolateral portal, and a shaver is inserted through the proximal anteromedial portal for resection. While there is no significant clinical difference between osteocapsulectomy and osteocapsulotomy, complete capsular release and partial brachialis release (Fig. 24.6) are often preferred for restoring elbow extension in cases of post-traumatic stiffness.

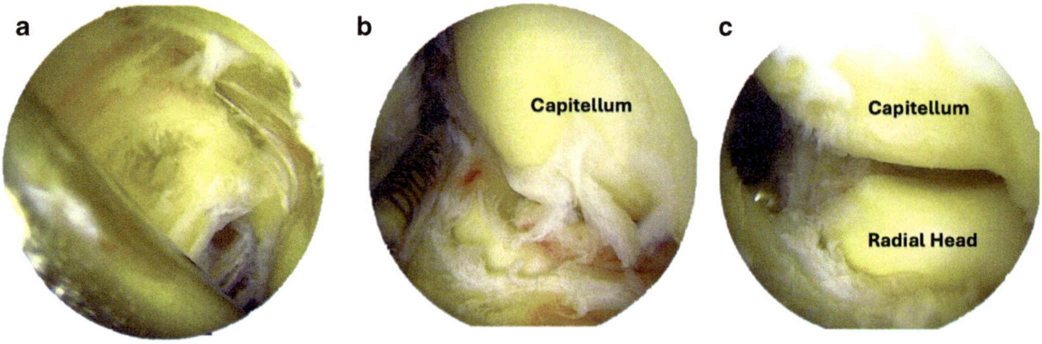

Fig. 24.5 Arthroscopic images of anterolateral compartment in posttraumatic stiff elbow. (**a**) Fibrotic thickened anterolateral capsule from anteromedial viewing portal. (**b**) Debridement process of hyperplastic synovium covering the radial head. (**c**) Exposure of radial head after debridement process

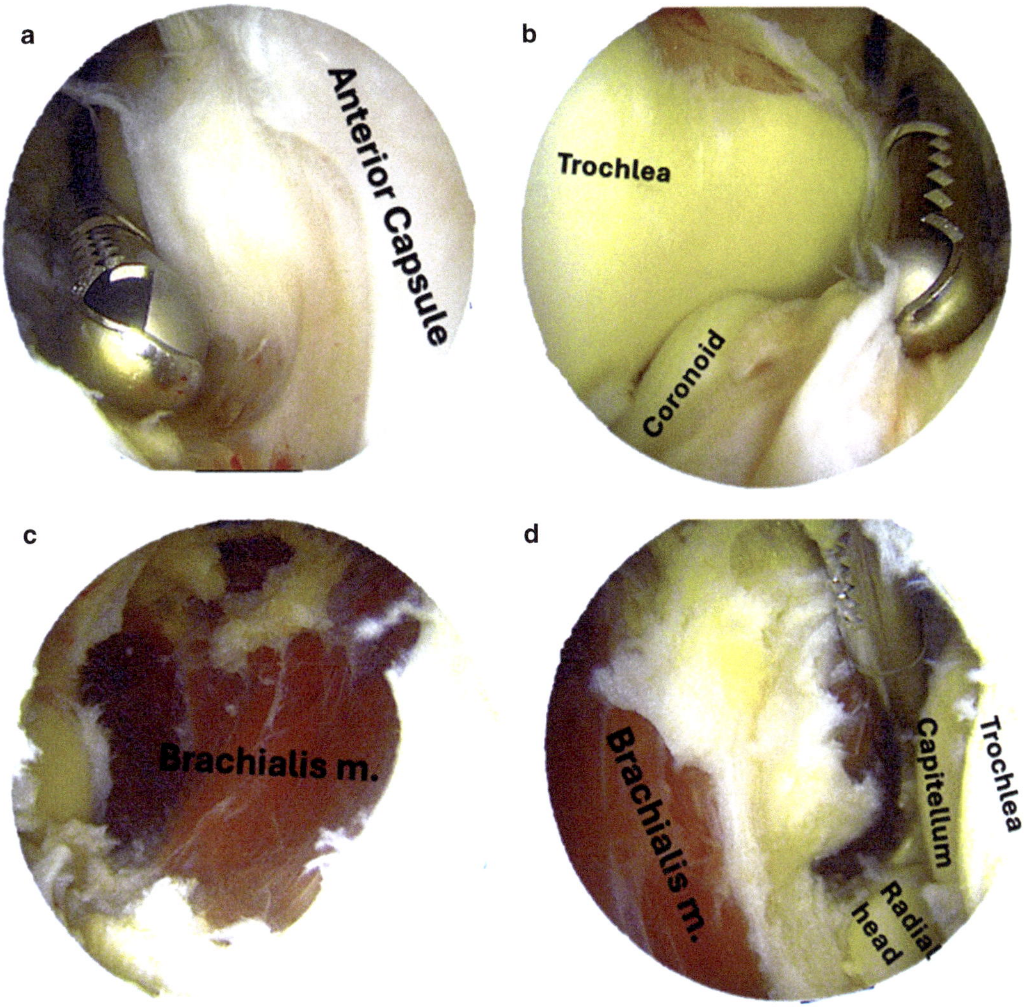

Fig. 24.6 Arthroscopic images of anteromedial compartment in posttraumatic stiff elbow. (**a**) thickened anterior capsule. (**b**) Exposure of coronoid and anterior capsulectomy. (**c**) Anterior capsulectomy state. (**d**) Exposure of brachialis muscle

5 Outcomes and Treatment Goals

Current literature indicates that arthroscopic capsular release yields comparable outcomes to open surgery (Table 24.2). However, severe elbow stiffness may require conversion to open surgery, which should be taken into account when interpreting Table 24.2. The primary treatment goal is to restore a functional range of motion of 30° ~ 130°.

6 Complications

6.1 Nerve Injury

Nerve injury is the most concerning complication of arthroscopic surgery. To minimize the risks, the ulnar nerve can be marked preoperatively using ultrasound and, if necessary, dissected via a mini-open approach and protected with a nerve sling. However, delayed-onset neuropathy may still occur, requiring ongoing monitoring [2, 3]. If

Table 24.2 Arthroscopic Surgery vs. Open Surgery Outcomes in posttraumatic stiff elbow

		Arthroscopic							Open						Comments
		PreOP		Post OP		ROM			PreOP		PostOP		ROM		
	N	Mean ROM	MEPS	Mean ROM	MEPS	Mean Gain	Complication	N	Mean ROM	MEPS	Mean ROM	MEPS	Mean Gain	Complication	
Lanzerath et al. [5]	1059	68.1	63.1	108.0	88.8	39.2	1.6%	607	42.7	61.4	113.2	89.7	70.4	6.3%	Comprehensive 1998 ~ 2019
Kodde et al. [6]	100	84		124		40	5%	637	52		103		51	23%	Comprehensive 1989 ~ 2012
Williams et al. [7]	45	87.2		113.4		26.2		110	64.8		106.1		41.3		Single Center Study
Kwak et al. [8]	13	72	52.3	107	80.8	34	22.5%	31	52	48.9	96	80.0	43	29%	Intra/Extra-articular Fractures

symptoms such as progressive pain, motion restriction, tingling, sensory loss, or muscle weakness develop, revision surgery with ulnar nerve transposition may be necessary. For patients at risk of delayed ulnar neuropathy, early ulnar nerve decompression should be considered, especially in the presence of heterotopic ossification, neurological symptoms, or severe preoperative stiffness.

The posterior interosseous nerve, a branch of the radial nerve, is at risk during excessive coagulation or capsular excision around the radial head. Using intra-articular retractors can help reduce nerve injury.

6.2 Heterotopic Ossification

According to the authors' research, the incidence of heterotopic ossification following elbow arthroscopy is 6.3%, primarily occurring medially [4]. Due to the nature of heterotopic ossification being common after ulnar nerve decompression, postoperative monitoring for at least 8 weeks is recommended. Other risk factors include young age, prolonged tourniquet time, and prolonged surgery time, all of which should be considered when performing elbow arthroscopy.

6.3 Other Complications

Due to the proximity of elbow to superficial skin, the risk of postoperative infection exists but can be minimized with preoperative patient evaluation and perioperative antibiotics.

Additional complications include nonhealing arthroscopic portals, aseptic fistulas, and recurrent fractures at previously healed trauma sites.

References

1. Morrey BF. Post-traumatic contracture of the elbow. Operative treatment, including distraction arthroplasty. J Bone Joint Surg Am. 1990;72(4):601–18.
2. Blonna D, Huffmann GR, O'Driscoll SW. Delayed-onset ulnar neuritis after release of elbow contractures: clinical presentation, pathological findings, and treatment. Am J Sports Med. 2014;42(9):2113–21. https://doi.org/10.1177/0363546514540448.
3. Haapaniemi T, Berggren M, Adolfsson L. Complete transection of the median and radial nerves during arthroscopic release of post-traumatic elbow contracture. Arthroscopy. 1999;15(7):784–7. https://doi.org/10.1016/s0749-8063(99)70015-0.
4. Ben H, Kholinne E, Zeng CH, Alsaqri H, Lee JB, So SP, et al. Prevalence, timing, locational distribution, and risk factors for heterotopic ossification after elbow arthroscopy. Am J Sports Med. 2023;51(13):3401–8. https://doi.org/10.1177/03635465231198862.
5. Lanzerath F, Wegmann K, Hackl M, Uschok S, Ott N, Müller LP, et al. Surgical arthrolysis of the stiff elbow: a systematic review. Arch Orthop Trauma Surg. 2023;143(5):2383–93. https://doi.org/10.1007/s00402-022-04442-0.
6. Kodde IF, van Rijn J, van den Bekerom MP, Eygendaal D. Surgical treatment of post-traumatic elbow stiffness: a systematic review. J Shoulder Elb Surg. 2013;22(4):574–80. https://doi.org/10.1016/j.jse.2012.11.010.
7. Williams BG, Sotereanos DG, Baratz ME, Jarrett CD, Venouziou AI, Miller MC. The contracted elbow: is ulnar nerve release necessary? J Shoulder Elb Surg. 2012;21(12):1632–6. https://doi.org/10.1016/j.jse.2012.04.007.
8. Kwak JM, Sun Y, Kholinne E, Koh KH, Jeon IH. Surgical outcomes for post-traumatic stiffness after elbow fracture: comparison between open and arthroscopic procedures for intra- and extra-articular elbow fractures. J Shoulder Elb Surg. 2019;28(10):1998–2006. https://doi.org/10.1016/j.jse.2019.06.008.

Septic Arthritis of the Elbow: Arthroscopic Management

25

Ji-Ho Lee

1 Background

Septic arthritis of the elbow presents unique challenges due to its subcutaneous anatomy and proximity to critical neurovascular structures. With an annual incidence of 12.0 per 100,000 individuals and mortality rates reaching 11% in untreated cases, prompt and effective management is critical [1, 2]. Over the past two decades, arthroscopic synovectomy has emerged as a gold-standard treatment for acute cases without osteomyelitis, achieving infection resolution rates of 94–96% compared to 84–88% with open arthrotomy [1–4]. This review synthesizes evidence from clinical studies, microbiological data, and technical refinements to establish evidence-based guidelines for managing septic elbow arthritis, with particular emphasis on arthroscopic techniques.

2 Epidemiological and Pathophysiological Insights

The elbow's susceptibility to septic arthritis stems from its limited soft-tissue coverage and frequent exposure to trauma. Epidemiological studies demonstrate that *Staphylococcus aureus* causes 56–70% of cases, with methicillin-resistant strains (MRSA) accounting for 5–10% in endemic regions [5]. Gram-negative organisms (8–12%) and *Mycobacterium tuberculosis* (<2%) require tailored antimicrobial strategies [5].

While less common than hip or knee infections, elbow involvement carries disproportionate risks: logistic regression analyses identify septic elbow as an independent mortality risk factor (odds ratio: 2.01) [1].

Long-term functional outcomes remain suboptimal even with successful infection clearance. A retrospective analysis of 42 patients revealed persistent 30–40% reductions in flexion-extension arcs compared to contralateral elbows at 2-year follow-up. These deficits correlate strongly with delayed surgical intervention, emphasizing the importance of early diagnosis and treatment within 48 h of symptom onset.

Culture-directed therapy remains paramount, with synovial fluid analysis guiding antibiotic selection. Intraoperative synovial biopsies improve diagnostic yield by 25% compared to preoperative aspiration alone [1, 2]. PCR assays detect bacterial DNA in 92% of culture-negative cases, reducing time-to-targeted therapy by 72 h. For methicillin-sensitive *S. aureus* (MSSA), 4 ~ 6 weeks of β- lactams (e.g., cefazolin) achieve cure rates of 90%, while vancomycin remains first-line for methicillin-resistant *S. aureus* (MRSA). Fungal and tuberculous infections necessitate prolonged courses (6 ~ 12 months) alongside surgical excision [5] (Table 25.1).

J.-H. Lee (✉)
Department of Orthopaedic Surgery, Pohang SM Christianity Hospital, Pohang, Republic of Korea

I.-H. Jeon et al. (eds.), *Elbow Arthroscopy*, https://doi.org/10.1007/978-981-95-3732-7_25

Table 25.1 Pathogen-specific management strategies

Pathogen	Prevalence	Empirical therapy	Special considerations
MSSA, MRSA	56 ~ 70%	Cefazolin, Vancomycin	MRSA requires 6-week IV therapy
Streptococcus spp.	12 ~ 18%	Ceftriaxone	Synergistic with clindamycin
Gram-negative bacilli	8 ~ 12%	Piperacillin-tazobactam	Adjust based on local resistance

Table 25.2 Outcomes of open vs. arthroscopic synovectomy for septic elbow arthritis

Author (year)	Approach	Sample size	Infection resolution %	Postoperative ROM (°)	Complication rate (%)	Recurrence (%)
Weston et al. (1999) [1]	Open	42	88	85 ~ 120	24	12
Van den Ende et al. (2012) [4]	Arthroscopic	18	94	100 ~ 135	11	6
Moon et al. (2014) [3]	Arthroscopic	25	96	105 ~ 140	8	4
Mercer et al. (2024) [2]	Open	31	84	75 ~ 110	29	15

3 Surgical Approaches: Comparative Outcomes of Open Versus Arthroscopic Techniques

Arthroscopic approaches achieve superior infection control through enhanced visualization of synovial recesses, enabling targeted debridement of infected tissue. Meta-analyses confirm arthroscopy's superiority in reducing reinfection risk (OR 1.35; $p = 0.0002$) and complications (OR 1.32; $p = 0.001$) [6]. However, open arthrotomy remains indispensable for cases with extensive osteomyelitis or large soft-tissue abscesses requiring radical debridement (Table 25.2).

4 Indication of Arthroscopic Technique

Acute septic elbow, which typically presents with symptoms lasting less than 2 weeks and minimal joint damage, is an ideal candidate for arthroscopic treatment [7]. The minimally invasive approach of arthroscopy allows for prompt and adequate joint drainage, aiding in removing pus and inflammatory debris that fuel the infection. Additionally, arthroscopic synovectomy allows removal of the infected synovium, which is crucial for eradicating the infection source and preventing recurrence.

Patients with underlying comorbidities that elevate the risks of open surgery, such as older age, diabetes mellitus, or immunosuppression, may find arthroscopic synovectomy especially beneficial [2, 4]. The less-invasive nature of arthroscopy offers significant advantages for this group, reducing postoperative complications and allowing for early rehabilitation.

Choice of surgical approach should take into consideration the infecting organism. Arthroscopic synovectomy has proven effective for infections caused by common bacteria like *Staphylococcus aureus* and *Streptococcus* species, but its effectiveness against atypical pathogens, such as *Mycobacterium tuberculosis* or fungal infections, is less well established [1, 2]. In such cases, open arthrotomy may be preferred to ensure proper tissue sampling for culture and sensitivity testing and to manage any related bone or soft-tissue involvement (Fig. 25.1).

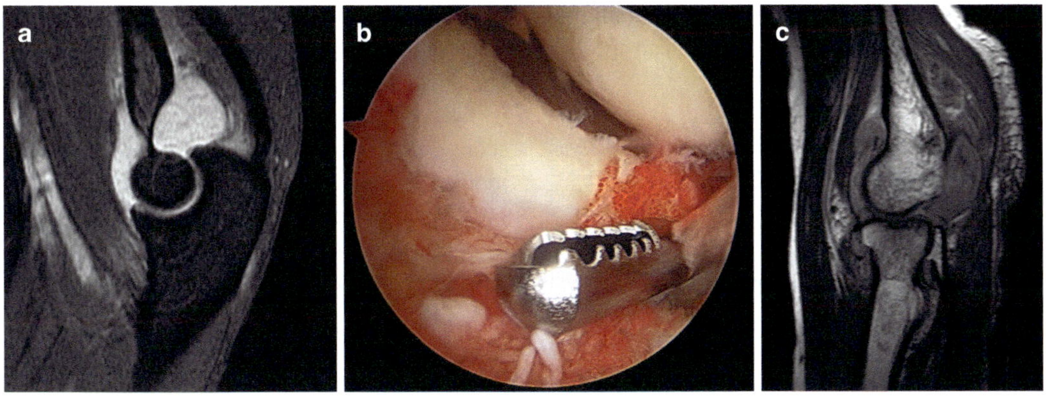

Fig. 25.1 MRI and surgical findings in septic elbow arthritis. (**a**) Typical MRI of septic elbow, showing joint effusion without other significant abnormalities. Clinical symptoms and hematological markers such as ESR and CRP are crucial for diagnosis. (**b**) Arthroscopic findings of the same patient, demonstrating synovitis around the radiocapitellar joint. (**c**) T2-weighted MRI image showing hypoechogenicity, suggesting a possibility of infections like Mycobacterium, which may necessitate open arthrotomy for proper management

5 Contraindications of Arthroscopic Technique

While arthroscopic synovectomy provides several benefits in treating septic arthritis of the elbow, specific contraindications require careful evaluation. Conditions such as extensive joint destruction, osteomyelitis, or large soft tissue abscesses may need open arthrotomy to ensure proper debridement and drainage [4, 8, 9]. Furthermore, patients with bleeding disorders or severe medical issues that restrict general or regional anesthesia may not be ideal candidates for arthroscopic procedures.

6 Procedures of Arthroscopic Synovectomy in Septic Elbow

The procedure of arthroscopic synovectomy for septic arthritis of the elbow involves several critical steps designed to remove infected tissue, drain purulence, and irrigate the joint while preserving function and minimizing invasive intervention. The process typically includes the following:

6.1 Patient Positioning and Anesthesia

The patient is placed in the lateral decubitus, prone position under general anesthesia, or supine position with positioning products under general or regional anesthesia. A tourniquet is applied to the upper arm to control bleeding.

6.2 Portal Establishment

The arthroscopic procedure starts with establishing standard portals, often including proximal anteromedial, anterolateral, posterior, and posterolateral portals, to access the anterior and posterior compartments of the elbow. Special care is taken to avoid damage to neurovascular structures, especially the ulnar and radial nerves.

6.3 Synovectomy and Debridement

The infected synovium is debrided using a motorized shaver. Loose bodies, scar tissue, and debris are removed from both the anterior and posterior compartments. Irrigation with saline (approximately 2 to 6 L) is performed to clean the joint thoroughly.

6.4 Intraoperative Culture and Irrigation

Purulent fluid is aspirated for culture and analysis before and during the procedure. This step is repeated to reduce the false-negative rate for bacterial cultures. Continuous saline irrigation is performed to reduce bacterial load.

6.5 Completion of Debridement

The working and viewing portals are swapped as necessary to ensure a complete debridement of the joint. The posterior compartment, including the medial and lateral gutters, is also debrided using the shaver. Depending on the extent of infection, suction drains may be placed postoperatively to allow further fluid outlet.

6.6 Closure and Postoperative Care

The portals are typically closed with sutures or skin tapes, and postoperative care includes intravenous antibiotics adjusted according to the culture results.

7 Postoperative Management

Postoperative management following arthroscopic synovectomy for septic elbow focuses on infection control, pain management, and early rehabilitation. Patients typically receive intravenous antibiotics for a duration determined by the causative organism and clinical response. Serial laboratory assessments, including WBC count, ESR, and CRP, are monitored twice a week until markers are stabilized to evaluate the effectiveness of treatment and identify any signs of recurrence.

Early mobilization of the elbow joint is crucial to prevent stiffness and promote functional recovery. Early mobilization within 48 h postoperatively correlates with 20% higher Quick DASH scores at 6 months [10]. Continuous passive motion devices improve flexion gains by 15° [10]. Pain management is typically achieved with a combination of oral analgesics and nonsteroidal anti-inflammatory drugs.

8 Conclusion

Arthroscopic synovectomy has become an essential option in treating septic elbow, providing a less-invasive approach to open arthrotomy. The minimally invasive approach allows for adequate joint debridement and drainage, leading to better patient outcomes such as reduced surgical trauma, fast recovery, and the preservation of joint function. As advancements in technology and surgical methods maintain, arthroscopic synovectomy plays a more noteworthy role in the management of septic elbow, helping to improve patient care and overall quality of life.

References

1. Weston VC, Jones AC, Bradbury N, Fawthrop F, Doherty M. Clinical features and outcome of septic arthritis in a single UK Health District 1982-1991. Ann Rheum Dis. 1999;58(4):214–9. https://doi.org/10.1136/ard.58.4.214.
2. Mercer HL, Rodriguez D, Mikola E, Mercer D. The septic elbow joint: treatment approaches for improved patient outcomes. Orthop Clin North Am. 2024;55(2):247–55. https://doi.org/10.1016/j.ocl.2023.09.007.
3. Moon JG, Biraris S, Jeong WK, Kim JH. Clinical results after arthroscopic treatment for septic arthritis of the elbow joint. Arthroscopy. 2014;30(6):673–8. https://doi.org/10.1016/j.arthro.2014.02.018.
4. van den Ende KI, Steinmann SP. Arthroscopic treatment of septic arthritis of the elbow. J Shoulder Elb Surg. 2012;21(8):1001–5. https://doi.org/10.1016/j.jse.2011.07.019.
5. Smith IDM, Milto KM, Doherty CJ, Amyes SGB, Simpson A, Hall AC. A potential key role for alpha-haemolysin of Staphylococcus aureus in mediating

chondrocyte death in septic arthritis. Bone Joint Res. 2018;7(7):457–67. https://doi.org/10.1302/2046-3758.77.Bjr-2017-0165.R1.
6. Acosta-Olivo C, Vilchez-Cavazos F, Blázquez-Saldaña J, Villarreal-Villarreal G, Peña-Martínez V, Simental-Mendía M. Comparison of open arthrotomy versus arthroscopic surgery for the treatment of septic arthritis in adults: a systematic review and meta-analysis. Int Orthop. 2021;45(8):1947–59. https://doi.org/10.1007/s00264-021-05056-8.
7. Earwood JS, Walker TR, Sue GJC. Septic arthritis: diagnosis and treatment. Am Fam Physician. 2021;104(6):589–97.
8. Finley ZJ, Savoie FH. Advanced elbow arthroscopy: tips and tricks. J Clin Orthop Trauma. 2021;20:101476. https://doi.org/10.1016/j.jcot.2021.101476.
9. Mehta P, Schnall SB, Zalavras CG. Septic arthritis of the shoulder, elbow, and wrist. Clin Orthop Relat Res. 2006;451:42–5. https://doi.org/10.1097/01.blo.0000229322.30169.29.
10. Hayashibara M, Hagino H, Hayashi I, Nagira K, Takasu Y, Mukunoki D, et al. A case of septic arthritis of the elbow joint in rheumatoid arthritis diagnosed by arthroscopic synovectomy. Mod Rheumatol Case Rep. 2023;7(1):24–7. https://doi.org/10.1093/mrcr/rxac048.

Rheumatoid Arthritis of the Elbow: Role of Arthroscopy

26

Sang-Pil So and In-Ho Jeon

1 Background

Rheumatoid arthritis (RA) is the most common chronic autoimmune disease characterized by symmetric inflammatory polyarthritis, affecting around 0.5% of adults [1]. Among patients diagnosed with rheumatoid arthritis, rates involving elbow joints are about 32% to 61% [2]. Major pathophysiology of RA is a chronic inflammation in the synovium, leading to destruction of the articular cartilage [3]. Larsen classification (Table 26.1) is one of the most commonly utilized radiographic classification of RA [4]. Symptoms and clinical manifestation could be differed by the severity of RA and control of the disease (from synovitis with minimal arthritic change to end-stage arthritis). Surgical indication and treatment for RA are basically not different from other arthritis; however, systemic disease control by medication including disease-modifying antirheumatic drugs is important and should precede before surgical treatment. Surgical treatment could be considered if systemic treatment and conservative treatment fail. By the severity of arthritis, surgical treatment options include synovectomy, osteocapsular arthroplasty, and total elbow replacement arthroplasty [5].

Table 26.1 Larsen classification for RA

Grade	Findings
0	Normal joint space and intact bony outlines
1	Slight abnormality (slight joint space narrowing, periarticular soft-tissue swelling, or osteoporosis)
2	Definite abnormality (one or several small erosions)
3	Medium destructive abnormality (marked erosions)
4	Severe abnormality (usually no joint space left, large erosions)
5	Gross deformity (bony outlines of joint have disappeared)

2 Arthroscopic Procedures for RA

Synovectomy is mainly performed for the early stage of RA including patients who are refractory to systemic treatment and have persistent pain and limitation of motion with minimal arthritic change. In RA patients, highly inflamed joint capsule with synovitis is observed at both the anterior and posterior compartments, and thorough synovectomy should be performed (Fig. 26.1, Video

Supplementary Information The online version contains supplementary material available at https://doi.org/10.1007/978-981-95-3732-7_26.

S.-P. So (✉)
Department of Orthopaedic Surgery, Armed Forces Capital Hospital, Seoul, Republic of Korea

I.-H. Jeon
Department of Orthopaedic Surgery, Asan Medical Center, University of Ulsan, College of Medicine, Seoul, Republic of Korea

I.-H. Jeon et al. (eds.), *Elbow Arthroscopy*, https://doi.org/10.1007/978-981-95-3732-7_26

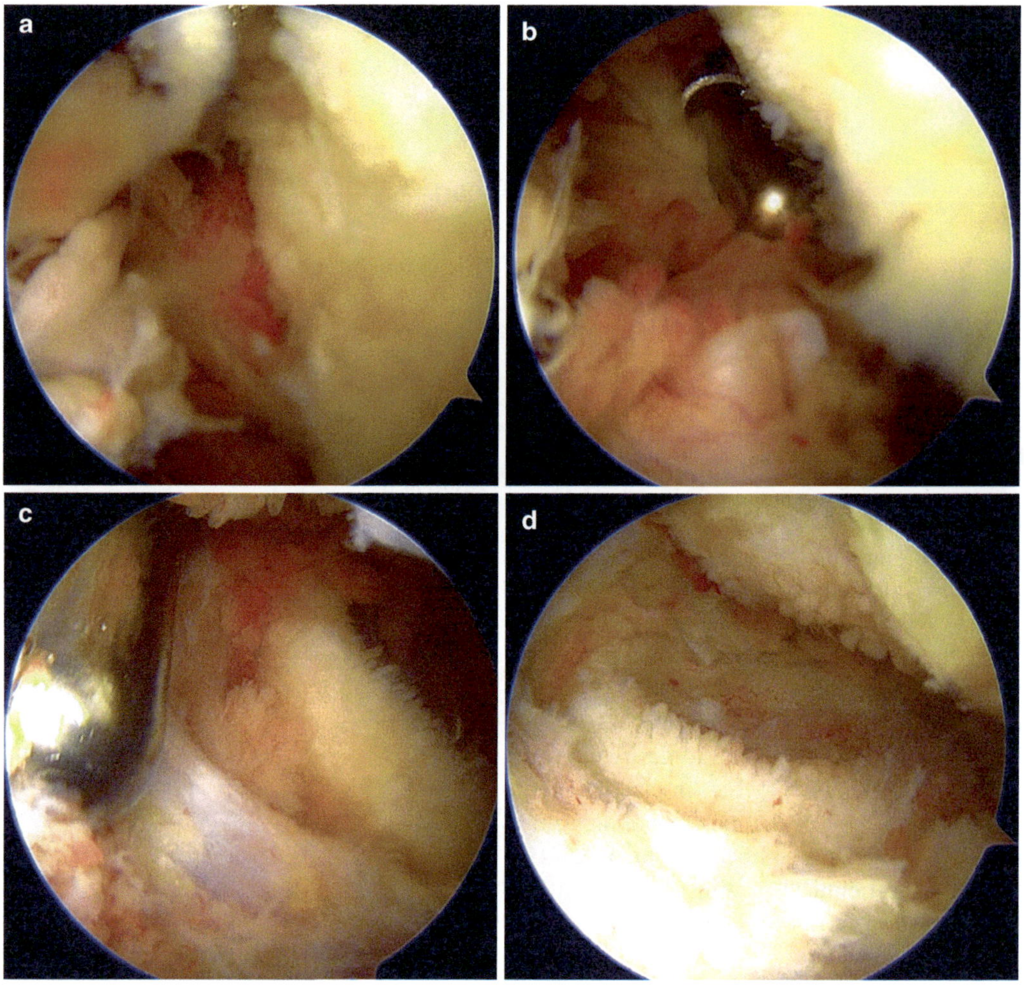

Fig. 26.1 Arthroscopic synovectomy performed for a 63-year-old male with RA. The viewing portal was proximal anteromedial portal. Severe synovitis was observed during diagnostic exam (**a**); arthroscopic synovectomy was performed using debrider from proximal anterolateral portal (**b**); further capsular release was performed (**c**); after synovectomy and capsular release, intra-articular structures were clearly visualized

26.1). Patients under consideration of surgery in early stage of RA commonly have limitation of motion and therefore a release procedure to gain better range of motion is mostly performed together with synovectomy. Chief complaints of the patient and thorough physical exam including range of motion should be evaluated before surgery to reach the best surgical outcome. If the patient has limitation of motion, release procedures in both anterior, and posterior compartments should be performed after arthroscopic synovectomy and postoperative range of motion should be checked and confirmed before finishing the surgery. Arthroscopic synovectomy for RA has shown favorable outcomes for early RA, leading to less pain and recovery of function [5–8] (Table 26.2).

In addition to synovectomy, osteocapsular arthroplasty could be performed to reshape the bone to remove the impingement between spurs, similar to osteoarthritis. Therefore, patients with arthritic change including bony spurs, leading to impingement and therefore limitation of motion are the right indication for the osteocapsular arthroplasty. Before surgery, establishing a detailed surgical plan is important by matching the patient's status (degree of limitation of motion) and radiographic imaging including plain radiograph and computed tomogra-

Table 26.2 Summary of the recent literature about outcomes after arthroscopic synovectomy for RA[a]

Author	Year	N[b]	Mean follow-up (mo)	Indication	Pain		ROM (°)		Function		Radiographic assessment	
					PreOP	PostOP	PreOP	PostOP	PreOP	PostOP	PreOP	PostOP
Lee and Morrey [8]	1997	14	42	Pain severity: moderate to severe and arc of flexion at least 45° and radiologic change Mayo Gr ≤ III	Moderate 12, Severe 2	None 5, Mild 4, Moderate 4, Severe 1	Flex[c]-ext[d] arc 91	Flex-ext arc 98	MEPS[e] 58	MEPS 78	NA[f]	NA
Horiuchi et al. [5]	2002	21	97	Unresponsive to conservative treatment (suggested indication: Larsen ≤2)	None 0, Mild 1, Moderate 11, Severe 9	None 2, Mild 14, Moderate 5, Severe 0	Ext 27 Flex 116	Ext 28 Flex 125	MEPS 48.3	MEPS 69.8*	Change (progression) by Larsen grading: No change, 4; One grade, 14; Two grade, 2; Three grade, 1.	
Tanaka et al. [10]	2006	23	156	Unresponsive to conservative treatment & Larsen ≤2	MEPS (pain) 12	MEPS (pain) 23*	Flex-ext arc 82	Flex-ext arc 103	MEPS (function) 13	MEPS (function) 15	Larsen 1.7	Larsen 3.1
									MEPS 50	MEPS 67*		
Kang et al. [7]	2010	26	33.9	Unresponsive to conservative treatment (at least 6 months) & Larsen ≤3	VAS[g] 6.5	VAS 3.1*	Flex-ext arc 98.1	Flex-ext arc 113.3*	MEPS 58.5	MEPS 77.4*	Radiologic change by Larsen grading: No change, 13; Improvement, 6; Progression, 7	

(continued)

Table 26.2 (continued)

Author	Year	N[b]	Mean follow-up (mo)	Indication	Pain		ROM (°)		Function		Radiographic assessment	
					PreOP	PostOP	PreOP	PostOP	PreOP	PostOP	PreOP	PostOP
Chung et al. [12]	2012	13	34	Unresponsive to conservative treatment (at least 6 months) and Larsen ≤3	VAS 9	VAS 1*	Flex-ext arc 75	Flex-ext arc 105*	DASH[h] score 82	DASH score 45*	NA	
Miyazaki et al. [13]	2015	18	39.1	NA	12/18 cases (66.6%) improved pain to the point without interference of active daily living		Ext 24 Flex 118	Ext 20 Flex 133	NA	AMA evaluation modified by Bruce et al.[i] 85.5	NA	
Shankar et al. [6]	2016	15	30	Unresponsive to DMARD[j] therapy AND Larsen ≤2	VAS 6.4	VAS 1.3*	Flex-ext arc 67.7	Flex-ext arc 85.0*	MEPS 53.3	MEPS 81.1*	Larsen 2.5	Larsen 2.5

[a]Outcomes at the final follow-up were compared with preoperative period
[b]Number of patients included
[c]Flexion
[d]Extension
[e]Mayo Elbow Performance Score
[f]Not applicable
[g]Visual Analog Scale
[h]Disabilities of arm, shoulder, and hand
[i]American Medical Association
[j]Disease modifying antirheumatic drug
*Statistically significant ($P < 0.05$)

phy scans [9]. If a patient has deficit in extension of the elbow, spurs at posterior compartment (olecranon process and fossa) should be observed and if a patient has deficit in further flexion of the elbow, spurs at anterior compartment (coronoid process/fossa and radial head/fossa) should be checked. Radial head excision could be considered for patients with limitation of rotation (supination or pronation). However, rotation of forearm could be affected by proximal, middle, and distal radioulnar joints, and each part should be thoroughly examined to confirm whether radial head excision is needed at the proximal radioulnar joint [7].

Due to a higher tendency for bleeding after synovectomy, drains are typically placed in the joint via portal postoperatively and should be monitored carefully. Postoperative rehabilitation protocols are generally similar to those following arthroscopic osteocapsular arthroplasty including early range of motion exercises. However, patients should be closely monitored for early postoperative complications such as neuropraxia caused by abrupt increase in range of motion (and subsequent nerve stretching), as well as infection or skin problems related to long-term use of steroids or anti-rheumatic drugs. Studies on long-term outcomes after arthroscopic synovectomy have reported overall favorable outcomes. Nonetheless, RA may continue to progress after arthroscopic synovectomy or osteocapsular arthroplasty, and further surgical intervention may be needed in cases of recurrent symptoms and radiographic progression.

Synovectomy and osteocapsular arthroplasty could be performed in both arthroscopic and open technique, and both techniques showed comparable clinical outcomes [10]. However, a recent study, which compared complications between arthroscopic and open arthrolysis for elbow RA utilizing a nationally representative database, reported higher risk of infection and wound complications in open arthrolysis compared to arthroscopic arthrolysis [11]. As a major concern after surgery in RA patients is wound problems and infection due to long-term steroid use, and since open surgery for elbow RA usually needs a large incision, the arthroscopic technique is more preferred than the open technique in terms of reducing wound complications and infection. However, patient-by-patient approach is required for the decision of surgical technique. Here, we attach our preferred treatment algorithm for RA elbow patients (Fig. 26.2).

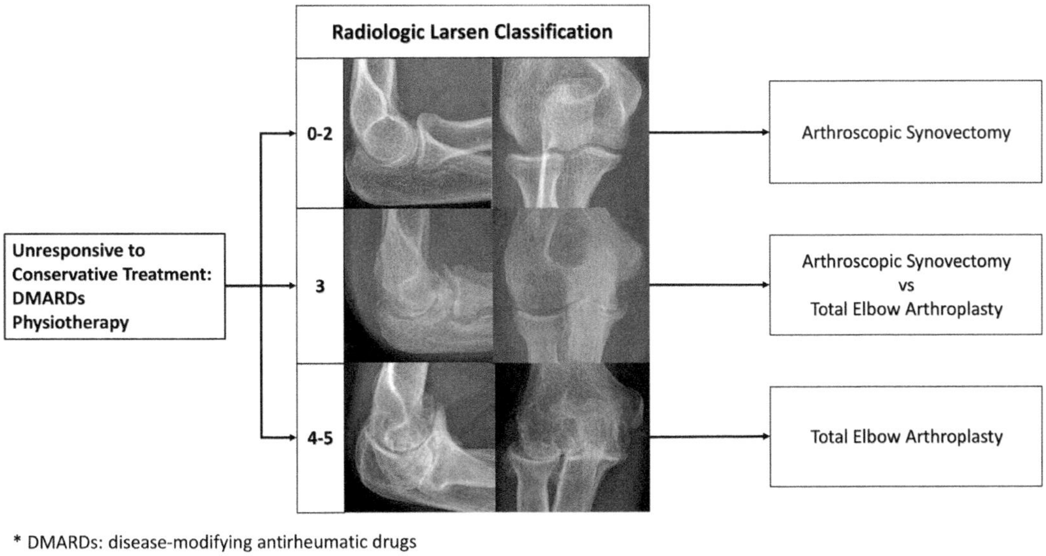

Fig. 26.2 Author's suggested treatment algorithm for RA patients unresponsive to conservative treatment

References

1. Almutairi KB, Nossent JC, Preen DB, Keen HI, Inderjeeth CA. The prevalence of rheumatoid arthritis: a systematic review of population-based studies. J Rheumatol. 2021;48(5):669–76. https://doi.org/10.3899/jrheum.200367.
2. Del Core MA, Koehler D. Elbow arthritis. J Hand Surg Am. 2023;48(6):603–11. https://doi.org/10.1016/j.jhsa.2022.12.014.
3. Stolt P, Källberg H, Lundberg I, Sjögren B, Klareskog L, Alfredsson L. Silica exposure is associated with increased risk of developing rheumatoid arthritis: results from the Swedish EIRA study. Ann Rheum Dis. 2005;64(4):582–6. https://doi.org/10.1136/ard.2004.028465.
4. Larsen A, Dale K, Eek M. Radiographic evaluation of rheumatoid arthritis and related conditions by standard reference films. Acta Radiol Diagn. 1977;18(4):481–91. https://doi.org/10.1177/028418517701800415.
5. Horiuchi K, Momohara S, Tomatsu T, Inoue K, Toyama Y. Arthroscopic synovectomy of the elbow in rheumatoid arthritis. J Bone Joint Surg Am. 2002;84(3):342–7. https://doi.org/10.2106/00004623-200203000-00002.
6. Shankar V, Sharma P, Mittal R, Mittal S, Kumar U, Gamanagatti S. Effectiveness of arthroscopic elbow synovectomy in rheumatoid arthritis patients: long-term follow-up of clinical and functional outcomes. J Clin Orthop Trauma. 2016;7(Suppl 2):230–5. https://doi.org/10.1016/j.jcot.2016.05.011.
7. Kang HJ, Park MJ, Ahn JH, Lee SH. Arthroscopic synovectomy for the rheumatoid elbow. Arthroscopy. 2010;26(9):1195–202. https://doi.org/10.1016/j.arthro.2010.01.010.
8. Lee BP, Morrey BF. Arthroscopic synovectomy of the elbow for rheumatoid arthritis. A prospective study. J Bone Joint Surg Br. 1997;79(5):770–2. https://doi.org/10.1302/0301-620x.79b5.7466.
9. So SP, Kwak JM, Lee JB, Ben H, Alsaqri H, Kim KH, et al. Clinical outcomes of revision arthroscopic osteocapsular arthroplasty in primary elbow osteoarthritis: a retrospective cohort study. Am J Sports Med. 2023;51(8):2050–6. https://doi.org/10.1177/03635465231171542.
10. Tanaka N, Sakahashi H, Hirose K, Ishima T, Ishii S. Arthroscopic and open synovectomy of the elbow in rheumatoid arthritis. J Bone Joint Surg Am. 2006;88(3):521–5. https://doi.org/10.2106/JBJS.E.00472.
11. Remily EA, Bains SS, Dubin J, Chen Z, Hameed D, Livesey MG, et al. Open versus arthroscopic treatment of the rheumatoid elbow arthritis: a comparison of complications at two years utilizing a nationally representative database. Eur J Orthop Surg Traumatol. 2024; https://doi.org/10.1007/s00590-024-03835-7.
12. Chung CY, Yen CH, Yip ML, Koo SC, Lao WN. Arthroscopic synovectomy for rheumatoid wrists and elbows. J Orthop Surg (Hong Kong). 2012;20(2):219–23. https://doi.org/10.1177/230949901202000217.
13. Miyazaki AN, Fregoneze M, Santos PD, da Silva LA, Ortiz RT, Mariz Pinto EC, et al. Assesment of arthroscopic elbow synovectomy outcomes in patients with rheumatoid arthritis. Rev Bras Ortop. 2009;44(6):491–5. https://doi.org/10.1016/s2255-4971(15)30146-4.

Part VI

Cartilage, Overuse, and Tendon Ruptures

Osteochondritis Dissecans and Loose Bodies of the Elbow: Pathology and Indications

27

E. D. Steenbeek, J. W. Colaris, D. Eygendaal, and A. E. van der Windt

1 Background

Capitellar osteochondritis dissecans (OCD) is a rare, localized disease of the subchondral bone of the humeral capitellum, most commonly affecting children between 10 and 15 years old (range 10–24 years) who participate in overhead or upper extremity weight-bearing sport activities. Examples of high-risk sports are baseball, tennis, gymnastics, and weightlifting [1]. Patients typically present with vague, insidious, activity-related lateral elbow pain [2]. Timely recognition and treatment are crucial for the prognosis. Unfortunately, diagnostic delay is common due to its specific clinical presentation and because the lesion is missed on simple radiographs in 50% of cases [3]. Therefore, low threshold for obtaining computed tomography (CT) or magnetic resonance imaging (MRI) in teenagers with lateral elbow pain will help clinicians. Osteochondritis dissecans should be differentiated from an osteochondral defect, which in general has an acute onset after a traumatic event.

2 Etiology

The precise etiology of capitellar OCD has not been elucidated to date. A multifactorial pathophysiological mechanism is assumed, where an interplay of (micro)traumatic, biomechanical, anatomic, and vascular factors is deemed most important. An epidemiological association between participation in activities with high demands of the elbow joint and occurrence of OCD is undeniable. A recent U.S. population study showed that the dominant arm is affected in seven out of ten cases and that eight out of ten patients participate in overhead sports activities, where throwing athletes are at risk especially [1]. Therefore, a single traumatic event or multiple microtraumas are thought to initiate OCD development. While trochlear and radial head OCD has been described [4, 5], the capitellum is the most common anatomic location within the elbow by far, the central part in particular [6]. There are several possible explanations for this specific location in the elbow.

From a biomechanical point of view, the capitellum is both relatively weak and exposed to high forces in overhead sports activities. The relative weakness of the capitellar condyle is shown in Fig. 27.1. The subchondral bone plate at this location consists of only one trabecular layer that is 0.1 mm thick, in contrast to the multiple layers

E. D. Steenbeek · J. W. Colaris · D. Eygendaal (✉) · A. E. van der Windt
Erasmus MC, University Medical Center Rotterdam, Department of Orthopaedics and Sports Medicine, Rotterdam, The Netherlands
e-mail: denise@eygendaal.nl

I.-H. Jeon et al. (eds.), *Elbow Arthroscopy*, https://doi.org/10.1007/978-981-95-3732-7_27

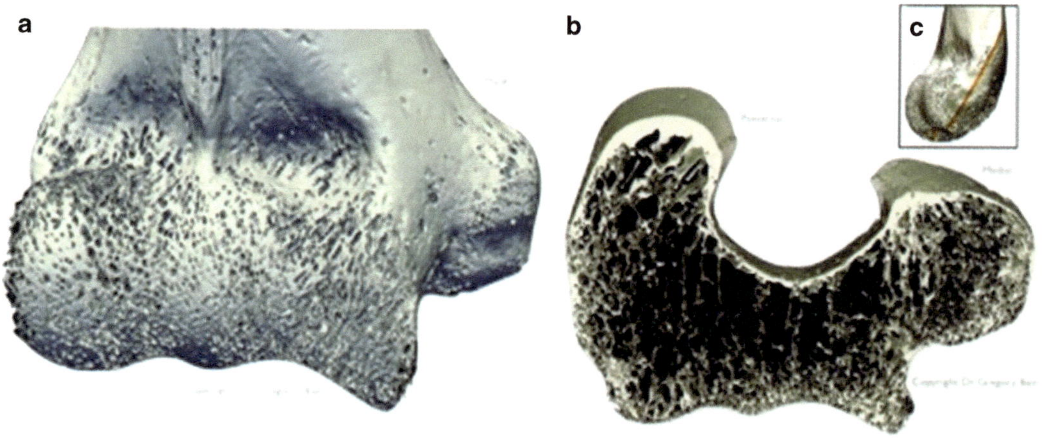

Fig. 27.1 The convex part of the capitellum only consists of one trabecular layer in contrast to the rest of the distal humerus. (Copyright Gregory Bain, reprint with permission. Reproduced from: Bain and MacLean [11])

of the remaining distal humerus [2]. This thin layer is prone to stress fractures. Furthermore, the relatively high stress on the capitellum during overhead sports activities has been explained by two theories. The first theory of the "radial head lag" was proposed by Rotman and recently substantiated with simulations on cadavers [7]. This theory implies that the radial head lags behind during the throwing movement as it is dragged along passively by the ulna, causing radiocapitellar incongruence and edge loading with high shear forces on the capitellum. The second theory links greater medial collateral ligament (MCL) laxity to greater stress on the capitellum. The elbow undergoes valgus stress during the throwing movement, and greater MCL laxity has been shown to cause greater compression of the capitellum in computer models (Fig. 27.2) [8]. Once a defect occurs, the radial head falls into the defect repeatedly, further increasing the damage.

From a histological point of view, the capitellum is susceptible to localized avascular necrosis (AVN) [2]. In understanding the mechanism of AVN, it helps to view the condition as an "osseous compartment syndrome" with three contributing variables: arterial inflow, venous outflow, and contents of the compartment (i.e., the capitellum), as illustrated in Fig. 27.3. Firstly, arterial inflow is relatively easily compromised. While richly vascularized in young children, the capitellum develops a poor arterial supply as it matures and ossifies [2]. Anatomically, vascular supply comes from two small end arteries only [9]. These are branches of the interosseous and radial recurrent arteries that enter the capitellum posteriorly [10]. If one of these branches is disrupted—for instance, due to trauma—ischemia is likely to occur, as there is no supply from medullary vessels (Fig. 27.4) [2]. The gradual development of poor vascularization together with the peak height velocity phase and increase in physical demands of the elbow may explain the peak incidence of capitellar OCD in the early second decade of life, just prior to the closing of the growth plates [2]. Secondly, the venous plexus is especially vulnerable in the capitellum because it is located directly beneath the thin subchondral bone plate [11]. Moreover, its venules have a parallel orientation to this bone plate with few interconnections (Fig. 27.5), so that minor trauma can have a great impact [2]. Impaired outflow leads to increased pressure in the compartment, causing hypoperfusion and thus, ischemia. Thirdly, the fat tissue in the compartment itself is highly susceptible to ischemia, and the resultant necrosis causes edema, which further increases the compartmental pressure [11].

In addition to these biomechanical and vascular mechanisms, more factors may play a role in the etiology of OCD. Twin studies suggest a possible genetic predisposition [12]. Metabolic, inflammatory, and endocrine factors have been

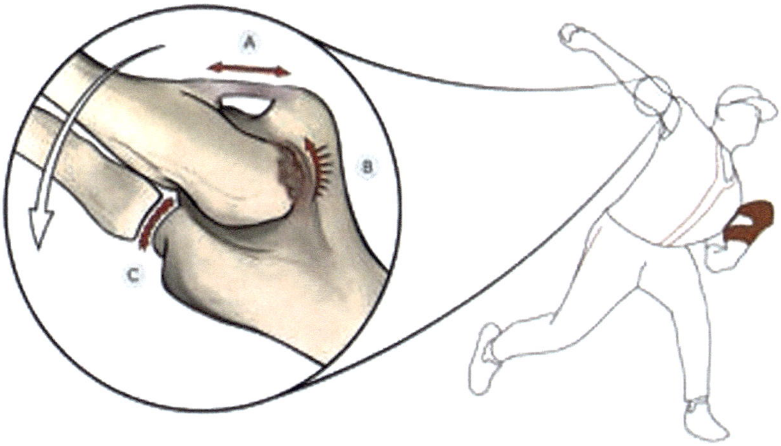

Fig. 27.2 Valgus stress on the elbow during throwing movement. A, traction forces on medial collateral ligament; B, possible concomitant ulnar neuropathy; C, compression forces on capitellum. (Copyright Rik Molenaars, reprint with permission. Reproduced from Molenaars [34])

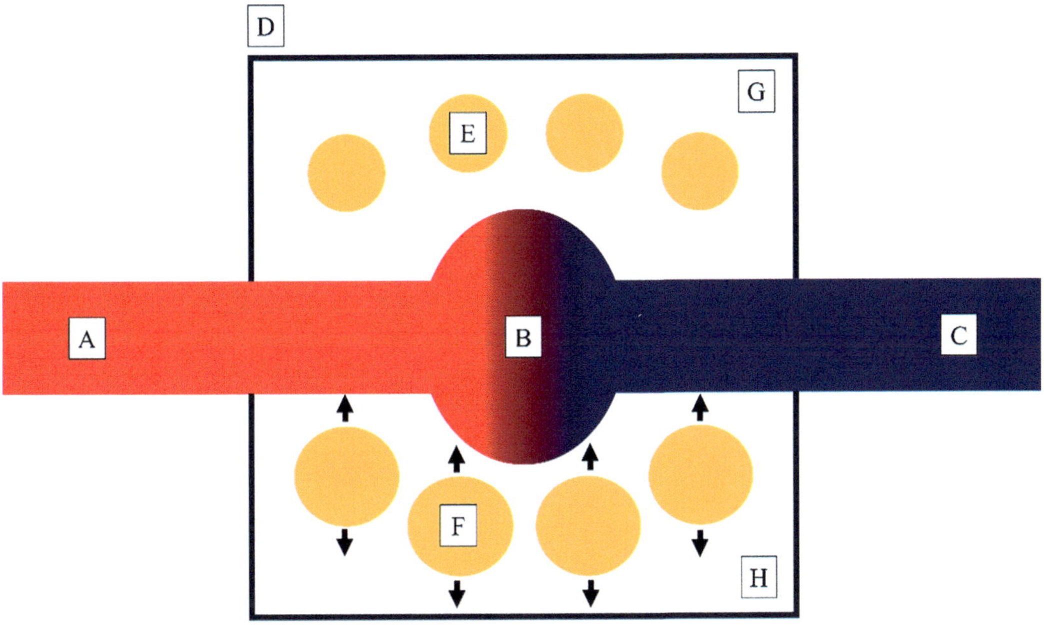

Fig. 27.3 Compartment syndrome of the capitellum, influenced by reduced arterial inflow, impaired venous outflow and further increase of compartmental pressure due to fat cell ischemia. A, arterial inflow; B, sinusoid; C, venous outflow; D, capitellum; E, normal fat cell; F, ischemic fat cell; G, normal compartmental pressure; H, increased compartmental pressure

suggested as well [2], although their precise contribution to OCD development remains to be elucidated.

Histologically, OCD typically progresses through three stages [2]. The first stage entails soft tissue edema and increased osseous blood flow. The second stage involves localized epiphyseal necrosis, sometimes accompanied by fragmentation, where the overlying cartilage loses its mechanical support. By the third stage, granulation tissue forms, and the articular surface may separate, potentially causing loose bodies.

Capitellar OCD patients are likely predisposed to early-onset osteoarthritis. Although the quality of evidence is limited, this causal link is supported by the following three long-term fol-

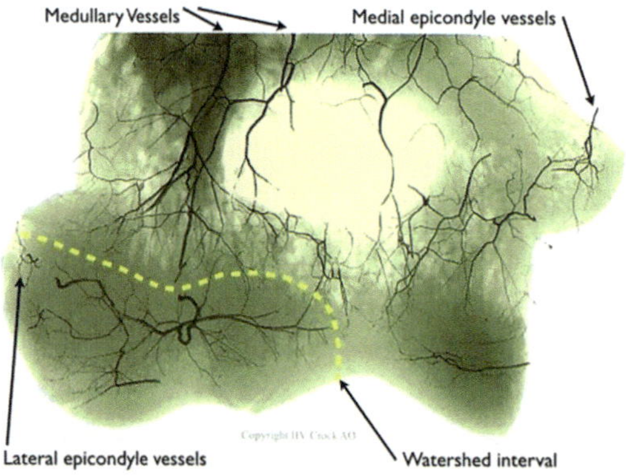

Fig. 27.4 Arterial supply of the humeral capitellum only arises posteriorly. There is no supply from medullary vessels, illustrated by the watershed interval. (Copyright HV Crock, modified by GI Bain. Reproduced with permission from: Bain and MacLean [11])

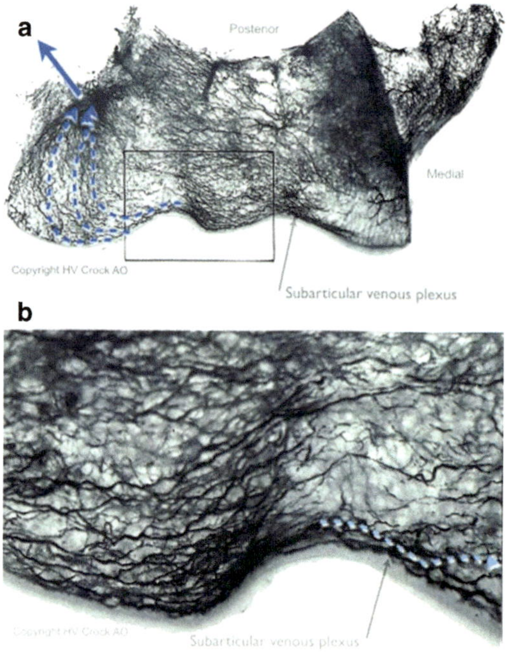

Fig. 27.5 The venous plexus is located directly beneath the subchondral bone plate. Note the orientation of the venules which is parallel to the cortex, as well as the lack of between-venule connections. (Copyright HV Crock. Reproduced with permission from: Bain and MacLean [11])

low-up studies. Bauer et al. followed 30 elbows (75% treated surgically) for an average of 23 years [13]. One-third displayed degenerative changes on radiographs, and four out of ten patients had complaints, where younger patients at presentation had better outcomes, with less pain and fewer signs of degeneration on radiographs. Takahara et al. followed 50 elbows (75% treated surgically) for an average of 13 years, and half of the patients had residual symptoms, regardless of treatment [14]. Braig et al. followed 50 elbows (85% treated surgically) for an average of 11 years and found better pain scores, fewer mechanical symptoms and better elbow flexion in the surgically treated group compared to the conservative group [15], although baseline between-group comparability is doubtful.

3 Indications and Contraindications for Arthroscopic Debridement

Nonoperative treatment is recommended for younger children with stable OCD and involves pausing all activities that stress the elbow for 6 months [16]. One may consider additional nonsteroidal anti-inflammatory drug therapy or cast immobilization, the latter of which seemed to have a beneficial effect in observational research [17].

Surgical intervention is indicated in patients with unstable lesions, symptomatic loose bodies, or failed nonoperative treatment. Stability is assessed with either a preoperative CT or MRI scan. It is recommended to base this assessment on individual imaging characteristics rather than published classification systems, as many different CT and MRI classifications have been proposed in the previous years and all failed to attain sufficient interobserver agreement [18, 19]. Some clinicians prefer preoperative CT over MRI, because it has a higher sensitivity to detect subchondral fracture nonunion, fragmentation, fragment tilting, loose bodies, and osteophytes [6, 20]. Sensitivity may further improve with photon-counting CT: a promising novel CT technique that enables higher spatial resolution while reducing radiation dosage [21]. Other clinicians prefer preoperative MRI without contrast; in a recent Delphi study, the following five MRI features were deemed to be most suggestive of unstable lesions: cartilage disruption, subchondral bone disruption, displaced progeny bone, high signal fluid beneath the cartilage, and loose bodies [22].

Over the past two decades, several surgical techniques have been developed, including arthroscopic debridement, retrograde drilling, microfracture, fragment fixation, and osteochondral autologous transplantation (OAT). The choice of surgical treatment depends on various factors that are assessed on preoperative imaging, as well as intraoperative visualization and tactile feedback during probing arthroscopically. The International Cartilage Repair Society (ICRS) classification is used intraoperatively to aid decision making (Table 27.1) [23]. In ICRS grade 1 lesions, retrograde drilling instead of debridement is recommended [23]. In (sub)acute ICRS grade 2 or 3 lesions with a large viable fragment, consider fixation [24]. In more advanced ICRS stage lesions with fragmentation, poor cartilage quality on the fragment or empty defects, debridement of the defect followed by microfracture is recommended (Table 27.2) [25]. In case of large lesions (>50% of capitellum surface) or lateral wall involvement, OAT can be considered, but donor-site morbidity is a drawback [2]. This chapter focusses on the surgical technique of debridement.

The goal of arthroscopic debridement is to create a stable lesion and enhance nutrient supply through chondral abrasion. Microfracturing may be an additional step to further boost nutrient flow and maximize the formation of fibrocartilaginous tissue [23]. During the debridement procedure, loose bodies are removed. While concomitant posteromedial impingement is rare in young OCD patients, it is more common in the older group, and arthroscopic debridement also facilitates removal of any impinging olecranon osteophytes [23].

Table 27.1 Indications and contraindications for arthroscopic debridement

Indications for arthroscopy	Contraindications for debridement during arthroscopic surgery
1. Symptomatic unstable OCD (a) On CT: subchondral fracture nonunion, fragmentation, tilting, loose bodies, and/or degenerative changes like osteophytes (b) On MRI: cartilage disruption, subchondral bone disruption, displaced progeny bone, high signal fluid beneath the cartilage, and/or loose bodies 2. Failure of nonoperative treatment for 6 months	1. ICRS grade 1 lesions 2. (Sub)acute ICRS grade 2–3 lesions where fragment fixation is possible

Table 27.2 International Cartilage Repair Society (ICRS) classification system for intraoperative assessment of osteochondritis dissecans lesions

ICRS	Description
Grade 1	Stable lesions with a continuous but softened area covered by visually and elastically normal cartilage
Grade 2	Lesions with partial discontinuity, stable when probed
Grade 3	Lesions with a complete discontinuity, not yet dislocated ("dead in situ")
Grade 4	Empty defects or defects with a dislocated or loose fragment within the bed

4 Arthroscopic Debridement: Step-by-Step Surgical Procedure

Step 1. Patient preparation

- Conduct a "time-out procedure" and provide prophylactic antibiotics.
- Place the patient in a lateral decubitus position on a beanbag mattress, with the arm

supported on a U-shaped holder to enable free elbow movement during the procedure. Ensure that the elbow is free from external pressure, particularly on the anterior capsule, to safeguard neurovascular structures. Position the opposite arm cranially in a "sleeping position," resting on the patient's pillow and secured with a sheet and clamp. This setup eliminates the need for additional arm support for the unaffected arm, providing more workspace for arthroscopy.

- Mark the bony landmarks, ulnar nerve trajectory and portal locations (Fig. 27.6).

Step 2. Assessment under anesthesia

Examine the elbow for MCL and lateral ulnar collateral ligament (LUCL) stability. Assess range of motion for flexion and extension, as well as pronation and supination.

Step 3. Further preparation and nerve management

- Exsanguinate the arm using an elastic bandage before inflating the tourniquet.

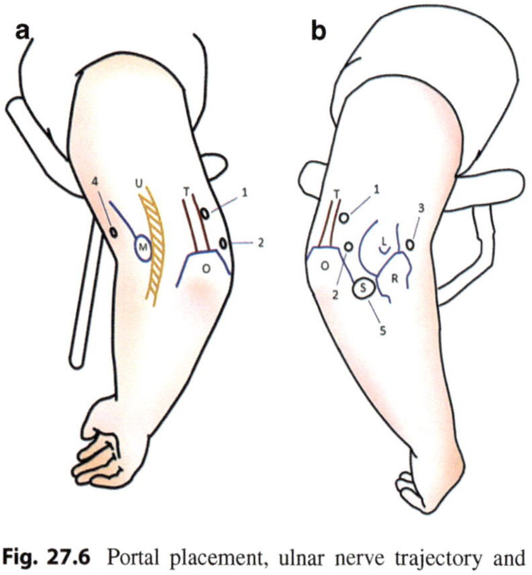

Fig. 27.6 Portal placement, ulnar nerve trajectory and bony landmarks. U, ulnar nerve; M, medial epicondyle; T, triceps central band; O, olecranon; L, lateral epicondyle; R, radial head; S, soft spot; 1, straight posterior portal; 2, posterolateral portal; 3, anterolateral portal; 4, anteromedial portal; 5, soft spot portal. (Reprint of Siemensma et al. EFORT open reviews. 2023)

- Inject 20 ml of saline into the olecranon fossa from posterior.
- In case of prior ulnar nerve symptoms, difficulty of locating the nerve or previous open surgeries, it is advisable to perform an open ulnar nerve release before initiating arthroscopy.

Step 4. Posterior compartment

- Introduce a straight posterior (i.e., midtricipital location, just lateral from the central band of the triceps) viewing portal and posterolateral working portal (see portals 1 and 2, respectively, in Fig. 27.6).
- Inspect the posterior compartment and remove any loose bodies with a grasper if present. These are usually located in the olecranon fossa or medial gutter.
- Remove any impinging posteriomedial osteophytes until the anatomic contour is restored. Be aware of the ulnar nerve running just outside of the posteromedial capsule. When osteophyte debridement was necessary, reassess UCL integrity for latent insufficiency, which may become clear at this stage only [26].
- Assess the elbow for posterolateral instability by first placing the arthroscope in the lateral gutter via the posterior portal, and then attempting to move it along the ulnohumeral articulation into the medial gutter. In a stable elbow, there is insufficient space to make this maneuver. If it is possible, however, the "drive-through sign of the elbow" is positive, indicating posterolateral instability [27].

Step 5. Visualization of the OCD lesion

- In order to properly visualize the capitellar OCD lesion, which has a central location on the capitellum but is mostly visible from the posterolateral compartment as the elbow is 90° flexed during the surgery, introduce a direct lateral (soft spot) portal for the arthroscope (portal 5 in Fig. 27.6). This enables visualization of 80% of the capitellum [28]. A second lateral working portal can be made to perform the debridement. Make sure to place this second lateral portal ulnarly to the first portal to stay proximally and posteriorly to the lateral ligamentous complex and prevent iatrogenic posterolateral instability.

- Grade the OCD lesion using the ICRS system (Table 27.1) using a probe via the direct lateral portal to assess lesion stability [29]. Indications for debridement, among others based on the ICRS grade, were discussed above.

Step 6. Debridement

- First remove any loose necrotic fragments with a grasper.
- Introduce a 4.5 mm or 5.5 mm shaver or a Volkmann curette to remove fibrotic tissue, necrotic bone, and the unstable rim of the cartilage until only viable and stable-looking cartilage remains, with blood seeping from the subchondral bone.
- Additional techniques like microfracture may be utilized to promote the healing response of fibrocartilaginous tissue [25]. Use an awl to create 4 to 7 microfractures in the subchondral bone, depending on the size of the defect.

Step 7. Anterior compartment

- Introduce a proximal anteromedial portal (portal 4 in Fig. 27.6).
- After placement of the first proximal anteromedial portal, take care to protect the posterior interosseous nerve and other fragile structures by placing all subsequent portals under direct arthroscopic view, following initial outside-in needle placement for orientation.
- Inspect the anterior capitellum. Please note that this site may look normal. In case of lateral trochlear OCD lesions, which are located inferiorly, these may be partly visible.
- Inspect the coronoid fossa and the coronoid.
- Introduce an anterolateral working portal with the outside-in needle technique to minimize the risk of iatrogenic injury of the radial nerve. Remove any loose bodies or osteophytes if present.
- Assessment of the MCL can be an option and is performed using an arthroscopic valgus stress test in the anterior compartment [30].
- Inspect the intra-articular radial collateral ligament and the annular ligament. Test laxity of these ligaments with the lateral-pivot-shift test as well as the annular drive-through sign [27].

5 Postoperative Care and Outcomes

In the first weeks following arthroscopic debridement, patients should begin unrestricted range-of-motion exercises if the pain is tolerated. In order to reduce swelling and achieve early full range of motion, gravity-assisted exercises are useful. After 2 months, strength exercises against resistance are introduced. Only after 4 months, axial loading of the capitellum is allowed. Before returning to their sports, overhead athletes should follow a prevention program that is tailored to the demands of their specific sport. In this program, it is important to target the entire kinetic chain from the wrist up until the trunk with a focus on gradually building strength, maintaining mobility and improving neuromuscular control, thereby aiming to minimize lateral compressive forces on the elbow [31]. Return of elbow range of motion and healing on postoperative imaging are widely accepted criteria for initiating return to sport with a timeline around 4 to 6 months [32].

Outcome reporting following debridement and microfracture is heterogenous in the literature [33]. In the largest patient series to date, 75 elbows were followed for a mean follow-up of 3.5 years in the Netherlands [25]. The postoperative Oxford Elbow Score was 41/48, where higher scores indicate better function. Regarding complications, a recent systematic review including 7 studies with a total of 80 elbows, showed a recurrence rate of loose bodies of 10%, all of which required reoperation [33].

6 Tips and Tricks

- Avoid diagnostic delay. Any child participating in overhead sports activities with lateral elbow pain or locking symptoms has capitellar OCD until proven otherwise!
- Care should be taken to distinguish capitellar OCD from capitellar osteochondrosis, also named Panner's disease. The latter presents in younger children between the ages of 4 and 12 [2]. While there may be some etiological similarities, there is no clear link with sports activities and the disease is generally self-limiting. Spontaneous necrosis of the capitellar epiphysis occurs due to ischemia, after which the epiphysis regenerates [2]. Radiographically, subchondral stress fractures of the capitellum can be seen in contrast to the isolated localized lesion which characterizes OCD [9].
- Although capitellar OCD lesions can also be viewed through a posterolateral portal, the consequent orientation of the scope in the direction of the surgeons is unpractical. Using the direct lateral soft spot viewing portal, as described above, enables better visualization of the capitellum, simplifies instrumentation and avoids "sword fighting."
- Reserve fixation for large, viable osteochondral lesions; fixation of necrotic lesions is not useful.

References

1. Uvodich ME, Braig ZV, Reinholz AK, Till SE, O'Driscoll SW, Morrey ME, et al. Incidence and epidemiology of symptomatic capitellar osteochondritis dissecans of the elbow: a United States population-based study over a 25-year period. Orthop J Sports Med. 2022;10(11):23259671221135933. https://doi.org/10.1177/23259671221135933.
2. Eygendaal D, Bain G, Pederzini L, Poehling G. Osteochondritis dissecans of the elbow: state of the art. J ISAKOS. 2017;2(1):47–57. https://doi.org/10.1136/jisakos-2015-000008.
3. Kijowski R, De Smet AA. Radiography of the elbow for evaluation of patients with osteochondritis dissecans of the capitellum. Skeletal Radiol. 2005;34(5):266–71. https://doi.org/10.1007/s00256-005-0899-6.
4. Malik SS, Rasidovic D, Saeed A, Jordan RW, Maclean S, G IB. Management of osteochondritis dissecans (OCD) of the elbow trochlea in the adolescent population: a systematic review. Should Elb. 2022;14(4):415–25. https://doi.org/10.1177/17585732221079585.
5. Tatebe M, Hirata H, Shinohara T, Yamamoto M, Morita A, Horii E. Pathomechanical significance of radial head subluxation in the onset of osteochondritis dissecans of the radial head. J Orthop Trauma. 2012;26(1):e4–6. https://doi.org/10.1097/BOT.0b013e318214d678.
6. van den Ende KIM, Keijsers R, van den Bekerom MPJ, Eygendaal D. Imaging and classification of osteochondritis dissecans of the capitellum: X-ray, magnetic resonance imaging or computed tomography? Should Elb. 2019;11(2):129–36. https://doi.org/10.1177/1758573218756866.
7. Rotman D, Kwak JM, Rojas Lievano J, Hooke A, Camp CL, Fitzsimmons JS, et al. Radial head lag: a possible biomechanical mechanism for osteochondritis dissecans of the capitellum in baseball pitchers. Am J Sports Med. 2021;49(12):3226–33. https://doi.org/10.1177/03635465211033971.
8. Kamei K, Sasaki E, Fujisaki K, Harada Y, Yamamoto Y, Ishibashi Y. Ulnar collateral ligament dysfunction increases stress on the humeral capitellum: a finite element analysis. JSES Int. 2021;5(2):307–13. https://doi.org/10.1016/j.jseint.2020.10.022.
9. van den Bekerom MP, de Klerk HH, van Riet R. Update in diagnosis, treatment, and prevention of osteochondritis dissecans of the capitellum. Should Elb. 2024;16(1 Suppl):24–34. https://doi.org/10.1177/17585732231190011.
10. Yamaguchi K, Sweet FA, Bindra R, Morrey BF, Gelberman RH. The extraosseous and intraosseous arterial anatomy of the adult elbow. J Bone Joint Surg Am. 1997;79(11):1653–62. https://doi.org/10.2106/00004623-199711000-00007.
11. Bain G, MacLean S. Osteochondritis dissecans of the elbow: introduction. In: Bain G, Eygendaal D, van Riet RP, editors. Surgical techniques for trauma and sports related injuries of the elbow. Berlin, Heidelberg: Springer Berlin Heidelberg; 2020. p. 671–6.
12. Kenniston JA, Beredjiklian PK, Bozentka DJ. Osteochondritis dissecans of the capitellum in fraternal twins: case report. J Hand Surg [Am]. 2008;33(8):1380–3. https://doi.org/10.1016/j.jhsa.2008.05.008.
13. Bauer M, Jonsson K, Josefsson PO, Linden B. Osteochondritis dissecans of the elbow. A long-term follow-up study. Clin Orthop Relat Res. 1992;284:156–60.
14. Takahara M, Ogino T, Sasaki I, Kato H, Minami A, Kaneda K. Long term outcome of osteochondritis dissecans of the humeral capitellum. Clin Orthop Relat Res. 1999;363:108–15. https://doi.org/10.1097/00003086-199906000-00014.

15. Braig ZV, Uvodich ME, Till SE, Reinholz AK, Morrey ME, Sanchez-Sotelo J, et al. Osteochondritis dissecans of the capitellum of the elbow: improved outcomes in surgically treated versus nonoperatively treated patients at long-term follow-up. Arthrosc Sports Med Rehabil. 2023;5(2):e435–e44. https://doi.org/10.1016/j.asmr.2023.01.011.
16. Bexkens R, Hilgersom NFJ, Eygendaal D. Osteochondritis dissecans of the elbow: classification and treatment rationale. In: Bain G, Eygendaal D, van Riet RP, editors. Surgical techniques for trauma and sports related injuries of the elbow. Berlin, Heidelberg: Springer Berlin Heidelberg; 2020. p. 677–81.
17. Takahara M, Uno T, Maruyama M, Harada M, Mitachi R, Ono H, et al. Conservative treatment for stable osteochondritis dissecans of the elbow before epiphyseal closure: effectiveness of elbow immobilization for healing. J Shoulder Elb Surg. 2022;31(6):1231–41. https://doi.org/10.1016/j.jse.2022.01.148.
18. Claessen FM, van den Ende KI, Doornberg JN, Guitton TG, Eygendaal D, van den Bekerom MP, et al. Osteochondritis dissecans of the humeral capitellum: reliability of four classification systems using radiographs and computed tomography. J Shoulder Elb Surg. 2015;24(10):1613–8. https://doi.org/10.1016/j.jse.2015.03.029.
19. Bexkens R, Simeone FJ, Eygendaal D, van den Bekerom MP, Oh LS, et al. Interobserver reliability of the classification of capitellar osteochondritis dissecans using magnetic resonance imaging. Should Elb. 2020;12(4):284–93. https://doi.org/10.1177/1758573218821151.
20. Muller SA, Muller-Lebschi JA, Shotts EE, Bond JR, Tiegs-Heiden CA, Collins MS, et al. Advantages of CT versus MRI for preoperative assessment of osteochondritis dissecans of the capitellum. Am J Sports Med. 2022;50(14):3941–7. https://doi.org/10.1177/03635465221129598.
21. Mourad C, Gallego Manzano L, Viry A, Booij R, Oei EHG, Becce F, et al. Chances and challenges of photon-counting CT in musculoskeletal imaging. Skeletal Radiol. 2024;53(9):1889–902. https://doi.org/10.1007/s00256-024-04622-6.
22. Kostyun RO, Nguyen JC, Chhabra B, Todd RLJ, Polousky JD, Saper M, et al. MRI features that contribute to decision-making for treatment of capitellar OCD lesions: an expert consensus using the Delphi Method. Orthop J Sports Med. 2024;12(6):23259671241252813. https://doi.org/10.1177/23259671241252813.
23. Hilgersom NFJ, Bexkens R, van den Bekerom MPJ, Eygendaal D. Osteochondritis dissecans of the elbow: arthroscopic debridement. In: Bain G, Eygendaal D, van Riet RP, editors. Surgical techniques for trauma and sports related injuries of the elbow. Berlin, Heidelberg: Springer Berlin Heidelberg; 2020. p. 683–6.
24. Sayani J, Plotkin T, Burchette DT, Phadnis J. Treatment strategies and outcomes for osteochondritis dissecans of the capitellum. Am J Sports Med. 2021;49(14):4018–29. https://doi.org/10.1177/03635465211000763.
25. Bexkens R, van den Ende KIM, Ogink PT, van Bergen CJA, van den Bekerom MPJ, Eygendaal D. Clinical outcome after arthroscopic debridement and microfracture for osteochondritis dissecans of the capitellum. Am J Sports Med. 2017;45(10):2312–8. https://doi.org/10.1177/0363546517704842.
26. Kamineni S, ElAttrache NS, O'Driscoll SW, Ahmad CS, Hirohara H, Neale PG, et al. Medial collateral ligament strain with partial posteromedial olecranon resection. A biomechanical study. J Bone Joint Surg Am. 2004;86(11):2424–30. https://doi.org/10.2106/00004623-200411000-00010.
27. O'Brien MJ, Savoie FH 3rd. Arthroscopic and open management of posterolateral rotatory instability of the elbow. Sports Med Arthrosc Rev. 2014;22(3):194–200. https://doi.org/10.1097/JSA.0000000000000029.
28. Davis JT, Idjadi JA, Siskosky MJ, ElAttrache NS. Dual direct lateral portals for treatment of osteochondritis dissecans of the capitellum: an anatomic study. Arthroscopy. 2007;23(7):723–8. https://doi.org/10.1016/j.arthro.2007.01.029.
29. Brittberg M, Winalski CS. Evaluation of cartilage injuries and repair. J Bone Joint Surg Am. 2003;85-A Suppl 2(Suppl 2):58–69. https://doi.org/10.2106/00004623-200300002-00008.
30. Field LD, Altchek DW. Evaluation of the arthroscopic valgus instability test of the elbow. Am J Sports Med. 1996;24(2):177–81. https://doi.org/10.1177/036354659602400210.
31. Wilk KE, Reinold MM, Andrews JR. Rehabilitation of the thrower's elbow. Clin Sports Med. 2004;23(4):765–801, xii. https://doi.org/10.1016/j.csm.2004.06.006.
32. George A, Holderread BM, Phelps BM, Erwin ER, Singer W, Jack RA 2nd. Rehabilitation and return to sport criteria following surgical treatment of osteochondritis dissecans of the capitellum: a systematic review. JSES Int. 2024;8(2):355–60. https://doi.org/10.1016/j.jseint.2023.11.003.
33. Leal J, Hones KM, Hao KA, Slaton PT, Roach RP. Arthroscopy and microfracture for osteochondritis dissecans of the capitellum in adolescent athletes shows favorable return to sport: a systematic review. Arthroscopy. 2024;40(4):1325–39. https://doi.org/10.1016/j.arthro.2023.08.075.
34. Molenaars RJ. Introduction and thesis outline. In: Molenaars RJ, editor. Ulnar collateral ligament insufficiency of the elbow in overhead athletes: history, workup, and pathoanatomy. Drukkerij Luxor Nijmegen; 2024. p. 10–25.

Osteochondritis Dissecans and Loose Bodies of the Elbow: Arthroscopic Debridement, Bone Grafting, and Fixation

28

Kozo Shimada

1 Background

Osteochondritis dissecans (OCD) of the elbow is a common sports-related disorder involving humeral capitellum in young athletes with overhead activity. If the osteochondral lesion progresses, the damaged articular cartilage detaches from the capitellum, producing painful osteochondral loose bodies and resulting in irreversible osteoarthritis. Arthroscopic debridement for a progressive lesion is widely accepted because of its technical simplicity and early functional recovery. But the debrided articular surface is covered with reproduced fibrous tissue, so the long-term results are not reliable and sometimes develop irreversible osteoarthritis especially in a large lesions [1]. We have described reconstructive surgery with satisfactory results; however, it can be done on the victim of donor site such as the patient's posterior humerus, knee, or the costal rib [2–4]. Several authors tried in situ repairing procedure by bone pegs, pull-out wires, and compression screws [5–7]. They showed good outcomes in selected cases but in a case of progressed lesion, the results were not reliable. We indicated bone pegs fixation for early stage OCD (usually for ICRS OCD-II) to aim complete cure of the lesion with open method in former days and arthroscopically recently. If it can be done arthroscopically, the blood supply to the lesion is preserved, better clinical results can be expected, and surgical indication can be expanded to early ICRS OCD-III. We describe our treatment protocol and technique of arthroscopic procedure for capitellum OCD.

Supplementary Information The online version contains supplementary material available at https://doi.org/10.1007/978-981-95-3732-7_28.

K. Shimada (✉)
Department of Orthopaedic Surgery, Japan Community Healthcare Organization (JCHO) Osaka Hospital, Osaka, Fukushima, Japan
e-mail: k-shimada1960@nifty.com

2 Treatment Protocol (Fig. 28.1)

Clinical findings including pain, tenderness, catching/locking phenomenon, and range of motion are checked. Radiography is obtained including routine two-direction views and a 45° flexion view (tangential view). In case the view is complex or progressed, CT or MRI is added for precise evaluation. For a radiographically lucent lesion at the first visit, suspicious ICRS OCD-I, rest and conditioning exercises are prescribed. For patients whose lesion remains radiographically lucent after more than 6 months conservative treatment suspicious ICRS OCD-II, arthroscopic evaluation and bone pegs fixation are indicated. For more progressive lesions such as ICRS OCD-III or -IV, arthroscopic debridement with or without reconstruction of the lesion is indicated.

I.-H. Jeon et al. (eds.), *Elbow Arthroscopy*, https://doi.org/10.1007/978-981-95-3732-7_28

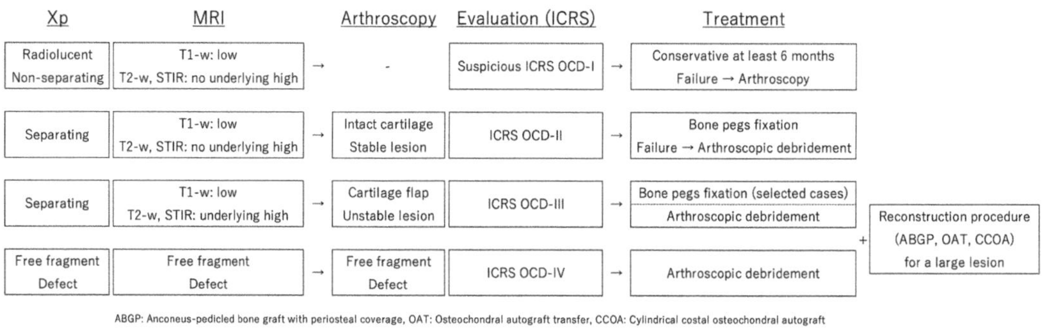

Fig. 28.1 Treatment protocol of capitellum OCD

3 Technical Steps

3.1 Positioning. Prone (or Lateral Decubitus) Position with the Forearm Suspended or in Full-Flexion “Salute” Position
3.2 Anterior Space Viewing at First to Remove Hypertrophic Synovitis and Loose Bodies If Existed
3.3 Direct Lateral Viewing to Identify the OCD Lesion and Following Procedure Decision
 ① In case the lesion diagnosed as stable [ICRS OCD-I and II (intact articular cartilage)] or early OCD-III (undetached lesion with minimum crack of cartilage), fixation is indicated.
 ② Complete debridement of the lesion if the lesion progressed (ICRS OCD-III or IV). Measurement of the lesion size after debridement. The procedure is finished if the lesion is small (smaller than 10 mm in diameter).
 ③ Open reconstructive procedure is followed if the lesion progressed (ICRS OCD-III or IV) and large (more than 10 mm). The open reconstruction method was described in other articles [2–4].
3.4 Bone Pegs Harvesting and Shaping After 3.3-①
3.5 The First 2.4 mm K-Wire Insertion to Keep the Elbow in “Salute” Position
3.6 Arthroscopic Bone Pegs Fixation
3.7 Pull-Out Sutures (Optional)
3.8 Finishing
3.9 Postoperative Care

4 Procedures

4.1 Positioning (Fig. 28.2)

Positioning is important. Operation is started as usual elbow arthroscopy at prone or lateral decubitus position and wide clearance around the patient’s shoulder must be secured in order to keep the forearm in full flexion (so to speak “salute” position).

4.2 Anterior Arthroscopic Synovectomy, Loose Bodies Resection, and Observation (Fig. 28.3, Video 28.1)

Arthroscopic observation is started from anterior to evaluate the OCD lesion. Routine arthroscopic procedure for capitellum OCD such as synovectomy and loose bodies resection are performed through anterior portals.

4.3 Evaluation and Debridement of OCD Lesion Through Direct Lateral (Soft Spot) Portal (Fig. 28.4, Video 28.2)

Arthroscopy is switched to the posterior viewing through direct lateral portal.

① After further observation of the OCD lesion, arthroscopic OCD fixation is indicated for the stable OCD (ICRS OCD-II) with intact

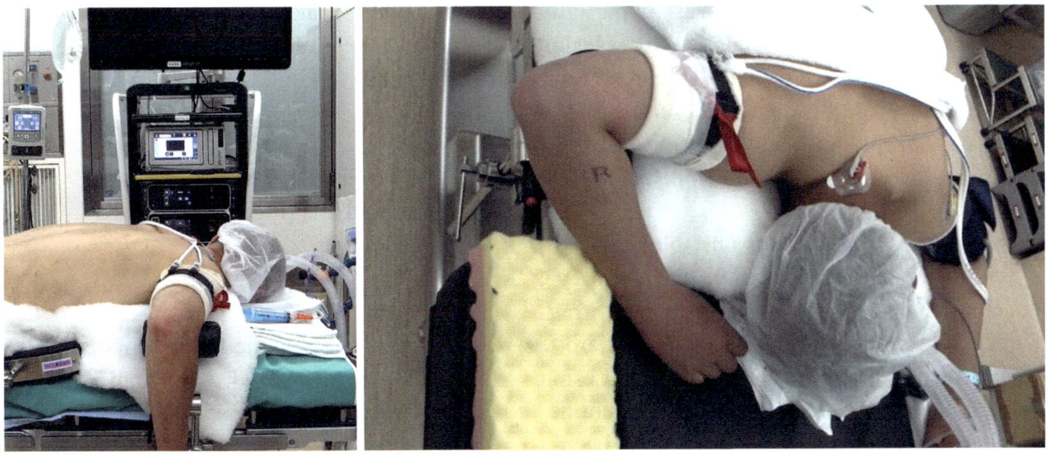

Fig. 28.2 Positioning of arthroscopic surgery of the elbow. Forearm suspended prone position (left) and full-flexion "salute" position (right)

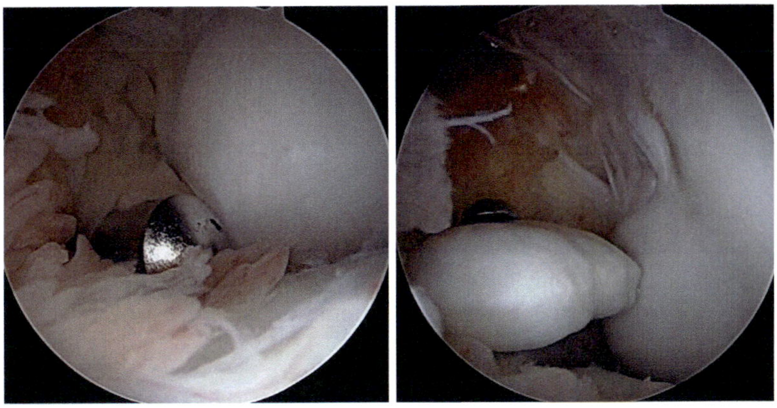

Fig. 28.3 Video 1 Anterior view of the elbow OCD. Arthroscopic synovectomy (left) and free body removal (right)

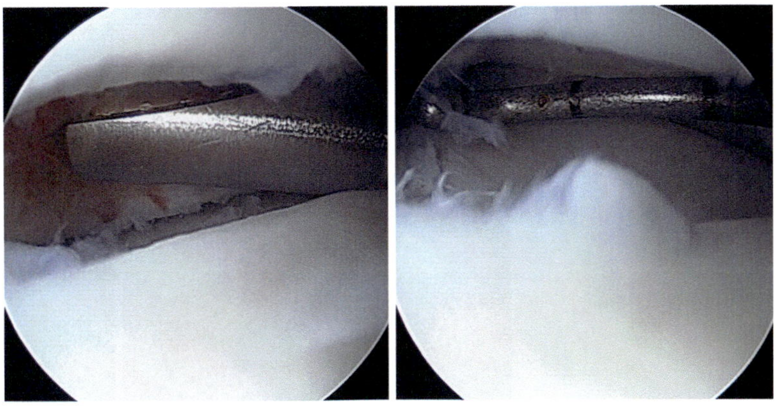

Fig. 28.4 Video 2 Direct lateral (soft-spot) view of the elbow OCD. Debridement to the subchondral bone of OCD lesion (left) and measurement of the lesion diameter (right)

articular cartilage. Some cases of partially detached lesion (minimal flap-like lesion suspicious mild ICRS OCD-III) can be indicated; however, it is dependent on the operator's skill. Optional pull-out sutures (Procedure 3.7) are recommended for those cases.

② In case the OCD lesion is unstable (flap-like) or already detached (ICRS OCD-III and IV), complete debridement of osteochondral fragment is performed under arthroscopy. Sclerotic subchondral bone is also debrided. Lesion diameter is measured after complete debridement. When the lesion is smaller than 10 mm in diameter, procedure is finished.

③ In case the OCD lesion is larger than 10 mm after debridement, reconstruction procedure is followed usually by open method (Fig. 28.5).

4.4 Bone Pegs Harvesting and Shaping (Fig. 28.6)

If the indication of arthroscopic OCD fixation is applied, 3 cm incision on the posterior olecranon or lateral humeral condyle is applied. After sharp dissection to the posterior cortex, 5 × 30 mm strut bone is harvested and cut into four pieces of 2.5 × 15 mm bone pegs. The donor site is buried with artificial bone substitute such as beta TCP.

4.5 The First 2.4 mm K-Wire Insertion (Fig. 28.7, Video 28.3)

Lateral (soft-spot) portal is applied to obtain direct visualization of the OCD lesion, and the elbow is maximally flexed. A 2.4 mm K-wire is inserted into the OCD lesion just above the radial head to keep the elbow in full-flexed "salute" position.

4.6 Drilling and Fixation with Bone Pegs (Fig. 28.8, Video 28.4)

A 2.4 ~ 3.2 mm diameter bony hole is drilled, and a sleeve is inserted to keep the position. A piece of bone peg is inserted in the bony hole of the lesion through the sleeve. This procedure is repeated three times to obtain stable fixation of the OCD lesion. A transparent canula is useful for the sleeve.

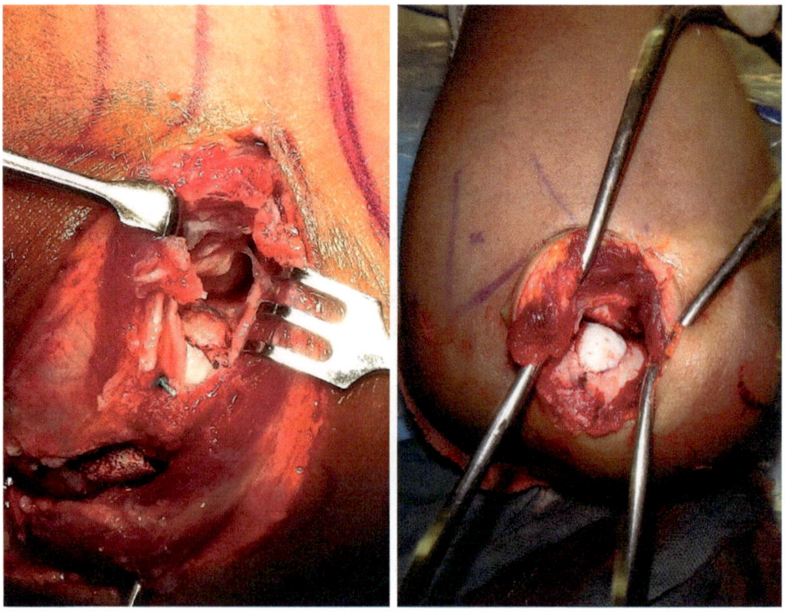

Fig. 28.5 Open reconstruction for the moderate-sized OCD lesion by anconeus-pedicled bone graft with periosteal coverage (ABGP, left) and cylindrical costal osteochondral autograft (CCOA, right)

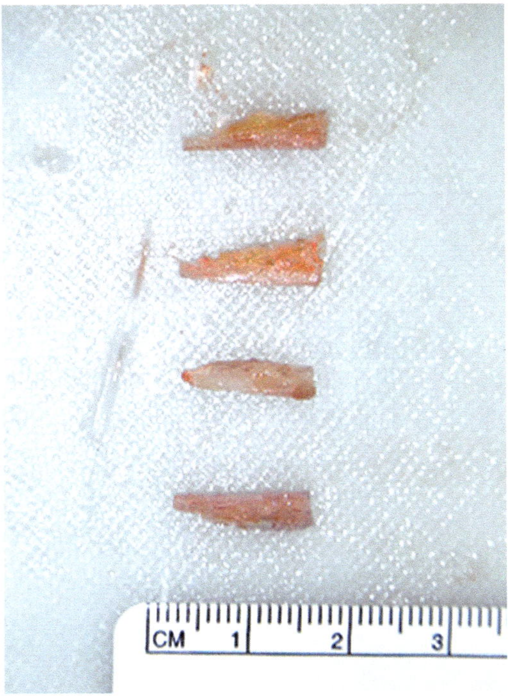

Fig. 28.6 Bone pegs harvested and shaped from the posterior olecranon

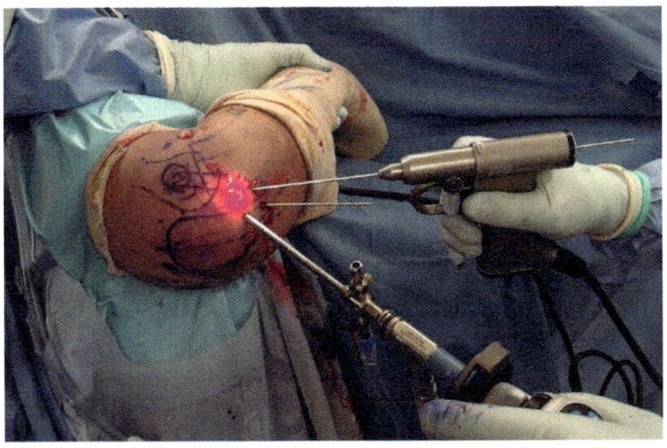

Fig. 28.7 Video 3 A 2.4 mm K-wire is introduced under direct lateral arthroscopic vision to keep salute position, and the second K-wire is drilled in the lateral area of OCD lesion

4.7 Pull-Out Sutures (Optional) (Fig. 28.9)

Additional pull-out sutures are applied in some ICRS OCD-III cases. Through anterior visualization, two bony tunnels are created just anterior to the lesion by 1.5 ~ 2.0 mm K-wire inserted from the posterior humeral lateral condyle near the harvested site of bony pegs. 2–0 nylon loop is introduced through each of the tunnel and pulled out to the direct lateral portal. Next, through lateral arthroscopy in salute position, the OCD lesion is identified and 2.4 mm bony tunnel is drilled at inferior part of the lesion from posterior lateral humeral condyle. A suture retriever is introduced through the tunnel, and the former sutures are pulled out. They are tightened on the posterior lateral humeral condyle. The hole can be buried with a residual bony peg.

4.8 Finishing

Finally, the K-wire keeping the salute position is removed, and a bony peg is inserted into the hole. The tips of the bony pegs are pushed by a bony tamp or shaved arthroscopically to flatten the articular surface. Stability of the OCD lesion is identified.

4.9 Postoperative Care

Two to three weeks immobilization is applied, followed by range of motion and strengthening exercises. Bony union of the lesion is usually identified by radiography in 3 months, and limiting sports activity is allowed. Full activity is allowed in 6 months including overhead sports.

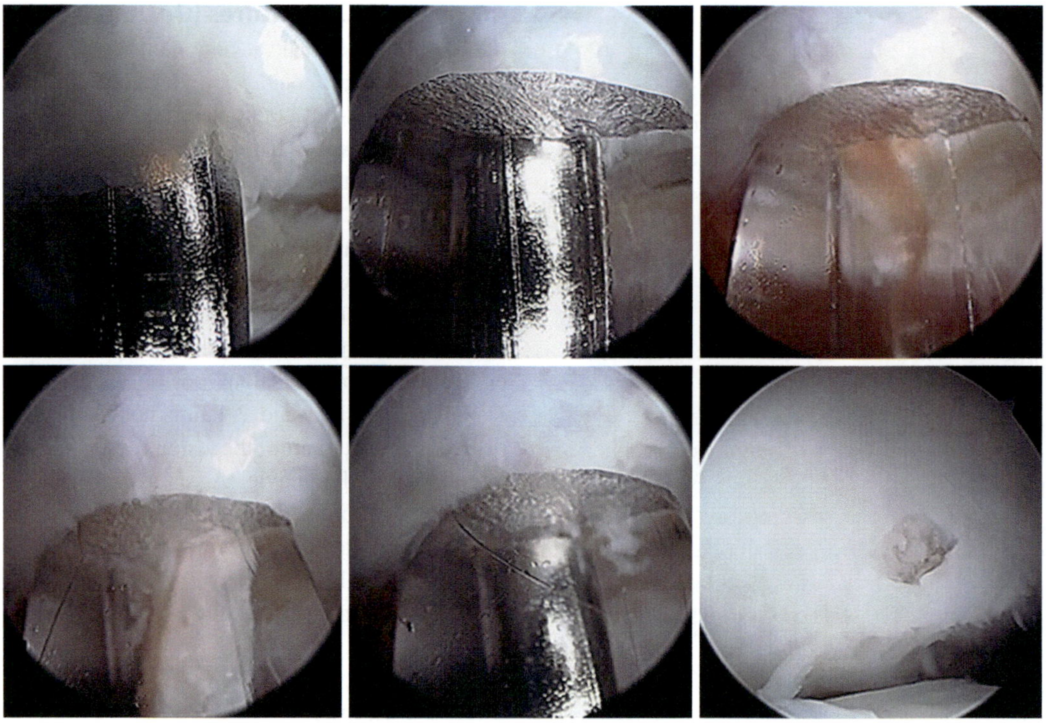

Fig. 28.8 Video 4 Arthroscopic bone peg fixation. OCD lesion is drilled at first. A bone peg is introduced through transparent canula, and the tip is shaved. This procedure is repeated three or four times

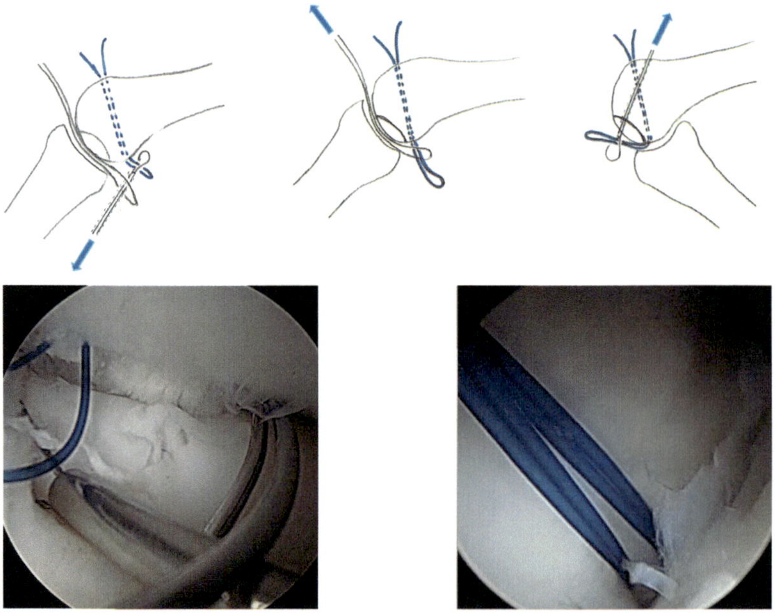

Fig. 28.9 Pull-out technique for flap-like lesion. At anterior arthroscopy, 2–0 Nylon or PDS loop is introduced through 18 G needle or canula in the anterior space and pulled back to the soft spot (left and center). Next, at direct lateral arthroscopy in salute position, posterior part of the OCD lesion is drilled. A suture retriever pulled the strings through the drill hole, and the sutures are tightened on the posterior area of the lateral condyle (right)

5 Clinical Outcomes (Table)

We treat the patients of nonprogressive elbow OCD conservatively and followed for 6 months at least. Surgical treatment is indicated for the patients who do not respond to the conservative treatment or whose lesion is already progressed at the first visit. As a result, we surgically treated more than 200 cases of elbow OCD in last 20 years (Fig. 28.1). Half of them were already progressed cases and were treated with reconstructive procedure such as osteochondral autograft [2–4], and a quarter of the cases were treated with arthroscopic debridement alone because the lesion was small. Fixation procedures were performed for 28 patients with stable OCD whose lesion did not respond to conservative treatment; these patients were operated on and followed for more than 24 months (24 to 169 with mean of 43 months). Most of the lesion stages at arthroscopic observation were ICRS OCD-II, and four cases were a combination of II and III, which means that most of the lesion was stable, but small part of the lesion showed crack between the lesion and the healthy capitellum. Open bone pegs fixation was followed after arthroscopic evaluation in former days, and arthroscopic bone pegs fixation was applied since 2019 in 10 cases. Half of the cases were accomplished arthroscopically, and the other half were switched to open surgery because of technical difficulty such as thick strong muscles or limitation of flexion.

Results were generally good either arthroscopically or by open method. Preoperative clinical status of these patients was generally good; however, radiographic lucent and fragile subchondral bone was observed. We strictly limited surgical indication of bone peg fixation for those nonprogressed lesion (ICRS OCD-II) at first, and have now slightly widened the indication to early ICRS OCD-III, so the results were good or excellent in most of the cases. All of them returned the former sports activity, and a small loose body was recurred in three patients. It was treated arthroscopic removal alone and quickly returned to the full sports activity again. Overall results were shown in the Table.

References

1. Takahara M, Ogino T, Sasaki I, Kato H, Minami A, Kaneda K. Long term outcome of osteochondritis dissecans of the humeral capitellum. Clin Orthop Relat Res. 1999;363:108–15. https://doi.org/10.1097/00003086-199906000-00014.
2. Shimada K, Temporin K, Oura K, Tanaka H, Noguchi R. Anconeus muscle-pedicle bone graft with periosteal coverage for osteochondritis dissecans of the humeral capitellum. Orthop J Sports Med. 2017;5(9):2325967117727531. https://doi.org/10.1177/2325967117727531.
3. Shimada K, Tanaka H, Matsumoto T, Shima H, Kitamura T, Yamada H, et al. Cylindrical costal osteochondral autograft for reconstruction of large defects of the capitellum due to osteochondritis dissecans. J Bone Joint Surg Am. 2012;94(11):992–1002. https://doi.org/10.2106/JBJS.K.00388.
4. Shimada K, Yoshida T, Nakata K, Hamada M, Akita S. Reconstruction with an osteochondral autograft for advanced osteochondritis dissecans of the elbow. Clin Orthop Relat Res. 2005;435:140–7. https://doi.org/10.1097/01.blo.0000160025.14363.f9.
5. Oshiba H, Itsubo T, Ikegami S, Nakamura K, Uchiyama S, Kato H. Results of bone peg grafting for capitellar osteochondritis dissecans in adolescent baseball players. Am J Sports Med. 2016;44(12):3171–8. https://doi.org/10.1177/0363546516658038.
6. Takeda H, Watarai K, Matsushita T, Saito T, Terashima Y. A surgical treatment for unstable osteochondritis dissecans lesions of the humeral capitellum in adolescent baseball players. Am J Sports Med. 2002;30(5):713–7. https://doi.org/10.1177/03635465020300051501.
7. Kuwahata Y, Inoue G. Osteochondritis dissecans of the elbow managed by Herbert screw fixation. Orthopedics. 1998;21(4):449–51. https://doi.org/10.3928/0147-7447-19980401-10.

Valgus Extension Overload Syndrome of the Elbow

29

Maxwell J. McKay, Ronald J. Shamus, Kassem Ghayyad, and Luke S. Oh

1 Background

Valgus extension overload syndrome (VEOS) frequently affects athletes engaged in repetitive rotational and compounding stress on the elbow joint. This condition typically arises when rapid valgus torque is applied to a flexed elbow, exerting significant compression and tension on the medial aspect of the joint. These forces are most pronounced during the acceleration phase of throwing motions and activities involving gripping or wrist flexion [1].

Prolonged strain on the joint can lead to inflammation and tenderness in the tendinous and ligamentous structures, as well as chondral deficiencies that impair mechanical function (Fig. 29.1) [1]. Chronic wear may also predispose individuals to osteoarthritis or acute injuries, such as osteochondral dissecans, which can produce loose bodies within the joint. These foreign bodies often restrict elbow range of motion, resulting in symptoms such as locking, mechanical dysfunction, and impingement-related pain.

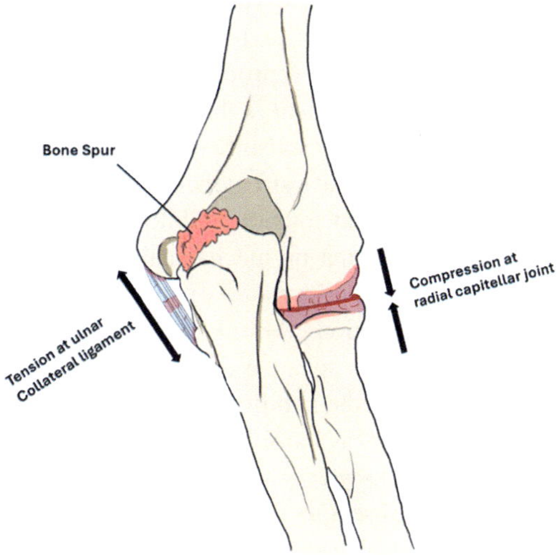

Fig. 29.1 Biomechanical visualization of medial valgus tension and radiocapitellar compression caused by olecranon bone spurs. (Courtesy of Hyunki Lee, MD)

Valgus extension overload syndrome primarily affects overhead-throwing athletes and is characterized by posterior or posteromedial elbow pain. The chief complaint often arises from posterior pain at ball release, particularly when the elbow approaches terminal extension [2]. Evaluation requires a thorough history and physical examination, focusing on range of motion and symptoms such as pain with forced terminal extension, mechanical issues like locking or catching, and ulnar collateral ligament (UCL) laxity. UCL laxity leads to micromotion of the olecranon tip within the

Supplementary Information The online version contains supplementary material available at https://doi.org/10.1007/978-981-95-3732-7_29.

M. J. McKay · R. J. Shamus · K. Ghayyad · L. S. Oh (✉)
Rothman Orthopaedics Florida at AdventHealth, Orlando, FL, USA
e-mail: LOH@partners.org

I.-H. Jeon et al. (eds.), *Elbow Arthroscopy*, https://doi.org/10.1007/978-981-95-3732-7_29

fossa, increasing medial compression on the olecranon-olecranon fossa articulation during forced extension, resulting in abnormal tracking [2].

This compression impinges the posteromedial olecranon process on the medial wall of the olecranon fossa with shear forces, which stimulates osteophyte formation as a compensatory mechanism to regain stability [2]. Diagnostic imaging modalities, including radiographs, CT, and MRI, are useful for detecting osteophytes, loose bodies, and related pathologies. Additionally, the "valgus extension overload test," which combines valgus stress with elbow extension, serves as a key diagnostic tool to reproduce symptoms [1].

Nonsurgical treatment is the initial approach, focusing on rest, ice, anti-inflammatory medications, and a progressive strengthening program to improve elbow and forearm stability. However, persistent symptoms or mechanical issues that impair athletic performance may necessitate surgical intervention. Arthroscopic techniques are preferred over open surgery due to superior visualization and their ability to address common pathologies, such as loose bodies, synovitis, and posterior osteophytes, while preserving joint function. Arthroscopic valgus stress testing during surgery can also evaluate UCL integrity, with ligament reconstruction indicated for significant instability [1].

Postoperative outcomes vary. Arthroscopic techniques frequently allow athletes to return to competition, though recurrence and reoperation remain challenges, particularly if underlying UCL insufficiency is not adequately managed. Limited long-term studies exist regarding UCL integrity following osteophyte resection. Future research is essential to clarify the relationship between osteophyte removal and UCL stress, ensuring optimal outcomes for athletes [1].

2 Indications and Contraindications

Indications	Contraindications
Trauma-related	*Relative*
Fractures of the radial head, capitellum, and coronoid	Prior elbow surgery
Post-traumatic contractures	Previous elbow trauma
Loose bodies	Previous subcutaneous transposition of the ulnar nerve
Inflammatory	Severe post-traumatic/degenerative arthritis
Olecranon bursitis	Ulnar nerve entrapment distal to elbow joint
Synovectomy	*Absolute*
Rheumatoid arthritis	Previous submuscular/intramuscular transposition of the ulnar nerve
Degenerative	
Osteoarthritis	
Osteochondritis dissecans of the capitellum	
Mechanical	
Posterior/posteromedial elbow impingement	
Lateral/medial epicondylitis	
Restricted range of motion due to post-traumatic or degenerative changes	
Mechanical abnormalities (locking)	
Osteochondritis dissecans of the capitellum	
Posterolateral synovial plica syndrome	
Septic arthritis lavage and debridement	
Functional	
Elbow instability	
Elbow discomfort secondary to overuse	
Fixation of fractures	

3 Arthroscopic Procedure

3.1 Surgical Equipment

The preparatory phase begins with ensuring the availability of relevant equipment to guarantee stability and precise joint manipulation throughout the procedure. Essential tools include saline (30 mL), a Wissinger rod, a 4.5 mm arthroscope with a scope sheath, motorized burrs and shavers, Metzenbaum scissors, a pituitary rongeur for larger loose body removal, and an osteotome with a mallet for addressing bony impingement.

3.2 Patient Evaluation

Thorough patient evaluation is critical to prevent complications. Preoperative assessment should confirm a valid indication for surgery, based on symptoms and medical history, to avoid unnecessary interventions and mitigate risks such as nerve damage. Conditions like prior trauma, previous surgeries, rheumatoid arthritis, burns, or congenital deformities can complicate surgery by altering normal anatomy and making neurovascular identification challenging. Advanced imaging techniques, such as CT, MRI, or ultrasound, are often necessary for accurate diagnosis and surgical planning, especially in cases involving subluxating or transposed ulnar nerves (Figs. 29.2 and 29.3) [1, 3]. The combined use of 2D and 3D CT scans allows precise localization of bony impingement, ensuring meticulous surgical planning. Preoperative precautions, such as examining the patient under anesthesia, marking anatomical landmarks, and carefully identifying nerve pathways, are vital for safe surgical outcomes. When the ulnar nerve anatomy is unclear, open approaches may be the safest option (Figs. 29.3 and 29.4).

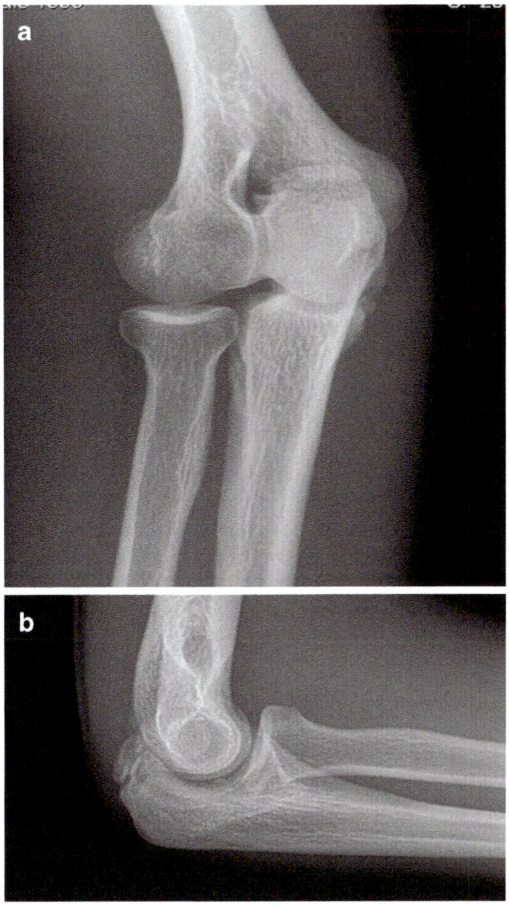

Fig. 29.2 Elbow X-ray imaging presenting osteophytes within the anterior compartment of the elbow. Posterior (**a**) and lateral (**b**) images with elbow flexion

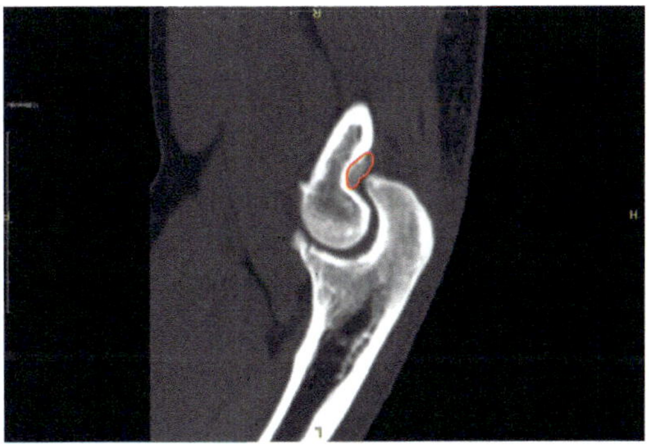

Fig. 29.3 Sagittal CT scan of osteophyte located on the olecranon fossa within the posteromedial space

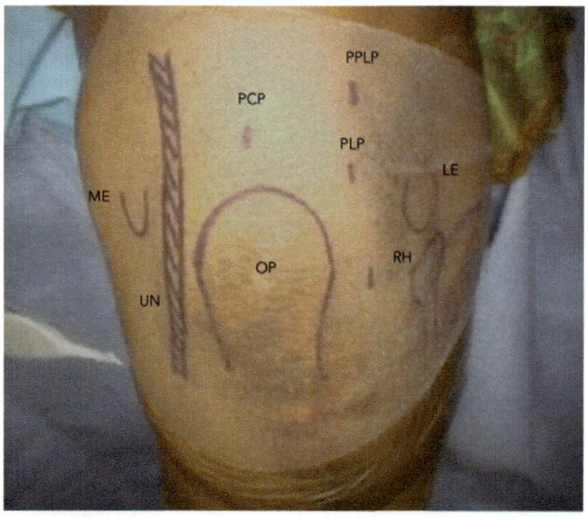

Fig. 29.4 Anatomical landmark drawing prior to elbow arthroscopic procedure, with the patient in the lateral decubitus position on a short bean bag, and the elbow draped and prepared for surgery: ME medial epicondyle, RH radial head, OP olecranon process, UN ulnar nerve, PCP posterocentral portal, PLP posterolateral portal, PPLP proximal posterolateral portal

3.3 Patient Preparation

Patient preparation emphasizes proper positioning and joint preparation for optimal access and safety [3]. Gravity assists in displacing neurovascular structures away from the anterior capsule and working field, improving safety. The lateral decubitus position offers significant advantages, as gravity displaces neurovascular structures away from the anterior capsule, creating a safer working environment. This position is both comfortable for the patient and ideal for accessing all relevant compartments. The arm is stabilized using an arthroscopic arm holder, and a proximal tourniquet serves as both a cushion and support. Adequate padding of bony prominences and preoperative marking of the surgical area are essential for precision (Fig. 29.5) [3]. Joint insufflation with 30 mL of saline expands the working space, improves visualization of anatomical landmarks, and reduces neurovascular risk [3]. Flexing the elbow to 90° further increases the safety margin by distancing the brachial artery and anterior nerves from the joint capsule.

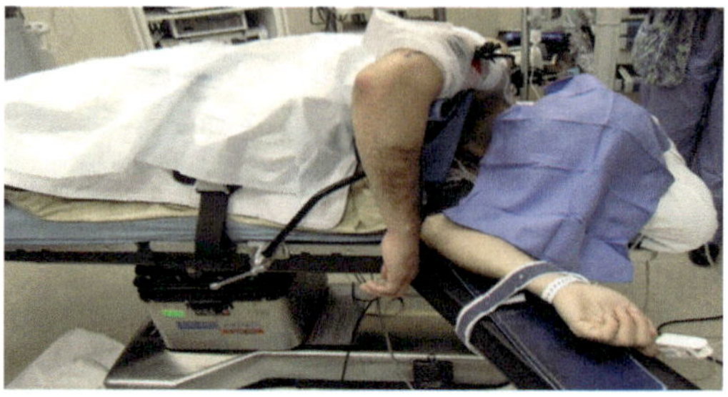

Fig. 29.5 Preoperative placement of patient in the lateral decubitus position on a short beanbag, with padding materials

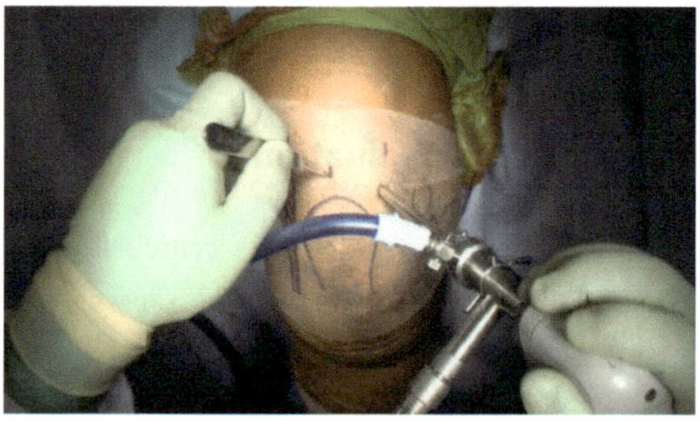

Fig. 29.6 Incision of the posterocentral portal with visualization of the posterior compartment from the posterolateral portal

3.4 Compartment Access and Removal of Foreign Bodies

Accessing the posterior compartment begins with the creation of a posterolateral portal. An incision approximately 3 cm proximal to the olecranon, lateral to the center of the anconeus triangle, is carefully made to avoid damaging the brachial artery and radial nerves (Figs. 29.1 and 29.6) [4]. A Wissinger rod is used to perform a blunt dissection to the capsule, after which the sheath of the arthroscope is slid over the rod to facilitate posterior compartment visualization. A posterocentral portal is then created midline over the triceps, 3 cm proximal to the olecranon (Figs. 29.1 and 29.6) [4]. Using a straight snap to elevate tissues and release capsular adhesions enhances visualization, enabling efficient removal of loose bodies with a grabber or pituitary rongeur. Larger loose bodies may require portal enlargement for effective retrieval.

Loose body removal in the posterior compartment uses either the posterocentral or posterolateral portals for retrieval (Fig. 29.6). Loose bodies are then removed using a grasper or pituitary rongeur, with portal access adjusted as needed for visualization and removal.

3.5 Compartment Access and Removal of Bone Spurs

For bony impingement and osteophyte removal, a proximal posterolateral viewing portal is created to access posteromedial structures (Figs. 29.1 and 29.7). Preoperative CT imaging aids in identifying osteophyte locations on or around the olecranon fossa (Fig. 29.3). An osteotome is positioned at the interface between the osteophyte and the posterior cortex of the distal humerus, and a mallet is used to gently detach the osteophyte under dynamic arthroscopic visualization. The fragment is then removed through the proximal posterolateral portal. Using a motorized burr, the olecranon fossa is recontoured to restore its concavity, minimizing disruption to joint anatomy. Similarly, anterior impingement can be alleviated by excising osteophytes from the coronoid fossa and process, reshaping the area with a motorized burr.

Dynamic arthroscopy confirms the absence of residual impingement and ensures proper joint function before completing the procedure. Precise execution of each step, combined with preoperative planning and intraoperative adjustments, minimizes risks and optimizes outcomes for the patient (Fig. 29.8).

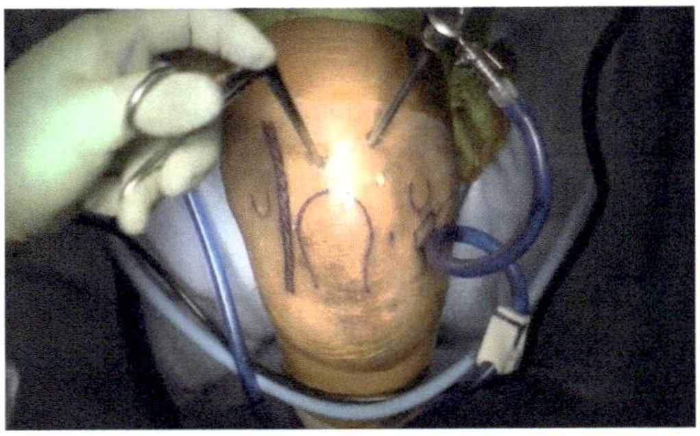

Fig. 29.7 Manipulation of the posteromedial space from the posterocentral portal with visualization of the osteophyte on the olecranon fossa from the proximal posterolateral portal

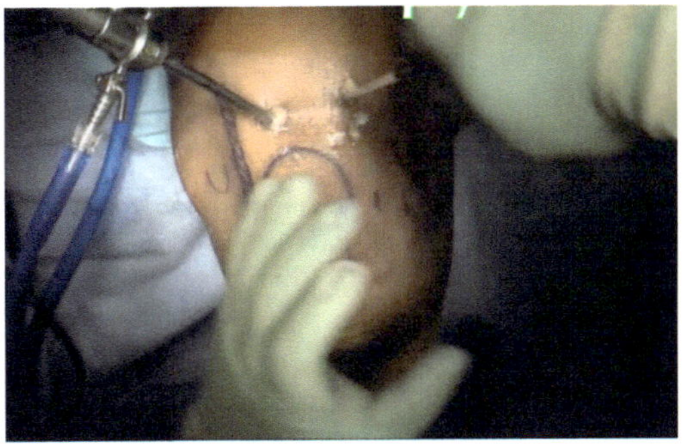

Fig. 29.8 Removal of osteophyte from the proximal posterolateral portal with visualization of the posteromedial space from the posterocentral portal

4 Pearls/Pitfalls of the Procedure

Pearls	Pitfalls
1. Proper patient positioning is essential to provide easy access to all elbow compartments	1. This technique is not suitable for novice elbow arthroscopists and should only be attempted by experienced surgeons
2. Prior surgical procedures, especially ulnar nerve transposition, increase the risk of nerve injury and may require preoperative imaging, such as ultrasound	2. Despite flexion increasing the distance between nerves and the joint capsule, nerves remain in close proximity, necessitating cautious technique
3. Control of fluid pressure is critical postcapsular release, as extracapsular fluid extravasation can limit visualization	3. Insufflation of approximately 30 mL of saline improves the working space but does not eliminate proximity of neurovascular structures
4. Performing bony procedures before capsular release can prevent early swelling and capsular collapse, ensuring better visualization	4. Failing to orient and grab larger loose bodies properly during extraction may lead to complications; use a pituitary rongeur for larger fragments
5. Elbow arthroscopy is best performed in a flexed position to increase safety by displacing neurovascular structures	5. Poor visualization in the posterior compartment can occur without properly releasing capsular adhesions using a straight snap
6. Utilizing both 2D and 3D CT imaging allows precise preoperative planning and accurate identification of bony impingements	6. Relying solely on imaging techniques like ultrasound or standard CT may miss critical structural details

References

1. Rossy WH, Oh LS. Pitcher's elbow: medial elbow pain in the overhead-throwing athlete. Curr Rev Musculoskelet Med. 2016;9(2):207–14. https://doi.org/10.1007/s12178-016-9346-7.
2. Ahmad CS, ElAttrache NS. Valgus extension overload syndrome and stress injury of the olecranon. Clin Sports Med. 2004;23(4):665–76, x. https://doi.org/10.1016/j.csm.2004.04.013.
3. Hilgersom NF, Oh LS, Flipsen M, Eygendaal D, van den Bekerom MP. Tips to avoid nerve injury in elbow arthroscopy. World J Orthop. 2017;8(2):99–106. https://doi.org/10.5312/wjo.v8.i2.99.
4. Schwab PE, Kelly S, DeFroda S. Elbow arthroscopy for posteromedial impingement and fixation of olecranon stress fracture. Arthrosc Tech. 2023;12(12):e2169–e74. https://doi.org/10.1016/j.eats.2023.07.040.

Acute Distal Biceps Tendon Rupture: Endoscopic Repair

30

Roger van Riet, Flynn van Riet,
and Pieter Caekebeke

1 Background

Distal biceps endoscopy is an effective technique for treating complete distal biceps ruptures and is especially beneficial for managing partial tears [1, 2]. This method provides a magnified view of the injury site without requiring manipulation of the tendon. Originally described by Eames et al. [3], the technique presented in this chapter is an adaptation of the original approach and is applicable for both partial tears and acute complete ruptures [1, 4].

R. van Riet (✉)
University of Antwerp, Antwerp, Belgium

Orthopaedic Surgery, University Hospital Antwerp, Antwerp, Belgium

AZ Monica, Orthoca, Antwerp, Belgium

F. van Riet
University of Antwerp, Antwerp, Belgium

P. Caekebeke
University of Antwerp, Antwerp, Belgium

University Hospital Antwerp, Orthopaedic Surgery, Antwerp, Belgium

AZ Monica, Orthoca, Antwerp, Belgium

Ziekenhuis Oost-Limburg, Orthopaedic Surgery, Genk, Belgium

University of Hasselt, Hasselt, Belgium

2 Indications and Contraindications for Biceps Endoscopy

Biceps endoscopy is particularly useful for diagnostic biceps exploration, where a thorough examination of the biceps tendon is needed to determine the extent of injury or pathology. The procedure is also indicated for the debridement of low-grade partial tears of the distal biceps tendon, allowing for precise removal of damaged tissue while preserving the tendon's overall structure. Anchor reinforcement of the insertion can be performed under direct endoscopic view. In cases of high-grade partial tears, where significant tendon compromise has occurred, biceps endoscopy facilitates both the detachment and repair of the tendon, ensuring effective healing and restoration of function. Additionally, the technique is employed in the repair of acute, complete ruptures of the distal biceps tendon, offering a minimally invasive approach with the advantage of direct visualization.

However, biceps endoscopy is contraindicated in chronic cases with severe retraction. In these situations, the tendon may require additional grafting, which, at the moment, cannot be adequately managed through endoscopy alone.

I.-H. Jeon et al. (eds.), *Elbow Arthroscopy*, https://doi.org/10.1007/978-981-95-3732-7_30

3 Step-by-Step Surgical Procedure

This procedure can be performed under either locoregional or general anesthesia, depending on the patient and surgeon preference. We typically use a tourniquet for both partial and acute complete tears. The patient is positioned supine with the arm placed on an arm table (Fig. 30.1). The elbow crease is identified by flexing the elbow, and a 2 cm incision is made approximately 3 cm distal to the elbow crease, centered on the forearm (Fig. 30.2). The lateral antebrachial cutaneous nerve (LABCN) is carefully protected throughout the procedure (Fig. 30.3).

For partial tears, the tendon is palpated and traced to its insertion. Retractors are used to minimize the risk of injury to the anterior neurovascular structures (Fig. 30.4). A small portal is created in the bicipital bursa, either by sharp dissection or by piercing with a trocar (Fig. 30.5). The scope is then inserted between the tendon and the bicipital tuberosity to assess the extent of the tear (Fig. 30.6). In cases where fraying obscures the view (Fig. 30.7), a shaver is introduced by gliding it along the scope's cannula to the tip (Fig. 30.8), allowing for debridement until the tear is clearly visible (Fig. 30.9).

In cases where there is no tear, but the tendon and bursa appear inflamed (Fig. 30.10), the bursa is excised. This excision can be performed either under direct view through the portal or using an arthroscopic technique with a shaver, depending on the surgeon's preference. The endoscopic procedure is also very useful to identify and possibly remove any osteophytes that may be present at the tuberosity (Fig. 30.11).

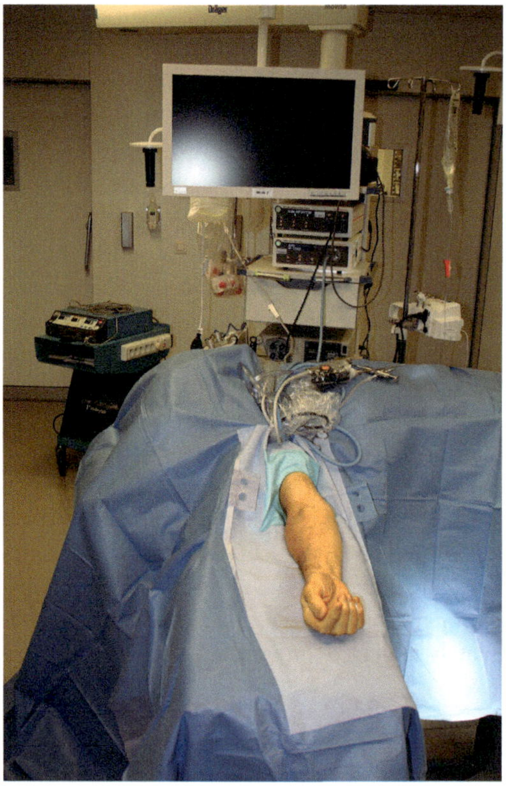

Fig. 30.1 The patient is placed supine with the arm on an arm table. Reproduced with permission ©MoRe Foundation 2026. All Rights Reserved

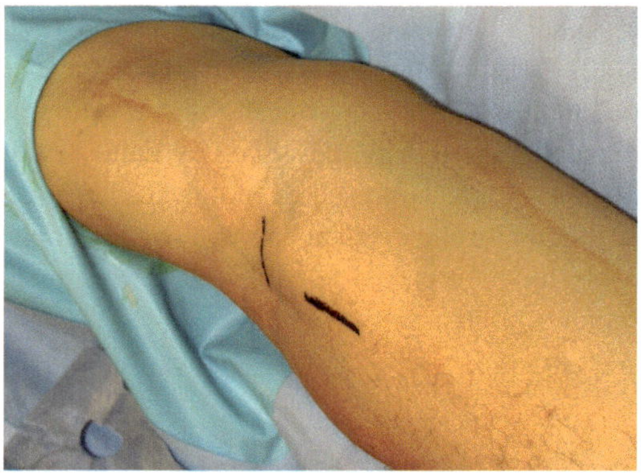

Fig. 30.2 The elbow crease and incision site are marked with a skin marker. A 2 cm incision is made approximately 3 cm distal to the elbow crease. Reproduced with permission ©MoRe Foundation 2026. All Rights Reserved

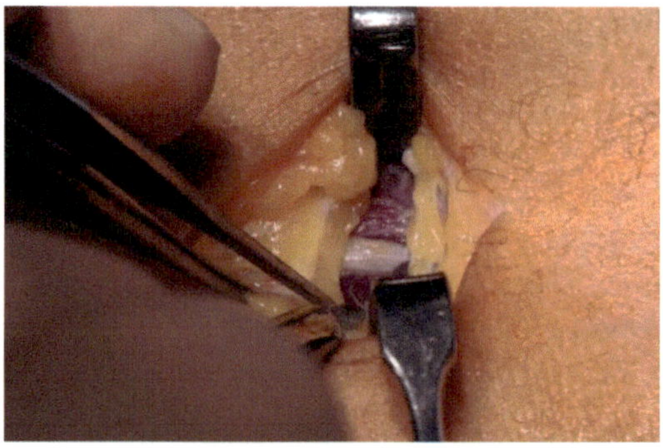

Fig. 30.3 The lateral antebrachial cutaneous nerve can be identified and needs to be protected throughout the procedure. Reproduced with permission ©MoRe Foundation 2026. All Rights Reserved

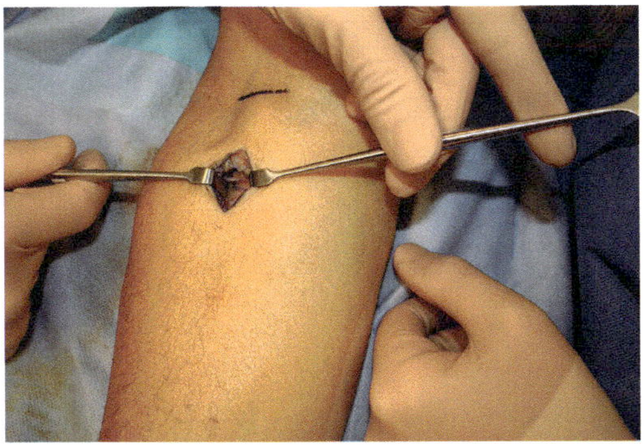

Fig. 30.4 Retractors are used to minimize the risk of injury to the anterior neurovascular structures. Reproduced with permission ©MoRe Foundation 2026. All Rights Reserved

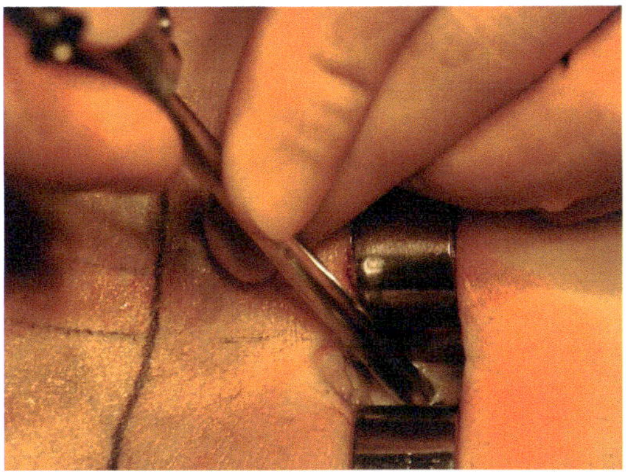

Fig. 30.5 The trocar is used to create a small portal in the bursa. Reproduced with permission ©MoRe Foundation 2026. All Rights Reserved

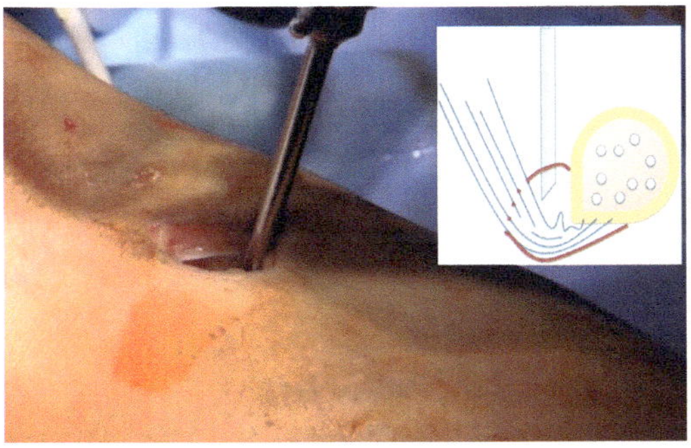

Fig. 30.6 The scope is placed between the tendon and the bicipital tuberosity. Reproduced with permission ©MoRe Foundation 2026. All Rights Reserved

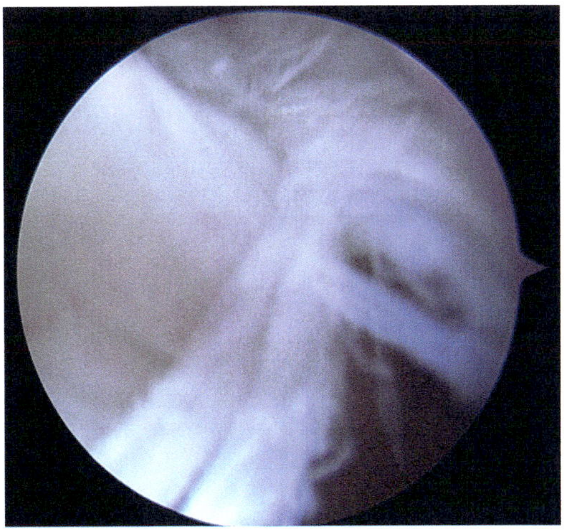

Fig. 30.7 The endoscopic view of the insertion of the tendon is obscured by fraying of the tendon. Reproduced with permission ©MoRe Foundation 2026. All Rights Reserved

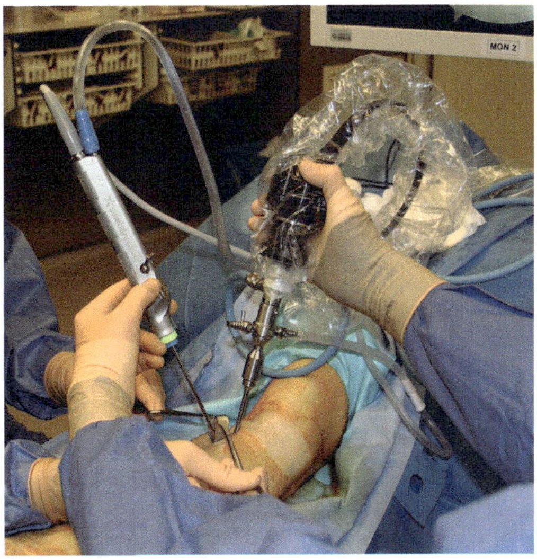

Fig. 30.8 A shaver can be used to debride the tendon or to remove the bursa. Note the placement of retractors to avoid damage to other anterior structures. Reproduced with permission ©MoRe Foundation 2026. All Rights Reserved

When dealing with partial tears, the extent of the tear determines the course of treatment. If the tear involves less than 25% of the tendon's width, simple debridement is typically sufficient (Fig. 30.12). However, if the tear affects between 25% and 50% of the tendon insertion, the tear should be debrided, and the tendon is reattached

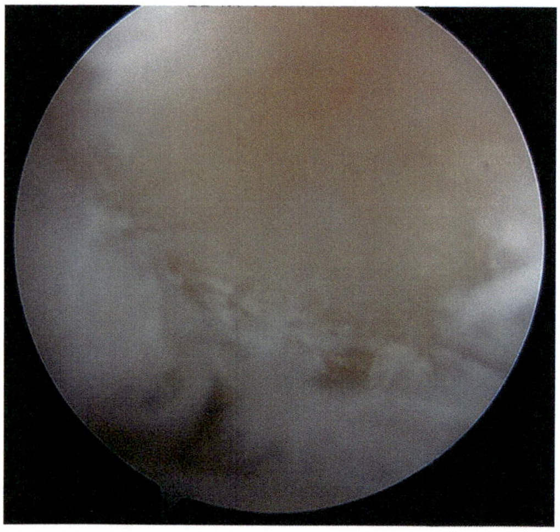

Fig. 30.9 The extent of the tear becomes apparent following debridement of the tendon. In this case, approximately 25% of the tendon had been torn. Reproduced with permission ©MoRe Foundation 2026. All Rights Reserved

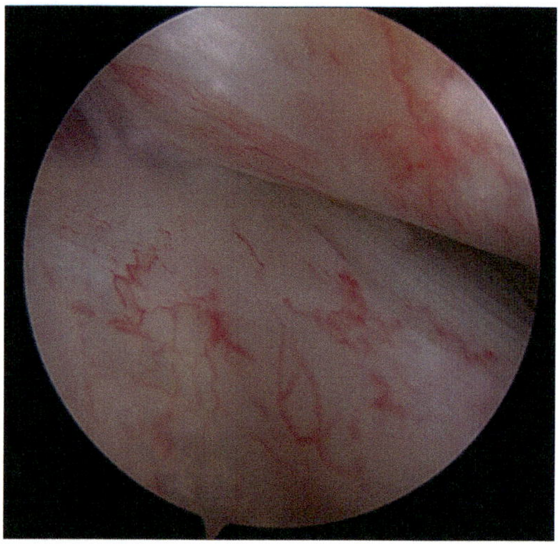

Fig. 30.10 A direct endoscopic view from within the bicipital bursa showing inflammation of bursa and tendon. Reproduced with permission ©MoRe Foundation 2026. All Rights Reserved

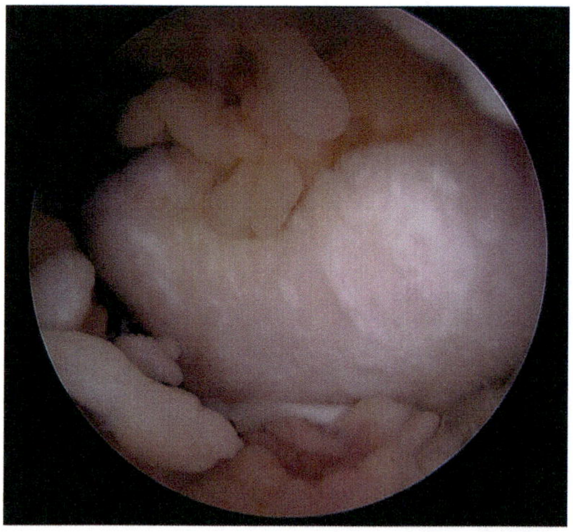

Fig. 30.11 Osteophytes at the tuberosity can be identified and removed endoscopically. Reproduced with permission ©MoRe Foundation 2026. All Rights Reserved

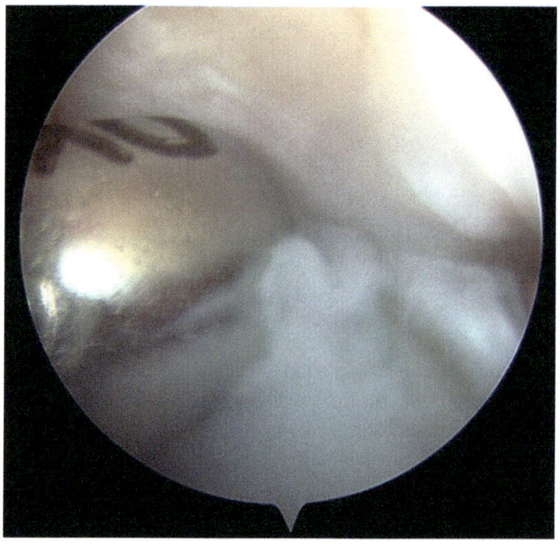

Fig. 30.12 Small tendon attritions can be debrided with a shaver. Reproduced with permission ©MoRe Foundation 2026. All Rights Reserved

using a bone anchor (Fig. 30.13). For tears that involve more than 50% of the tendon insertion or if the tendon is of poor quality, the entire tendon is best released completely and reinserted using the endobutton technique for optimal fixation (Fig. 30.14). The position of the guidepin can be determined endoscopically (Fig. 30.15).

In acute tears with significant retraction of the tendon, the procedure varies slightly. After identifying the bicipital tuberosity through palpation

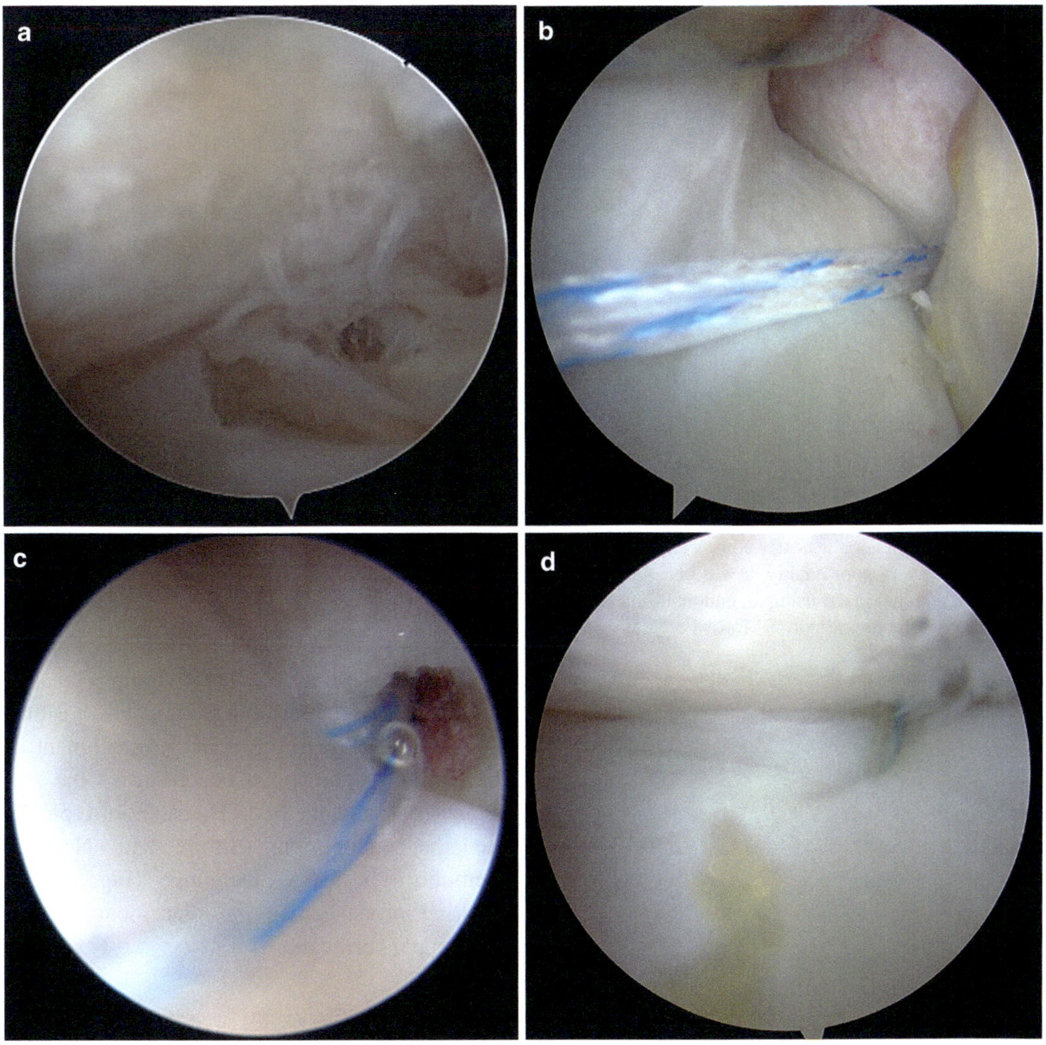

Fig. 30.13 (**a**) A tear of approximately 50% was found in this patient. (**b**) The tear is debrided, and a 1.4 mm all-suture anchor was placed at the base of the insertion. (**c**) Sutures of the anchor are inserted in the tendon. (**d**) The final view after arthroscopic suture anchor repair of a partial biceps tendon rupture. Reproduced with permission ©MoRe Foundation 2026. All Rights Reserved

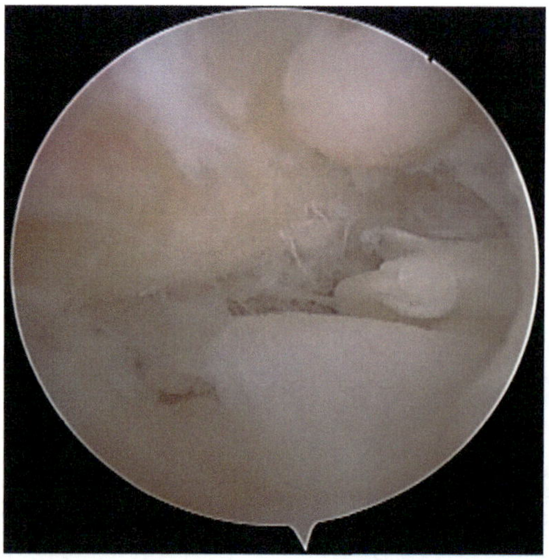

Fig. 30.14 The tendon is nearly completely torn, and the insertion is of very poor quality. It was decided to detach the tendon and to reinsert using an endobutton technique. Reproduced with permission ©MoRe Foundation 2026. All Rights Reserved

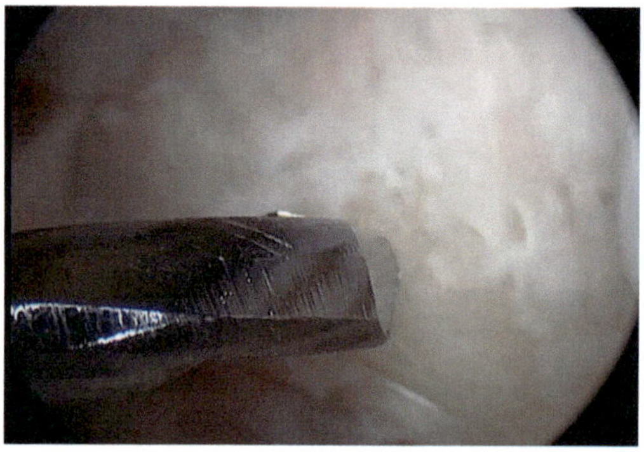

Fig. 30.15 The guidepin can be drilled under direct vision, improving accuracy of tunnel placement. Reproduced with permission ©MoRe Foundation 2026. All Rights Reserved

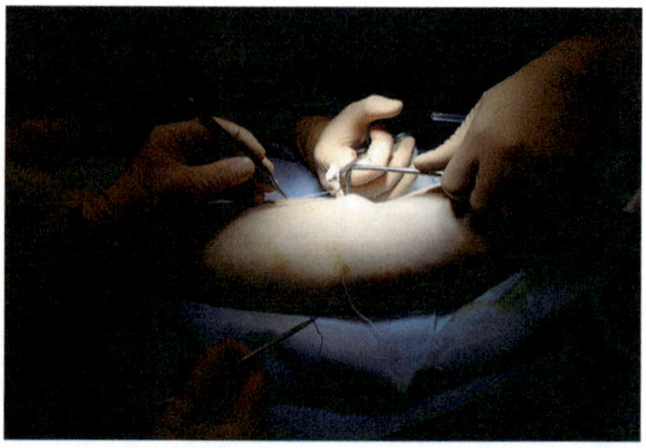

Fig. 30.16 The ruptured distal biceps tendon is pulled out of the portal and an endobutton is sutured to the stump. Reproduced with permission ©MoRe Foundation 2026. All Rights Reserved

and blunt dissection, the scope is used to directly visualize and debride the footprint. The scope is then employed to follow the retracted biceps tendon and find its stump. Once the stump is located, a clamp is used to grasp the tendon, which is then brought out through the skin. Reattachment of the tendon is performed according to the surgeon's preferred method. The authors typically use the endobutton (Smith and Nephew, Memphis TN, USA) technique (Fig. 30.16), ensuring proper guide pin placement through endoscopic verification.

4 Postoperative Care

A protective bandage removable splint (eXo elbow splint, JakeDesign, Belgium) are applied for the first postoperative day to avoid any unwanted movements while the patient is waking up from the general anaesthetic or while the locoregional block is still in effect after which the patient is encouraged to begin elbow mobilization immediately. If the endobutton technique is used, the patient is allowed full range of motion and is allowed to lift up to 20 kg from the first postoperative day. For partial tears that have been debrided or reinforced with an anchor, the elbow is protected with a removable splint for 2 weeks after which progressive lifting is allowed. Full activities are allowed after a minimum period of 3 months.

5 Break Down the Procedure into Clear, Sequential Steps

5.1 Anesthesia and Patient Positioning

- Locoregional or general anesthesia based on patient preference.
- Position the patient supine with the arm on an arm table (Fig. 30.1).
- Apply a tourniquet for partial and acute complete tears.

5.2 Incision and Nerve Identification

- Identify the elbow crease by flexing the elbow.
- Make a 2 cm incision, 3 cm distal to the elbow crease, centered on the forearm (Fig. 30.2).
- Identify and protect the lateral antebrachial cutaneous nerve throughout the procedure (Fig. 30.3).

5.3 Tendon Assessment and Bursa Access

- For partial tears, palpate the tendon and trace it to its insertion.
- Use retractors to protect anterior neurovascular structures (Fig. 30.4).
- Create a small portal in the bicipital bursa, either sharply or with a trocar (Fig. 30.5).
- Insert the scope between the tendon and bicipital tuberosity to evaluate the extent of the tear (Fig. 30.6).

5.4 Debridement and Treatment Algorithm

- Introduce a shaver by gliding it along the scope's cannula to the tip (Fig. 30.8).
- Debride the tendon to clear the view and assess the tear extent.
  - *If no tear:* Excise the bursa if inflamed, using direct view or arthroscopy (Fig. 30.10).
  - *If partial tear (<25%):* Debride the tear (Fig. 30.12).
  - *If partial tear (25–50%):* Debride the tear and reattach the tendon using a bone anchor (Fig. 30.13).
  - *If partial tear (>50%):* Release the entire tendon and reinsert using the endobutton technique (Fig. 30.16).
- Osteophytes can be removed endoscopically for all stages of tendon tearing (Fig. 30.11).

5.5 Acute Tear with Retraction (If Applicable)

- Use the scope to view and debride the tuberosity footprint.
- Trace the retracted biceps using the scope; flex the elbow to locate the stump.
- Clamp and pull the tendon out of the skin (Fig. 30.16).
- Reinsert the tendon using the endobutton technique, ensuring correct guide pin placement (Fig. 30.15).

5.6 Postoperative Care

- Apply a protective bandage for 2 weeks.
- Allow immediate elbow mobilization.
- Use a removable splint for 2 weeks in cases of partial tears that were debrided or reinforced with an anchor (Fig. 30.17).
- Follow the standard postoperative protocol for endobutton fixation.

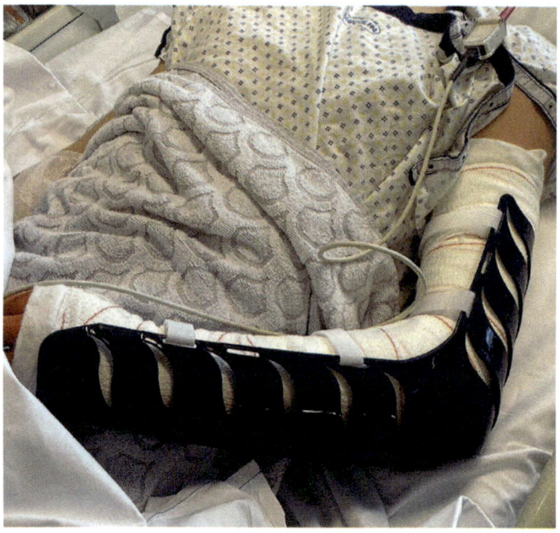

Fig. 30.17 A removable splint can be used in the direct postoperative period. Reproduced with permission

6 List Important Points to Watch Out for During the Surgery

Pearls

- Flex the elbow to 90° to easily identify the elbow crease used for placement of the incision.
- Utilize retractors throughout the procedure to protect the anterior neurovascular structures.
- Ensure that you can feel the bicipital tuberosity when inserting the trocar to confirm correct placement.
- Rotate the forearm to improve visualization of the tendon, particularly in challenging cases. Supination will increase the view on the footprint.
- Always keep the shaver tip fully visible during use to avoid unintended damage to surrounding tissues.

Pitfalls

- Be cautious with retraction, as excessive force can damage the lateral antebrachial cutaneous nerve.
- In chronic cases with tendon retraction, visualizing the tendon can be particularly challenging.

7 Key Procedure Highlight

- *Indications:* Biceps endoscopy is valuable for diagnosing and treating distal biceps tendon issues, including debridement of low-grade partial tears, repair of high-grade partial tears, and acute complete ruptures. We do not recommend this technique for chronic cases with retraction.
- *Visualization and protection:* Use retractors to protect the anterior neurovascular structures

and rotate the forearm to enhance tendon visualization.

- *Trocar and scope placement:* Insert the trocar at the bicipital tuberosity, ensuring contact with the bone; position the scope between the tendon and the bicipital tuberosity.
- *Tendon debridement:* Utilize a shaver to debride the tendon under direct view, maintaining full visibility of the shaver tip during use.
- *Tear management:* Apply an algorithm based on tear severity—debride for minor tears, reinsert with a bone anchor for moderate tears, or perform a full tendon release and endobutton fixation for large tears.
- *Postoperative care:* The elbow is protected with a compressive bandage and an eXo elbow splint. The splint can be removed from day one. Active and passive motion is allowed immediately. Loading may be delayed in patients with a partial bone-anchor repair, depening on the quality of the tissue. Patient with an endobutton fixation are allowed to lift up to 20kg from the first postoperative day.

References

1. Caekebeke P, van Riet RP. Distal biceps endoscopy. In: Bain GI, Eygendaal D, van Riet RP, editors. Surgical techniques for trauma and sports related injuries of the elbow. Berlin, Heidelberg: Springer Berlin Heidelberg; 2020. p. 419–22.
2. Caekebeke P, Verstreken F, van Riet RP. Distal biceps endoscopy at the elbow. Tech Should Elbow Surg. 2018;19(2):93–4.
3. Eames MHA, Bain GI. Distal biceps tendon endoscopy and anterior elbow arthroscopy portal. Tech Should Elbow Surg. 2006;7(3):139–42.
4. Caekebeke P, Galatz L, van Riet R. Accuracy and safety of the endoscopic repair of the distal biceps: a cadaveric study. Acta Orthop Belg. 2020;86(4):711–6.

31 Acute Distal Triceps Tendon Rupture: Endoscopic Repair

Jia Guo, Erica Kholinne, and In-Ho Jeon

1 Background

Distal triceps tendon ruptures are rare, comprising less than 1% of all tendon injuries in the upper extremity [1]. The typical mechanism of injury involves strong eccentric loading applied to a contracting triceps tendon, often following a fall on an outstretched hand.

Distal triceps tendon ruptures typically occur as insertional injuries at the olecranon rather than musculotendinous injuries, with detachment of the central third of the tendon being the most common lesion [2, 3].

The triceps footprint insertion is a dome-shaped area. A recent cadaveric study of the distal triceps tendon footprint identified three distinct insertional areas on the olecranon facet: capsular, deep muscular, and superficial tendinous [4] (Fig. 31.1).

The superficial layer contains a central tendon formed by the long and lateral heads, with an average length of 15.2 cm [5]. Kholinne et al. described the thickened tendinous portion at the center of this superficial tendon layer as the "central cord," identifying it as the most robust part of the distal triceps tendon, occupying half of the dorsal facet of the olecranon [4] (Fig. 31.1).

Distal triceps tendon ruptures can be classified as partial or complete ruptures. Surgical treatment is indicated for patients with high-grade partial ruptures (usually >50% of the tendon) (Figs. 31.2 and 31.3) or complete ruptures [2]. For cases involving less than 50% of the tendon, surgical repair is advised for individuals with significant weakness or high functional demands [6].

There have been reports of open trans osseous repair and repair with anchors showing good results [7, 8]. However, this chapter will focus solely on the endoscopic repair of partial tendon tears.

Supplementary Information The online version contains supplementary material available at https://doi.org/10.1007/978-981-95-3732-7_31.

J. Guo (✉) · I.-H. Jeon
Department of Orthopaedic Surgery, Asan Medical Center, University of Ulsan, College of Medicine, Seoul, Republic of Korea

E. Kholinne
Faculty of Medicine, Universitas Trisakti, Jakarta, Indonesia

I.-H. Jeon et al. (eds.), *Elbow Arthroscopy*, https://doi.org/10.1007/978-981-95-3732-7_31

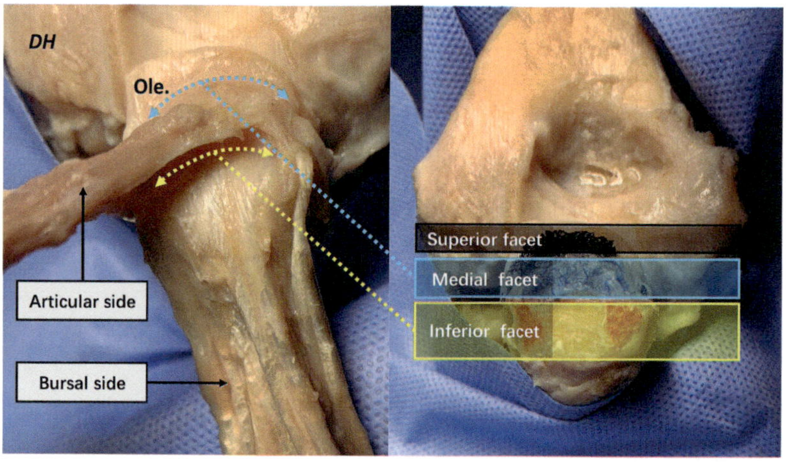

Fig. 31.1 Three distinct insertional areas of the distal triceps brachii on the olecranon facet: (1) Superficial facet (outlined with a black frame): capsular layer (black area on the bone), (2) medial facet (outlined with a blue frame): deep muscular layer (blue area on the bone), and (3) inferior facet (outlined with a yellow frame): superficial tendinous layer (red area on the bone), with the central cord shown as the region between the two red-marked areas

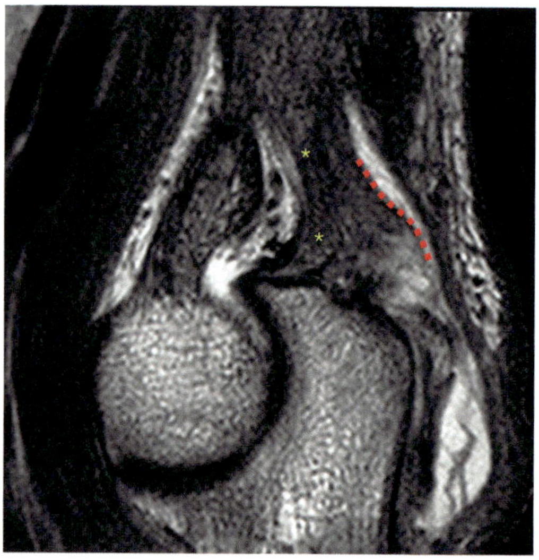

Fig. 31.2 T2-weighted sagittal MRI illustrating a partial-thickness tear confined to the superficial layer (*red dashed line*) of the distal triceps tendon, while the deep layer remains intact (*yellow double asterisks*). MRI magnetic resonance imaging

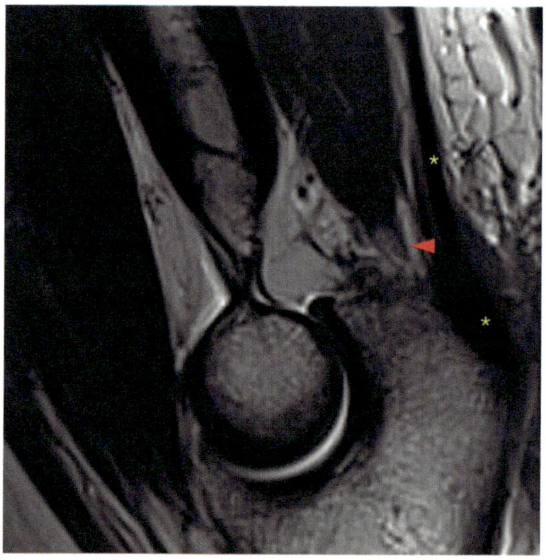

Fig. 31.3 T2-weighted sagittal MRI illustrating a partial-thickness tear involving only the deep layer *(red triangle)* of the distal triceps tendon, while the superficial layer remains intact *(yellow double asterisks)*. MRI magnetic resonance imaging

2 Step-by-Step Procedure

2.1 Patient Preparation

The patient is positioned in the lateral decubitus position under anesthesia, with the arm secured on an arm holder. A sterile tourniquet is applied proximally on the upper arm to ensure the elbow is flexed at 90°, allowing the forearm to hang freely. Key anatomical landmarks, such as the medial and lateral borders of the triceps, olecranon, medial epicondyle, and lateral epicondyle, are marked. Particular care is taken to identify and mark the ulnar nerve to ensure its protection throughout the procedure. 10 ml of saline solution is administered to insufflate the olecranon bursa.

2.2 Endoscopic Assessment and Footprint Preparation

A standard 4.0 mm 30° arthroscope was used. A direct posterior center portal is created 3 cm proximal to the olecranon tip and serves as the viewing portal. A posterolateral working portal is established along the lateral border of the triceps, 1 cm anterior to the midpoint of the line connecting the olecranon and the lateral epicondyle. A posteromedial working portal is created under endoscopic visualization, with careful attention to protect the ulnar nerve.

A bursectomy is performed using a shaver inserted through the posterolateral portal to expose the ruptured distal triceps tendon under endoscopic visualization. Special care is required when using the shaver in the posteromedial aspect of the elbow to avoid injury to the extraarticular ulnar nerve. The free end of the retracted triceps tendon is grasped and mobilized, followed by a trial reduction performed using a retriever. Residual soft tissue is debrided from the inferior facet of the olecranon to expose the insertional footprint of the superficial layer (bursal side) of the triceps tendon. The insertional area of the "central cord" should be identified to facilitate the subsequent positioning of anchors or creation of bone tunnels for fixation (Fig. 31.1).

2.3 Double Row Repair with Suture Anchors or Transosseous Technique

Either suture anchors or bone tunnels can be used for the endoscopic repair of the distal triceps tendon.

1. *Suture anchors fixation with double-row technique*

Two double-loaded knotless suture anchors are inserted into the predefined central cord insertion area (Figs. 31.4 and 31.5). The FiberWire sutures are shuttled through the distal triceps tendon, and gentle traction is applied to reduce the tendon onto the footprint. A lateral anchor is then positioned at the proximal ulna to secure the tendon with proper tension (Figs. 31.4 and 31.5).

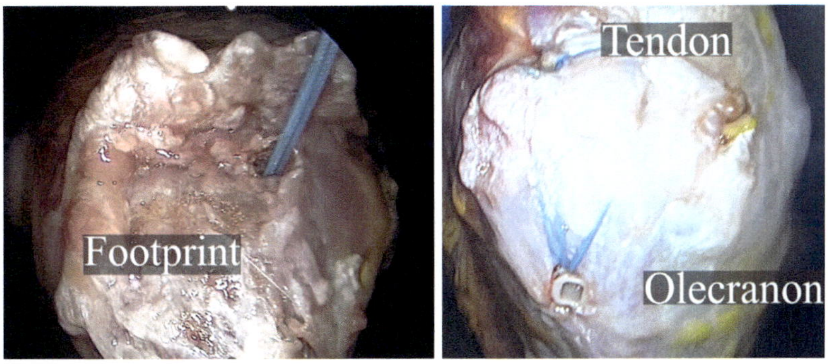

Fig. 31.4 One of the medial anchors is inserted into the footprint. After passing all sutures through the free end of the triceps tendon, a lateral anchor is placed at the proximal ulna to securely fix the tendon with proper tension

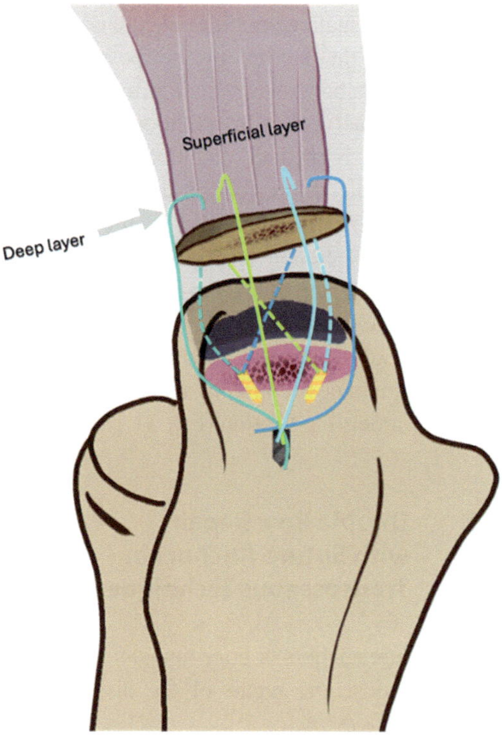

Fig. 31.5 Illustration of fixation with double row repair with suture anchors

2. *Transosseous technique*

Two transosseous cruciate bone tunnels are drilled in the predefined central cord insertion area, with two exits at the proximal ulna. Sutures are then shuttled through the ulnar bone tunnels (Figs. 31.6).

After temporarily securing the distal suture limbs at the tunnel exits on the ulna, the free limbs are passed through the distal tendinous portion of the triceps. The suture limbs are subsequently tied to their opposing pairs at the triceps tendon footprint (Fig. 31.7).

The strength of fixation and tension-free elbow motion must be assessed following each repair method.

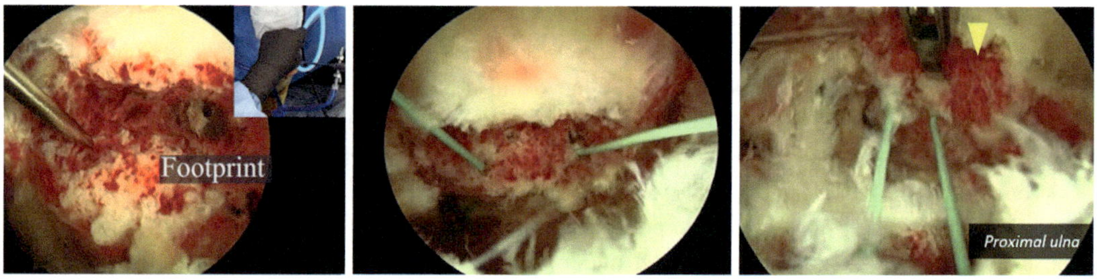

Fig. 31.6 Sutures shuttled through the transosseous cruciate bone tunnels on the footprint of the distal triceps tendon, subsequently passing through the distal triceps tendon (yellow triangle)

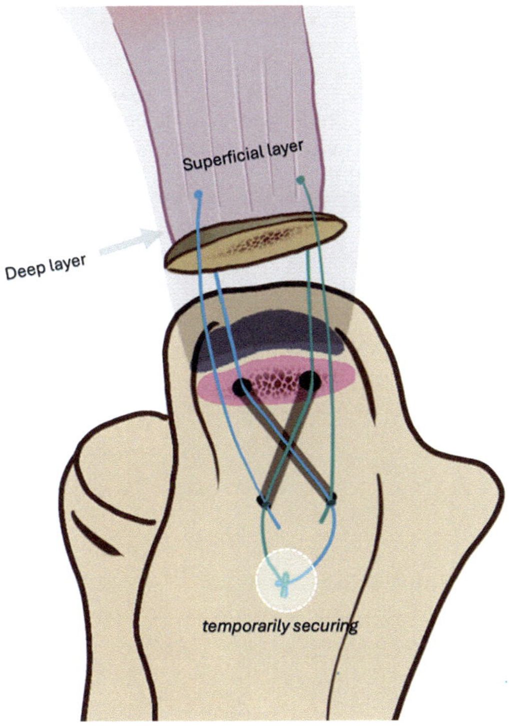

Fig. 31.7 Illustration of transosseous technique

3 Pitfalls of the Procedure

1	*Inadequate workspace and poor visualization*
	Ensure sufficient debridement soft tissue is performed on the triceps surface.
	Confirm adequate mobility of the free end of the triceps tendon.
2	*Poor exposure of the footprint*
	Thoroughly debride all soft tissue from the inferior facet of the olecranon.
	Clearly identify the insertional area of the central cord of the triceps tendon.
3	*Poor coverage of the tendon on the footprint*
	Ensure the repair achieves at least 50% coverage of the footprint on the inferior facet.

4 Key Procedure (Supplementary Video 31.1)

(1) Positioning: Lateral decubitus; arm secured; elbow flexed to ~90°; (2) Portals: Viewing portal, direct posterior center portal ~3cm proximal to olecranon tip; Working portals, posterolateral portal along the lateral border of the triceps, and posteromedial portal established under visualization with ulnar nerve protection; (3) Shaver bursectomy to expose ruptured tendon; (4) Trial reduction to confirm reducibility; (5) Footprint preparation; (6) Fixation using either the "Double-row Repair" technique or the "Transosseous" technique; (7) Confirmation of secure fixation and tension-free elbow range of motion.

References

1. Anzel SH, et al. Disruption of muscles and tendons; an analysis of 1, 014 cases. Surgery. 1959;45(3):406–14.
2. Kholinne E, et al. MRI overestimates the full-thickness tear of distal triceps tendon rupture. J Orthop Surg (Hong Kong). 2018;26(2):2309499018778364.
3. Demirhan M, Ersen A. Distal triceps ruptures. EFORT Open Rev. 2016;1(6):255–9.
4. Kholinne E, et al. The anatomic - magnetic resonance imaging study of distal triceps brachii tendon. J Orthop Surg (Hong Kong). 2022;30(3):10225536221122262.
5. Keener JD, et al. Insertional anatomy of the triceps brachii tendon. J Shoulder Elb Surg. 2010;19(3):399–405.
6. Mair SD, et al. Triceps tendon ruptures in professional football players. Am J Sports Med. 2004;32(2):431–4.
7. van Riet RP, et al. Surgical treatment of distal triceps ruptures. J Bone Joint Surg Am. 2003;85(10):1961–7.
8. Yeh PC, et al. The distal triceps tendon footprint and a biomechanical analysis of 3 repair techniques. Am J Sports Med. 2010;38(5):1025–33.

Part VII

Complications

32 Prevention and Management of Complications in Elbow Arthroscopic Surgery

Sang-Pil So and In-Ho Jeon

1 Background

Due to its less invasiveness and early recovery, the popularity of elbow arthroscopy is increasing, and the arthroscopic technique has substituted a large portion of the open technique [1]. However, complications could be generated after elbow arthroscopy and reported complication rates were from 0% to 27%, while median or mean rates ranged from 4.8% to 5.5% [2, 3].

Despite attempts to understand elbow anatomy and safe portal placement, transient nerve palsy was the most frequently observed complication, followed by postoperative stiffness, wound infection, and heterotopic ossification (HO). Further, a variety of general medical complications including deep venous thrombosis, pulmonary embolism, and cerebrovascular accident could occur during elbow arthroscopy and generate fatal situation; therefore, these should not be overlooked.

Supplementary Information The online version contains supplementary material available at https://doi.org/10.1007/978-981-95-3732-7_32.

S.-P. So (✉)
Department of Orthopaedic Surgery, Armed Forces Capital Hospital, Seoul, Republic of Korea

I.-H. Jeon
Department of Orthopaedic Surgery, Asan Medical Center, University of Ulsan, College of Medicine, Seoul, Republic of Korea

A recent systematic review demonstrated that complication rates could be stratified according to surgery complexity [2]. Low-complexity surgery including loose body removal and diagnostic examination showed lower complication rates, while high-complexity surgery including contracture release, scope-assisted fracture surgery, and osteocapsular arthroplasty showed relatively higher complication rates. Therefore, careful patient selection and proper surgical technique are required especially for high-complexity surgery (Table 32.1).

Table 32.1 Common complications in elbow arthroscopy and occurrence rate reported by de Klerk et al. [2]

	Occurrence (n = 18,892)
Nerve injury	
Transient	281 (1.49%)
Permanent	7 (0.04%)
Stiffness/contracture	149 (0.79%)
Wound infection	
Superficial	175 (0.93%)
Deep	17 (0.09%)
Heterotopic ossification (HO)	53 (0.28%)
Instability	4 (0.02%)
General medical complication[a]	120 (0.64%)

[a]Includes deep venous thrombosis, pulmonary embolism, myocardial infarction, cerebrovascular accident, urinary tract infection, acute renal failure, or respiratory failure

I.-H. Jeon et al. (eds.), *Elbow Arthroscopy*, https://doi.org/10.1007/978-981-95-3732-7_32

2 Neurovascular Injury

Nerve injury is the most common and critical complication in elbow arthroscopy. Reported overall incidence rate of nerve injury ranges from 0.5% to 5.3% in elbow arthroscopy [4]. Most of nerve injuries are transient palsy; however, permanent nerve injury or complete nerve transection are also reported in elbow arthroscopy [5]. Nerve injury could happen in all three peripheral nerves including ulnar nerve, radial nerve, and median nerve, which are located around the elbow joint. Transient nerve palsy could occur due to nerve compression by distension of the elbow joint or nerve stretching by sudden large gain of range of motion after surgery. Permanent nerve injury could be generated during portal placement or procedure including anterior capsular release and posteromedial gutter release. All of three nerves have different causes and situations for the nerve injury; therefore, precise understanding of each nerve anatomy and situation leading to nerve injury is important to prevent possible nerve injuries in elbow arthroscopy.

If nerve injury is detected or direct nerve injury is suspected during elbow arthroscopy, exploration should be performed without delay to minimize the neurologic sequelae. Target nerve should be explored enough for both proximally and distally and direct nerve procedure including repair is required if nerve injury is confirmed. If neurologic signs are detected after surgery, the patient should be examined thoroughly to specify the injured nerve. If there is any possibility for direct nerve injury, ultrasound should be performed to trace the course of nerve and exploration should be performed without delay, if needed.

2.1 Ulnar Nerve

The ulnar nerve is the most commonly affected nerve in both transient and permanent nerve injuries [6]. The presence of ulnar nerve subluxation and a previous history of ulnar nerve procedures, including release or anterior transposition, should be checked before surgery. Most transient ulnar nerve palsies can be attributed to stretching and compression of the ulnar nerve caused by an increased flexion arc after surgery. For example, if a patient had preoperative elbow flexion <90° and flexion arc increased to 140° after arthroscopic release surgery, sudden increase of flexion arc could generate ulnar nerve stretching and nerve compression within cubital tunnel, leading to indirect nerve injury. Therefore, prophylactic ulnar nerve decompression should be preceded in selected patients with decreased elbow flexion arc and under consideration of surgery for gaining flexion arc. There are no definite criteria for a preoperative flexion arc needing prophylactic ulnar nerve decompression; however, pressure on the ulnar nerve in cubital tunnel is increased, if elbow is flexed over 90° in a biomechanical study [7]. Therefore, patients with <90° of elbow flexion are recommended to have prophylactic ulnar nerve decompression to minimize indirect ulnar nerve injury [8]. Ulnar nerve is posteromedially located and considering the route of ulnar nerve, it is difficult to get injured or transected during routine posterior portal placement. Most direct ulnar nerve injuries occur during procedures at the posteromedial gutter, including posteromedial release, and locating the ulnar nerve by palpation during elbow arthroscopy is accurate only in the immediate vicinity of the epicondyle. Therefore, if a patient is under consideration of procedure at posteromedial gutter, ulnar nerve should be identified by a mini-open incision before main arthroscopic surgery and protected by moving ulnar nerve anteriorly to be further from posteromedial gutter [2, 9] (Fig. 32.1).

2.2 Radial Nerve

Radial nerve or posterior interosseous nerve injury could occur during portal placement and procedure at anterior compartment [5]. Radial nerve is especially vulnerable to direct injury due to its anatomy. Radial nerve could be within 4 mm of anterolateral portal and in terms of intra-articular procedure, radial nerve is placed just

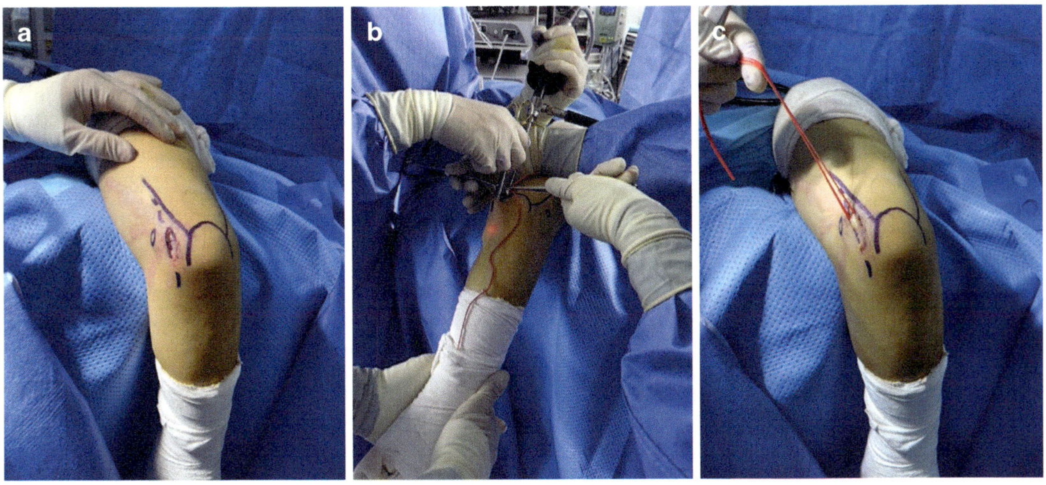

Fig. 32.1 Mini-open ulnar nerve release prior to main arthroscopic procedure. (**a**) skin incision of approximately 2 cm made along the ulnar nerve (between medial epicondyle and olecranon); (**b**) arthroscopic camera introduced into the skin incision for further release of the ulnar nerve (distally); (**c**) vessel loop for the protection of the ulnar nerve during remaining surgery

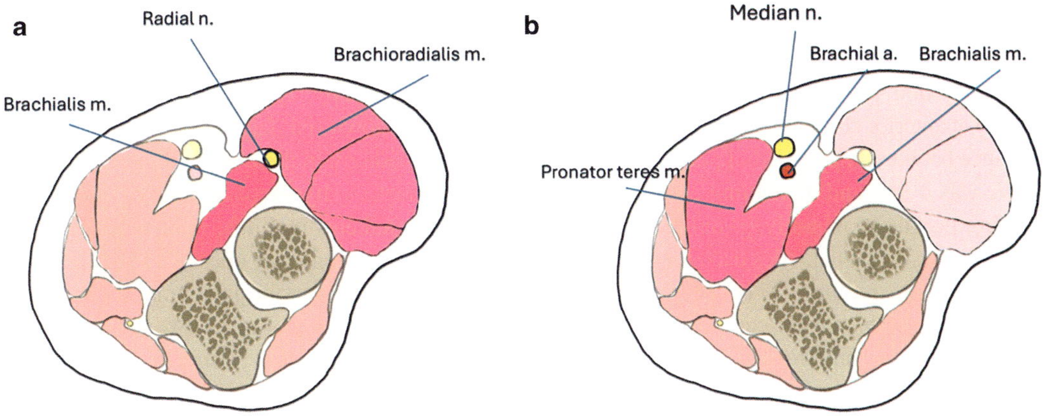

Fig. 32.2 Schematic illustration of the radial nerve (**a**) and median nerve (**b**) placement at the axial elbow. Radial nerve is placed just outside of anterior capsule without protection of other structures or muscles, while median nerve is placed above the brachialis muscle

outside of anterior capsule without protection of other structures, different from median nerve protected by brachialis muscle [10] (Fig. 32.2). To protect the radial nerve during anterolateral portal placement, distending the joint is necessary, if anterior compartment is operated prior to posterior compartment and making portals proximally (proximal anterolateral portal) helps increase safe distance from portal to radial nerve. Radial nerve is just above the anterior capsule without other protective structures; therefore, anterior capsular release should be performed cautiously, and further release should be stopped if fibers of brachioradialis overlying the capsule were observed (Fig. 32.3, Video 32.1).

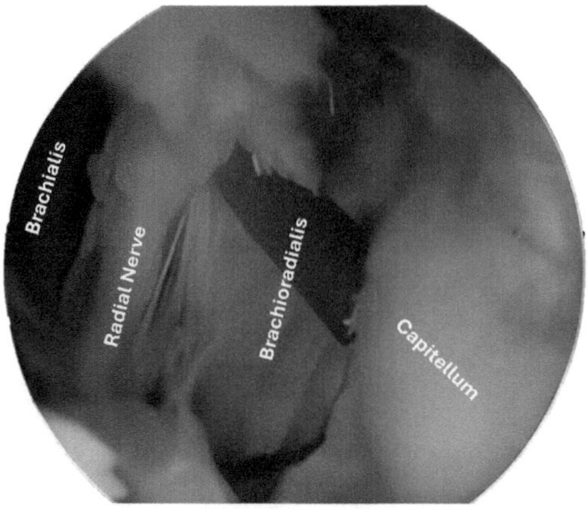

Fig. 32.3 Radial nerve exposure after anterior capsular release. If fibers of brachioradialis overlying the capsule were observed, further release should be stopped

2.3 Median Nerve

Median nerve or anterior interosseous nerve is the least injured nerve among three peripheral nerves due to its anatomy; however, it could be injured by both portal placement and during procedure at anterior compartment. Especially, mean distance between anteromedial portal and median nerve was 4 mm and distending elbow joint and making portals proximally (proximal anteromedial portal), similar to tactics used for radial nerve protection, are required [11]. Median nerve is protected by both anterior capsule and brachialis muscle; however, anterior capsule and brachialis muscle could be sometimes thin in certain conditions including rheumatoid arthritis (RA) or long-term steroid use and care must always be taken during anterior capsular release to avoid median nerve injury.

2.4 Vascular Injury

Vascular injuries has not been identified in elbow arthroscopy by current literature including recent systematic review of 18,892 arthroscopies [2]. However, due to its anatomy, the brachial artery always carries a risk of injury. The brachial artery is located lateral to the median nerve around the elbow joint and placed farther than the median nerve from the anteromedial portal, related to less chance of direct injury than the median nerve. While the median nerve was 5.97 mm farther from the proximal portal than the distal portal, the brachial artery was farther only less than 1 mm from the proximal portal than the distal portal [12]. However, still making portals proximally would help getting farther distance from the brachial artery. The brachial artery is placed over the anterior capsule and brachialis muscle, similar to the median nerve. Care should be taken during anterior capsular release, especially for RA patients or those with prolonged steroid use, which could lead to a thin capsule and brachialis layer.

3 Infection

According to a recent systematic review of 18,892 arthroscopies, overall infection rate after elbow arthroscopy was 1.02% (superficial: 0.93%, deep: 0.09%), while a comprehensive analysis of 2704 Medicare patients treated by elbow arthroscopy reported 1.5% of deep infection rate. Known risk factors for elbow infection after arthroscopy include alcohol use, inflammatory arthritis, hypercoagulability, age over 65 years, diabetes mellitus, intra-articular corticosteroid injection, and obesity [13–15]. Effect of preoperative steroid injection on infection remains unclear; however, a study showed preoperative steroid injection within 2 weeks before surgery increased the risk of infection after shoulder arthroscopy [16]. At least 2 weeks after the most recent steroid injection is required to minimize the risk of infection. Before surgery, past medical and social history should be taken, and higher risk of infection should be explained to patients with risk factors. If surgery is not performed in an emergent situation, control of blood glucose and body weight and quitting alcohol before the surgery should be prioritized. At the operating room, basic rules including sterile prepping and draping, and preoperative antibiotics within 60 min before surgical incision for infection prophylaxis, as outlined by the Surgical Care Improvement Project guidelines to minimize the chance of infection should be followed [17].

Classic symptoms and signs of infection include pain, heatness, redness, swelling, limitation of motion, and systemic symptoms like fever due to hyperinflammation. Symptoms could differ by the severity of infection and diagnosis could be sometimes difficult to distinguish from postoperative hyperinflammation. If infection is clinically suspected, history taking and physical examination should be preceded and inflammatory markers including leukocyte count, erythrocyte sedimentation rate (ESR), and C-reactive protein (CRP), and plain radiograph should be performed. Further imaging tests like magnetic resonance imaging with contrast enhancement could be considered for the precise diagnosis. Joint fluid aspiration and analysis should be considered if septic arthritis is suspicious. If diagnosis is not confirmed, careful monitoring of patient status and repetitive blood tests would help distinguish infection from hyperinflammation. Superficial infection could be initially treated with antibiotics, while deep infection requires consideration of both surgical therapy and antibiotics. Surgical treatment could be performed in either arthroscopic or open technique and patient-customized treatment based on the extent and severity of infection is required.

4 Postoperative Stiffness

Overall incidence of postoperative stiffness or contracture after elbow arthroscopy was 0.78% to 0.79% in a recent systematic review [2, 3]. Causes of postoperative stiffness could be various by the cause and type of surgery and include insufficient rehabilitation or prolonged immobilization, insufficient surgery for osteoarthritis or contracture, and recurrence of osteoarthritis or contracture after surgery, and heterotopic ossification [9]. Preoperative stiffness and radiologically severe osteoarthritis are risk factors for postoperative limited range of motion (ROM), and early active rehabilitation and minimal immobilization are most important to prevent postoperative stiffness [3, 18]. During arthroscopic osteocapsular arthroplasty for osteoarthritis and arthroscopic release surgery for contracture, insufficient surgery could lead to insufficient ROM, postoperatively. Therefore, sufficient recovery of ROM should be confirmed at the operating room, when performing surgery to gain the ROM.

Timing to recover ROM differs by the type of surgery and patient-customized approach is required. If a patient does not reach the ROM as wanted, active physiotherapy should be performed, and continuous nerve block could help control the pain; therefore, make ease to perform rehabilitation. If there is no improvement in ROM after intensive physiotherapy, manipulation under anesthesia (MUA) could be considered [19]. MUA increases the passive ROM and could help a patient increase motivation for rehabilitation by showing the ROM reached during MUA. Under sedation or general anesthesia, constant load in a gentle manner should be applied in one direction at a time (extension, flexion, pronation, supination). After MUA, temporary splint could be applied to maintain the ROM reached by MUA. For example, if a patient underwent MUA due to loss of extension (ROM: 60°–140°) and reached full ROM (0–140°) after MUA, an extension splint could be applied for the first few days to maintain the full extension, before patient could comfortably extend the elbow by him/herself. Timing of MUA is still under debate; however, a previous study showed that MUA within 3 months of original trauma or surgery showed significant increase of flexion-extension arc, while after 3 months, MUA did not show significant increase of ROM; therefore, if MUA is considered for the patient, it would be better to be performed within 3 months of original trauma or surgery [20].

Further release surgery could be considered for the refractory stiffness after conservative treatment or insufficient surgery for osteoarthritis or contracture. Release procedure could be performed by either arthroscopic or open technique. By dividing into anterior and posterior compartment, all structures should be thoroughly checked whether they are released enough [18]. Recovery of ROM should be confirmed at the operating room and early active physiotherapy and rehabilitation are required.

5 Heterotopic Ossification (HO)

Incidence rate of HO in elbow arthroscopy was between 0.28% and 0.38% in two review studies and was initially believed to rarely occur [2, 3]. However, a recent study assessing HO after elbow arthroscopy reported 6.3% rate of incidence [21]. Despite the development of HO, HO is not usually symptomatic and could present in different levels of symptoms including pain, decreased ROM, and functional impairment [22].

Prophylactic use of radiation therapy and nonsteroidal anti-inflammatory drugs (NSAIDs) is known to decrease the incidence of HO in the setting of hip arthroplasty and pelvis trauma; however, evidence for the prevention of HO in elbow injury or surgery is lacking [23]. A recent study showed a promising effect of prophylactic radiation therapy for prevention of HO after elbow injury or surgery; however, its evidence for clinical efficacy is still weak, and clinical use should be thoroughly considered due to possible complications [24]. Efficacy of NSAIDs for the prevention of HO in the elbow joint is controversial [25]. However, a retrospective study raised a possibility for the difference in incidence of HO by type of NSAIDs for the HO prophylaxis; celecoxib showed 20% of HO incidence (11/54), followed by ibuprofen (28%, 5/18), indomethacin (33%, 1/3), naproxen (50%, 1/2), and meloxicam (100%, 1/1) of HO incidence [25]. As one retrospective study to assess the effect of celecoxib for the prevention of recurrence of HO after open arthrolysis for post-traumatic elbow stiffness showed its effectiveness, further studies are required by different types of NSAIDs to assess their effectiveness for the prevention of HO in elbow injury or surgery [26].

Regular imaging checkup is important for the early detection of HO and if the patient has sudden pain or limitation during improvement of conditions, possibility for HO occurrence should be checked. If HO is confirmed by radiographs, customized management should be performed. At the early phase of HO, patient usually has pain and localized swelling, and treatment should be also focused on the pain control. At the later phase with HO maturation, main complaint is limitation of motion; therefore, active rehabilitation and physiotherapy should be prescribed. If patient has persistent limitation of motion after active rehabilitation or limitation of motion gets worse, excision of HO and contracture release could be considered. Excision of HO is generally performed at least 8 months after diagnosis of HO (after full maturation of HO). However, early HO removal (regardless of 8 months maturity of HO) was proposed to maximize the treatment effect by avoiding contracture and shortening of joint capsule, ligaments, tendons, and muscles around the joint [22, 27].

6 Deep Venous Thrombosis (DVT) and Pulmonary Embolism

DVT and pulmonary embolism are rare postoperative complications; however, different from localized complications, general medical complications could be life threatening. Studies of DVT or pulmonary embolism after elbow arthroscopy are lacking and studies of shoulder arthroscopy and upper extremity surgery have been reviewed to look for risk factors and prophylaxis methods.

Diabetes mellitus, rheumatoid arthritis and ischemic heart disease are known risk factors for DVT and pulmonary embolism following shoulder surgery and a longer operative time and obesity could be risk factors for DVT and pulmonary embolism after shoulder arthroscopy [28]. As a common position during elbow arthroscopy, lateral decubitus position during arthroscopy was considered to predispose to DVT in shoulder arthroscopy [29]. However, the main cause of this complication during shoulder arthroscopy is thought to be arm traction and reduced limb perfusion. Since arm traction is not applied during elbow arthroscopy, mechanism should be considered different from shoulder arthroscopy.

To minimize the risk for DVT and pulmonary embolism, preoperative patient evaluation and risk stratification are important. Except for emergent surgery, risk factors should be controlled before surgery and uncontrollable risk factors should be underlined for the patients. Mechanical thromboprophylaxis, including thromboembolic deterrent stockings and pneumatic compression foot pumps, could help reduce the risk of thromboembolic events, and early, active mobilization after surgery is important. Chemical or pharmacological thromboprophylaxis in orthopedic patients is still under debate and chemical thromboprophylaxis is not generally recommended and recommended only for selected patients after full assessment of risks and benefits of chemical thromboprophylaxis [30].

References

1. Mullett H, Sprague M, Brown G, Hausman M. Arthroscopic treatment of lateral epicondylitis: clinical and cadaveric studies. Clin Orthop Relat Res. 2005;439:123–8. https://doi.org/10.1097/01.blo.0000176143.08886.fe.
2. de Klerk HH, Verweij LPE, Sierevelt IN, Priester-Vink S, Hilgersom NFJ, Eygendaal D, et al. Wide range in complication rates following elbow arthroscopy in adult and pediatric patients: a systematic review. Arthroscopy. 2023;39(11):2363–87. https://doi.org/10.1016/j.arthro.2023.04.015.
3. Batko BD, Hakakian D, Norin JL, Tauro JC. Complications in elbow arthroscopy: management and prevention. Sports Med Arthrosc Rev. 2022;30(1):54–62. https://doi.org/10.1097/JSA.0000000000000334.
4. Temporin K, Miyoshi Y, Miyamura S, Oura K, Shimada K. Risk of nerve injury during elbow arthroscopy: ultrasonographic evaluation of preoperative patients. J Shoulder Elb Surg. 2023;32(3):486–91. https://doi.org/10.1016/j.jse.2022.11.002.
5. Mercer DM, Baldwin ED, Moneim MS. Posterior interosseous nerve laceration following elbow arthroscopy. J Hand Surg Am. 2015;40(3):624–6. https://doi.org/10.1016/j.jhsa.2014.05.036.
6. Hilgersom NFJ, van Deurzen DFP, Gerritsma CL, van der Heide HJL, Malessy MJA, Eygendaal D, et al. Nerve injuries do occur in elbow arthroscopy. Knee Surg Sports Traumatol Arthrosc. 2018;26(1):318–24. https://doi.org/10.1007/s00167-017-4431-8. PMID - 28184919.
7. Gelberman RH, Yamaguchi K, Hollstien SB, Winn SS, Heidenreich FP Jr, Bindra RR, et al. Changes in interstitial pressure and cross-sectional area of the cubital tunnel and of the ulnar nerve with flexion of the elbow. An experimental study in human cadavera. J Bone Joint Surg Am. 1998;80(4):492–501. https://doi.org/10.2106/00004623-199804000-00005.
8. Keener JD, Galatz LM. Arthroscopic management of the stiff elbow. J Am Acad Orthop Surg. 2011;19(5):265–74. https://doi.org/10.5435/00124635-201105000-00004.
9. So SP, Kwak JM, Lee JB, Ben H, Alsaqri H, Kim KH, et al. Clinical outcomes of revision arthroscopic osteocapsular arthroplasty in primary elbow osteoarthritis: a retrospective cohort study. Am J Sports Med. 2023;51(8):2050–6. https://doi.org/10.1177/03635465231171542.
10. Lynch GJ, Meyers JF, Whipple TL, Caspari RB. Neurovascular anatomy and elbow arthroscopy: inherent risks. Arthroscopy. 1986;2(3):190–7. https://doi.org/10.1016/s0749-8063(86)80067-6.
11. Andrews JR, Carson WG. Arthroscopy of the elbow. Arthroscopy. 1985;1(2):97–107. https://doi.org/10.1016/s0749-8063(85)80038-4.
12. Cushing T, Finley Z, O'Brien MJ, Savoie FH 3rd, Myers L, Medvedev G. Safety of anteromedial portals in elbow arthroscopy: a systematic review of cadaveric studies. Arthroscopy. 2019;35(7):2164–72. https://doi.org/10.1016/j.arthro.2019.02.046.
13. Intravia J, Acevedo DC, Chung WJ, Mirzayan R. Complications of elbow arthroscopy in a community-based practice. Arthroscopy. 2020;36(5):1283–90. https://doi.org/10.1016/j.arthro.2019.11.108.
14. Camp CL, Cancienne JM, Degen RM, Dines JS, Altchek DW, Werner BC. Factors that increase the risk of infection after elbow arthroscopy: analysis of patient demographics, medical comorbidities, and steroid injections in 2,704 medicare patients. Arthroscopy. 2017;33(6):1175–9. https://doi.org/10.1016/j.arthro.2017.01.035. PMID - 28342634.
15. Werner BC, Fashandi AH, Chhabra AB, Deal DN. Effect of obesity on complication rate after elbow arthroscopy in a medicare population. Arthroscopy. 2016;32(3):453–7. https://doi.org/10.1016/j.arthro.2015.08.025.
16. Bhattacharjee S, Lee W, Lee MJ, Shi LL. Preoperative corticosteroid joint injections within 2 weeks of shoulder arthroscopies increase postoperative infection risk. J Shoulder Elb Surg. 2019;28(11):2098–102. https://doi.org/10.1016/j.jse.2019.03.037.
17. Rosenberger LH, Politano AD, Sawyer RG. The surgical care improvement project and prevention of post-operative infection, including surgical site infection. Surg Infect. 2011;12(3):163–8. https://doi.org/10.1089/sur.2010.083.
18. So S-P, Kwak J-M, Lee J-B, Ben H, Alsaqri H, Koh KH, et al. Radiologically severe osteoarthritis is related to worse clinical outcomes after arthroscopic osteocapsular arthroplasty in primary elbow osteoarthritis at medium-term follow-up: a retrospective cohort study. J Shoulder Elbow Surg. 2023;32(11):2325–32. https://doi.org/10.1016/j.jse.2023.04.026. PMID - 37172808.
19. Rotman D, Factor S, Schermann H, Kadar A, Atlan F, Pritsch T, et al. Manipulation under anesthesia

for the postsurgical stiff elbow: a case series and review of literature. Eur J Orthop Surg Traumatol. 2019;29(8):1679–85. https://doi.org/10.1007/s00590-019-02492-6.
20. Spitler CA, Doty DH, Johnson MD, Nowotarski PJ, Kiner DW, Swafford RE, et al. Manipulation under anesthesia as a treatment of posttraumatic elbow stiffness. J Orthop Trauma. 2018;32(8):e304–e8. https://doi.org/10.1097/BOT.0000000000001194. PMID - 29762358.
21. Ben H, Kholinne E, Zeng CH, Alsaqri H, Lee JB, So SP, et al. Prevalence, timing, locational distribution, and risk factors for heterotopic ossification after elbow arthroscopy. Am J Sports Med. 2023;51(13):3401–8. https://doi.org/10.1177/03635465231198862.
22. Qi W, Jiang P, Aiyuan W, Wenjing X, Jinshu T, Jinshu T. Treatment and rehabilitation of post-traumatic elbow stiffness with heterotopic ossification. J Plast Surg Hand Surg. 2024;58:18–23. https://doi.org/10.1080/2000656X.2023.2231867. PMID - 37409920.
23. Board TN, Karva A, Board RE, Gambhir AK, Porter ML. The prophylaxis and treatment of heterotopic ossification following lower limb arthroplasty. J Bone Joint Surg Br. 2007;89(4):434–40. https://doi.org/10.1302/0301-620x.89b4.18845.
24. Ploumis A, Belbasis L, Ntzani E, Tsekeris P, Xenakis T. Radiotherapy for prevention of heterotopic ossification of the elbow: a systematic review of the literature. J Shoulder Elb Surg. 2013;22(11):1580–8. https://doi.org/10.1016/j.jse.2013.07.045.
25. Bochat K, Mattin AC, Ricciardo BJ. The efficacy of nonsteroidal anti-inflammatories in the prevention of heterotopic ossification following elbow trauma surgery. JSES Int. 2021;5(4):793–6. https://doi.org/10.1016/j.jseint.2021.04.004.
26. Sun Y, Cai J, Li F, Liu S, Ruan H, Fan C. The efficacy of celecoxib in preventing heterotopic ossification recurrence after open arthrolysis for post-traumatic elbow stiffness in adults. J Shoulder Elb Surg. 2015;24(11):1735–40. https://doi.org/10.1016/j.jse.2015.07.006.
27. Manske MC, Hanel DP. Postburn contractures of the elbow and heterotopic ossification. Hand Clin. 2017;33(2):375–88. https://doi.org/10.1016/j.hcl.2016.12.014.
28. Dattani R, Smith CD, Patel VR. The venous thromboembolic complications of shoulder and elbow surgery: a systematic review. Bone Joint J. 2013;95-B(1):70–4. https://doi.org/10.1302/0301-620X.95B1.29854.
29. Hennrikus WL, Mapes RC, Bratton MW, Lapoint JM. Lateral traction during shoulder arthroscopy: its effect on tissue perfusion measured by pulse oximetry. Am J Sports Med. 1995;23(4):444–6. https://doi.org/10.1177/036354659502300412.
30. Warwick D, Dahl OE, Fisher WD. International Surgical Thrombosis F. Orthopaedic thromboprophylaxis: limitations of current guidelines. J Bone Joint Surg Br. 2008;90(2):127–32. https://doi.org/10.1302/0301-620X.90B2.20106.

Part VIII

Conclusion and Future Perspectives

The Future of Elbow Arthroscopic Surgery

33

In-Ho Jeon

1 Background

Elbow arthroscopy has evolved into a cornerstone of minimally invasive orthopedic surgery; however, it continues to face challenges due to the limited intra-articular space, proximity to neurovascular structures, and variability in clinical outcomes. Emerging technologies—including high-definition imaging, artificial intelligence (AI), robotics, augmented reality (AR), and biologic therapies—offer promising avenues to improve procedural precision, safety, and patient-specific outcomes. This chapter examines the transformative potential of these innovations in advancing the field of elbow arthroscopy.

2 Technological Innovations

2.1 High-Definition Visualization and 3D Imaging

Advancements in 4 K imaging and three-dimensional (3D) reconstruction have significantly enhanced visualization within the elbow's confined joint space, facilitating more accurate detection of subtle intra-articular lesions and safer portal placement. Future innovations, such as hyperspectral imaging and 8 K-resolution arthroscopes, hold the potential to further refine intraoperative visualization and enable improved differentiation of soft tissue structures.

2.2 Artificial Intelligence in Elbow Surgery

Artificial intelligence (AI) is emerging as a valuable adjunct in elbow arthroscopy, offering capabilities in diagnostic support, surgical planning, intraoperative guidance (Fig. 33.1), and personalized rehabilitation protocols. Preoperatively, AI algorithms can assist in identifying critical anatomical structures and predicting potential complications. During surgery, AI may provide

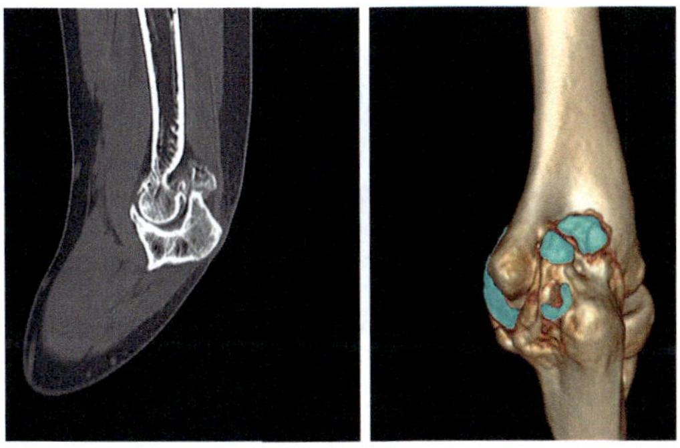

Fig. 33.1 A side-by-side comparison of traditional 2D imaging vs. a 3D reconstructed model for elbow surgical planning. The 3D model (right) provides enhanced spatial understanding of the joint, aiding in more precise portal placement and anticipating anatomical challenges

I.-H. Jeon (✉)
Department of Orthopaedic Surgery, Asan Medical Center, University of Ulsan, College of Medicine, Seoul, Republic of Korea

I.-H. Jeon et al. (eds.), *Elbow Arthroscopy*, https://doi.org/10.1007/978-981-95-3732-7_33

real-time alerts regarding anatomical "danger zones" and propose optimal procedural steps. Nonetheless, the integration of AI into surgical practice necessitates careful consideration of ethical and regulatory issues, including data privacy, algorithm validation, and the maintenance of appropriate surgeon oversight (Fig. 33.2).

2.3 Robotics and Precision Navigation

Robotic technologies contribute to improved surgical precision and stability, particularly in anatomically constrained spaces such as the elbow. Emerging concepts—such as continuum robots and instruments equipped with haptic feedback—may facilitate safer intra-articular navigation and enable automated portal placement. Although the application of robotics in elbow arthroscopy remains in its early stages, insights from robotic-assisted wrist and knee procedures underscore its substantial future potential.

2.4 Augmented Reality (AR) Guidance

AR technology enables the projection of critical anatomical structures—such as nerves and blood vessels—directly onto the surgeon's field of view, thereby enhancing safety during complex procedures such as capsular release. Additionally, AR can assist with spatial orientation and guide precise drilling trajectories, reducing dependence on mental mapping and potentially improving surgical accuracy and efficiency.

2.5 Biologics and Regenerative Approaches

Biologic therapies—such as platelet-rich plasma (PRP), stem cells, and cartilage scaffolds—serve as adjuncts to arthroscopy by enhancing tissue regeneration. Emerging strategies, including arthroscopic delivery of gene therapies and bioactive implants, are transforming the treatment of

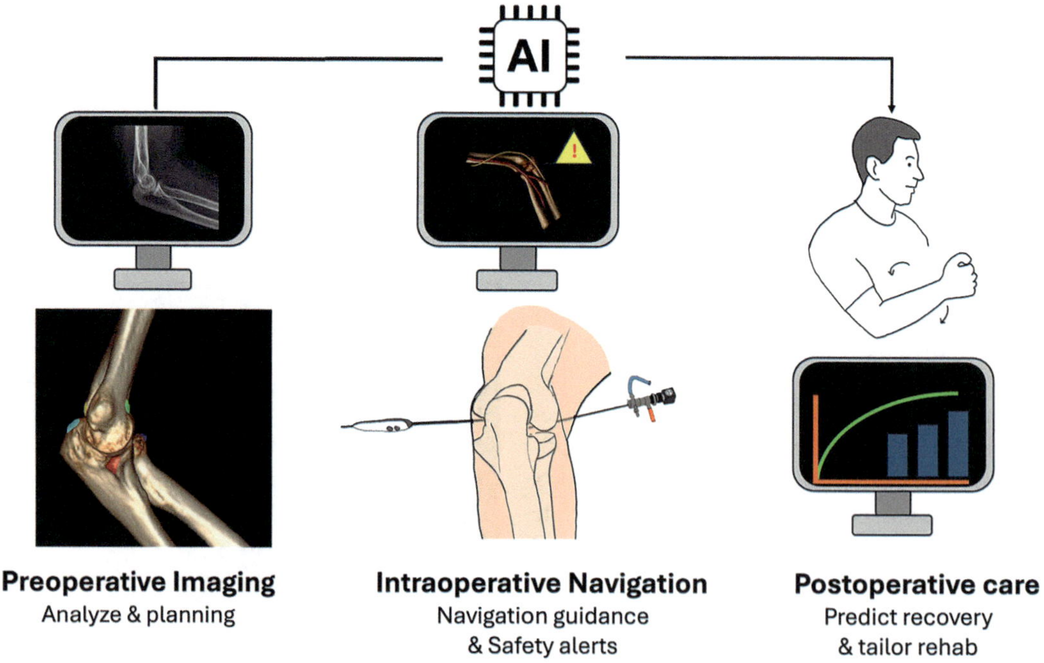

Fig. 33.2 Schematic of an AI-assisted elbow arthroscopy workflow. Preoperative imaging is analyzed by AI algorithms to identify pathology and plan the surgery (e.g., marking osteophytes to remove). During the procedure, the AI system provides real-time navigation guidance and safety alerts, and it continues into postoperative care by predicting recovery trajectories and customizing rehab protocols

cartilage defects, tendinopathies, and postoperative fibrosis.

3 Expanding Indications

3.1 Elbow Stiffness

Arthroscopic circumferential capsular release combined with ulnar nerve decompression has emerged as a reliable technique for restoring elbow range of motion, even in patients with prior surgical history or concomitant heterotopic ossification.

3.2 Instability and Ligament Reconstruction

With advancements in arthroscopic navigation and biologic augmentation, repairs of the lateral ulnar collateral ligament (LUCL) and ulnar collateral ligament (UCL) are becoming increasingly feasible. As techniques continue to evolve, arthroscopic ligament reconstruction may offer accelerated recovery, particularly for overhead athletes.

4 Technique Refinement and Safety

4.1 Portal Access

Patient-specific portal mapping utilizing 3D imaging and navigation systems aims to optimize surgical access and reduce the risk of nerve injury, particularly in cases involving complex deformities or revision procedures.

4.2 Circumferential Release

Comprehensive capsular release involving the anterior, medial, and lateral aspects effectively restores the flexion-extension arc of the elbow. In patient with high-risk of neuropathy, prophylactic ulnar nerve decompression is recommended to mitigate the risk of postoperative neuropathy.

5 Education, Simulation, and Global Adoption

Simulation platforms incorporating virtual reality (VR) and augmented reality (AR) are essential tools for training surgeons in the technically demanding field of elbow arthroscopy. Global collaboration is advancing standardized credentialing and lowering barriers to technology access, thereby promoting greater equity in surgical education and care worldwide.

6 Challenges and Considerations

Key challenges include the high costs of implementation, the necessity for long-term clinical validation, and ethical considerations surrounding the use of artificial intelligence and robotics. Comprehensive training programs and patient education are essential to ensure the safe and effective integration of these emerging technologies.

7 Vision for the Future

Future elbow arthroscopy is anticipated to evolve into a highly precise, AI-augmented, robot-assisted, and biologically optimized surgical modality. The integration of personalized preoperative planning, AR-guided navigation, and regenerative therapies will enable the management of complex elbow pathologies with improved safety, accuracy, and reproducibility. Furthermore, the implementation of telementoring and remotely assisted surgical platforms may significantly enhance global access to advanced arthroscopic care, bridging disparities in surgical expertise and infrastructure.

8 Conclusion

The convergence of visualization, AI, robotics, AR, and biologics is reshaping elbow arthroscopy. These innovations promise to improve precision, safety, and outcomes, expanding indications once considered too complex. With rigorous validation and thoughtful integration, the future of elbow arthroscopy is bright, accessible, and transformative.

GPSR Compliance

The European Union's (EU) General Product Safety Regulation (GPSR) is a set of rules that requires consumer products to be safe and our obligations to ensure this.

If you have any concerns about our products, you can contact us on ProductSafety@springernature.com

In case Publisher is established outside the EU, the EU authorized representative is:

Springer Nature Customer Service Center GmbH
Europaplatz 3
69115 Heidelberg, Germany

Batch number: 10683089

Printed by Printforce, the Netherlands